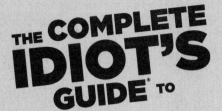

THE COMPLETE **IDIOT'S** GUIDE® TO

Vegan Living

Second Edition

by Beverly Lynn Bennett and Ray Sammartano

ALPHA

A member of Penguin Group (USA) Inc.

To all the creatures we share this world with.

ALPHA BOOKS

Published by Penguin Group (USA) Inc.

Penguin Group (USA) Inc., 375 Hudson Street, New York, New York 10014, USA • Penguin Group (Canada), 90 Eglinton Avenue East, Suite 700, Toronto, Ontario M4P 2Y3, Canada (a division of Pearson Penguin Canada Inc.) • Penguin Books Ltd., 80 Strand, London WC2R 0RL, England • Penguin Ireland, 25 St. Stephen's Green, Dublin 2, Ireland (a division of Penguin Books Ltd.) • Penguin Group (Australia), 250 Camberwell Road, Camberwell, Victoria 3124, Australia (a division of Pearson Australia Group Pty. Ltd.) • Penguin Books India Pvt. Ltd., 11 Community Centre, Panchsheel Park, New Delhi— 110 017, India • Penguin Group (NZ), 67 Apollo Drive, Rosedale, North Shore, Auckland 1311, New Zealand (a division of Pearson New Zealand Ltd.) • Penguin Books (South Africa) (Pty.) Ltd., 24 Sturdee Avenue, Rosebank, Johannesburg 2196, South Africa • Penguin Books Ltd., Registered Offices: 80 Strand, London WC2R 0RL, England

Copyright © 2012 by Beverly Lynn Bennett

International Standard Book Number: 978-1-61564-202-1
Library of Congress Catalog Card Number: 2012939810

14   13   12   8   7   6   5   4   3   2   1

Interpretation of the printing code: The rightmost number of the first series of numbers is the year of the book's printing; the rightmost number of the second series of numbers is the number of the book's printing. For example, a printing code of 12-1 shows that the first printing occurred in 2012.

Printed in the United States of America

Note: This publication contains the opinions and ideas of its authors. It is intended to provide helpful and informative material on the subject matter covered. It is sold with the understanding that the authors and publisher are not engaged in rendering professional services in the book. If the reader requires personal assistance or advice, a competent professional should be consulted.

The authors and publisher specifically disclaim any responsibility for any liability, loss, or risk, personal or otherwise, which is incurred as a consequence, directly or indirectly, of the use and application of any of the contents of this book.

Most Alpha books are available at special quantity discounts for bulk purchases for sales promotions, premiums, fund-raising, or educational use. Special books, or book excerpts, can also be created to fit specific needs. For details, write: Special Markets, Alpha Books, 375 Hudson Street, New York, NY 10014.

Publisher: *Mike Sanders*

Executive Managing Editor: *Billy Fields*

Executive Acquisitions Editor: *Lori Cates Hand*

Senior Development Editor: *Christy Wagner*

Senior Production Editor: *Janette Lynn*

Copy Editor: *Amy Borelli*

Cover Designer: *Rebecca Batchelor*

Book Designers: *William Thomas, Rebecca Batchelor*

Indexer: *Angie Bess*

Layout: *Brian Massey*

Senior Proofreader: *Laura Caddell*

Contents

Foreword

When I was first asked to write the foreword to a book titled *The Complete Idiot's Guide to Vegan Living*, I experienced two distinct feelings. On the one hand, I know how many people today are interested in vegan living, and having an easy-to-understand, simple-to-follow guide available seemed like a fine idea. And I knew Beverly Lynn Bennett and Ray Sammartano would do an excellent job.

At the same time, though, I am aware that most of the vegans I know are actually quite intelligent people who are sensitive to suffering and want to live healthy and compassionate lives. Something about "an idiot's guide" to the subject seemed a contradiction—not that being a vegan is like being a brain surgeon. Being a vegan is easy to do when you know how, and Beverly and Ray are wonderful guides to learning.

Why do people become vegans? For many reasons, but a common denominator seems to be an enhanced sensitivity to the cruelty inflicted upon animals in modern meat production. Compassion plays a large role in the experiences of most people who have an interest in vegan living. Vegans are people who want to see an end to cruelty to animals.

It can be hard to look at sometimes, and disturbing. I've been so blind myself. I remember watching the release of hundreds of beautiful white doves at the opening and closing ceremonies of the Olympic games, enthralled by the spectacle. I didn't think about the birds as animals and what they might be going through. I didn't know they had been trucked in, crowded underground, and then propelled upward. Nor did I know they were terrified and confused in completely strange surroundings. At the Korean games, many of the frightened and disoriented doves actually flew into the Olympic flame, and millions watching were treated to the far-from-inspiring spectacle of seeing the birds burned alive.

I remember, when I was a child, thinking that fur coats were fabulous. I never imagined that wild, fur-bearing animals who are caught in traps suffer slow, agonizing deaths. Or that when we purchase the products of fur farms, we support massive animal pain and death. But slowly it dawned on me that, as beautiful as furs are, they look a lot better on their original owners—the foxes, minks, and other animals from whom they were taken. Now I don't buy furs.

I also remember when I was a child going to a friend's house where there were deer heads on the walls. I thought they were cool. But comedian Ellen DeGeneres has a point when she says, "You ask people why they have deer heads on the wall. They always say, 'Because it's such a beautiful animal.' There you go. I think my mother's attractive, but I have photographs of her."

There's something about our society that makes it hard to see animals suffering, even when, or maybe particularly when, it's your own actions that are causing pain. It's not always easy to break through the wall of denial.

But many of the people who are drawn to a vegan way of life are doing so. And with this awareness comes the motivation to bring your life into greater alignment with your heart. If you are the kind of person who knows there is wisdom in your heart and wants to live by it, this book's for you.

—John Robbins

John Robbins is the author of numerous bestsellers, including *Diet For A New America*, *The Food Revolution*, and *No Happy Cows*. He is the recipient of the Rachel Carson Award, the Albert Schweitzer Humanitarian Award, Green America's Lifetime Achievement Award, the Peace Abbey's Courage of Conscience Award, and many other accolades.

Introduction

People are drawn to living a vegan lifestyle for various reasons, and this book explores many of them. Going vegan often stems from a love and compassion for animals and a deeper understanding that all creatures experience the same pain and suffering we humans do, along with a desire not to contribute to it anymore. That's what brought us to veganism. During the 20+ years we've been vegan, we've also discovered many of the positive effects veganism can have on our health and the environment.

Eliminating animal foods from your diet has gone from being thought of as a strange, "health nut" fad to receiving wide acclaim as a healthful, nutritionally sound, and even optimal way of eating. In comparison to the standard American diet (SAD), eating vegan is much richer in nutrients, lower in fat, and higher in fiber. It's definitely not just another fad diet that's here today and forgotten tomorrow.

Many people seem to think vegans are unhealthy, too thin, and have some pretty strange thoughts about things, but these stereotypes couldn't be further from the truth. Vegans come from all walks of life and are mothers, fathers, doctors, lawyers, teachers, preachers, politicians, actors, athletes, factory workers, students, and yes, some tree-hugging environmentalists and animal rights activists as well. We come in all shapes, sizes, and cultural backgrounds from all corners of the globe.

The one thing vegans really do all have in common is a desire to lessen humanity's negative impact on our fellow creatures and a willingness to try to do something about it. More and more people are becoming aware of how the things they buy, eat, wear, and do affect animals, other people, and the environment. They're making conscious decisions to eliminate animal cruelty from their lives, and positive changes are happening all over the place. The numbers of vegans are increasing every year—already in the millions—and there seems to be no stopping us!

In this book, we provide you with some tips to help you begin your transition into being, living, and not only surviving but thriving as a vegan. We also give you some practical advice on how to handle answering the many questions, from the ridiculous to the insightful, that most certainly will come your way. Remember, the word *vegan* and our approach to living and eating can be a new and confusing concept to some people. After we've filled you in on what it means to live as a vegan, maybe you can do your best to help spread the word to others.

As a new or aspiring vegan, be confident knowing you're one of millions of vegans out there in the world. We think and feel as you do. Find comfort in knowing you're not alone in your feelings or your decision to eliminate animal use and abuse from your life. Stand strong and proud as a vegan and know you're helping make a difference, and make a better world for all the creatures who inhabit it! By taking small steps, being true to yourself, and taking the time to analyze the various issues surrounding living a compassionate lifestyle, you are sure to be successful as a vegan and as a great human being!

How This Book Is Organized

This book is divided into seven parts. Each focuses on a different aspect of what it means to live as a vegan, from the philosophical and nutritional to the practical and functional. We provide you with the knowledge and tools necessary to transition into a vegan lifestyle and apply compassion and caring to all parts of your day-to-day life, including what you buy, eat, and wear.

Part 1, Venturing into Veganism, explains some of the spiritual, moral, and environmental issues behind being vegan. You learn the history of the vegetarian and vegan movements and take a quick quiz to determine if going vegan might be right for you. We also discuss some of the many added health benefits of a vegan diet, as well as some of the medical and dietary reasons that lead some people to eliminate animal products from their diet. We wrap up Part 1 with a few tips to get you started on your transition into becoming a vegan.

Part 2, Myths and Misconceptions About Veganism, alleviates any concerns you and your loved ones may have regarding the nutritional adequacy and healthfulness of a vegan diet. In these chapters, you discover the many delicious vegan foods you can enjoy that supply your body with all the protein, calcium, and carbohydrates it requires to stay healthy and fit. You also learn about the benefits of getting your calcium and protein from plant-based sources, as well as the importance of good carbs. Malnutrition and overconsumption are two opposite sides of the spectrum of the problem of world hunger; bet you didn't know eating vegan can greatly impact both of them in a positive way.

Part 3, A Vegan Survival Guide, gives you some essential information you need to be a healthy vegan. We start with a history and brief explanation of various food guidelines, as well as the development of the current USDA MyPlate and PCRM's vegan-friendly version the Power Plate. We also take a look at the standard American diet and all its drawbacks. To set you on course for eating right, we cover the basics of a proper, well-balanced vegan diet based on the New Four Food Groups, including how to eat wisely if you want to drop a few pounds. We help you cover your nutritional bases with supplementation, and for you mothers- and fathers-to-be, we offer you some advice and information you can use before, during, and after pregnancy. We also explore the topic of raw foods and their many benefits and give you some tips on incorporating more of them into your diet.

Part 4, Maintaining a Vegan Lifestyle, helps you with the various issues that arise after you've begun your journey into veganism. We give you some advice on handling the veg-curious you'll encounter. We share some tips on handling family get-togethers and holidays, eating out at restaurants, hosting your own gatherings, and even sharing kitchen space with meat-eaters. You'll also pick up a few traveling tips that will help you make the most out of your traveling experiences while not going hungry in the process. Being a wise shopper is important for saving time and money, getting your money's worth, and maybe even avoiding future problems with your health. To help you further embrace the vegan lifestyle, we offer tips on how and where to shop. We cover the advantages of buying in bulk, the joys of shopping at natural foods stores, the concept of fair trade, and the importance of reading food labels; plus, we look at a few vegan goodies that can make your life easier and tastier.

Part 5, Successful Substitutions, helps get you primed for vegan cooking and hopefully gets your creative culinary juices flowing. Starting with protein sources, you get the lowdown on how to cook and use beans, grains, and greens in your vegan dishes. You'll become soy savvy when it comes to using tofu, tempeh, and TVP, and we take a look at the versatile seitan, which you can use to create many a marvelous mock meat. We share the facts about fats, including which ones to use and avoid and why. You also learn how to use packaged alternatives like nondairy milks, yogurts, sour cream, cream cheeses, and assorted varieties of vegan cheese. We even offer some help in making your own "cheezy" creations! If vegan baking is your thing, you'll probably appreciate some vegan baking advice, including the various ways to replace butter, dairy, eggs, and gelatin or how to use tofu and fruit to make some spectacular baked goods.

Part 6, Vegan Food for the Soul, provides over 110 mouthwatering vegan recipe ideas for every meal of the day, from breakfast to dessert. The recipes are easy to follow, and most of them contain ingredients you may already have on hand or can easily obtain. We've included recipes to suit all tastes, food allergies, and sensitivities, and even some treats for you raw foodists. Several recipes take less than 5 minutes to prepare and contain only a few ingredients, which is perfect for when you need to dine and dash or eat on the go. If you're in need of a big meal with all the fixings, we've got you covered there, too.

Part 7, Vegan Lifestyle Choices, provides some information to further assist and empower you to live as a new vegan. We focus on the things you put on your body, from what you use to wash your face or brush your hair to how you cover your skin or feet. You learn about compassionate alternatives that can help you veganize your wardrobe and personal-care items. We also take a look around the house at some household items that may be derived from animal sources and offer some plant-based alternatives.

After Part 7, we include some appendixes we think you'll find helpful in your future vegan endeavors. Appendix A contains a list of defined terms used in the book, and Appendix B features lists of vegan books, websites, and contact information for various pro-veg organizations.

Extras

In every chapter you'll find sidebars that offer extra information, helpful tips, or just fun facts:

DEFINITION

These sidebars explain the meaning of some terms you might not be familiar with.

VEGAN VOICES

Check here for quotes and words of wisdom on a wide assortment of topics.

IN A NUTSHELL

These sidebars offer useful information or tips relating to the issues discussed in the text.

HOT POTATO

Heed the cautions in these sidebars that alert you to potential problems or pitfalls.

Acknowledgments

We wish to express our heartfelt appreciation to the people who helped make the first and now the second edition of this book possible: to BookEnds Literary Agency; to senior acquisitions editor Randy Ladenheim-Gil, executive acquisitions editor Lori Hand, and senior development editor Christy Wagner for their invaluable advice, input, and support; and to John Robbins for graciously agreeing to write the foreword to this book. Mr. Robbins has greatly influenced millions of people to go vegan and vegetarian through his work with EarthSave and his many books, including *Diet for a New America* and *The Food Revolution*. We would also like to thank our family and friends for their enthusiasm, guidance, and support while we were immersed in the writing and revising of this book. Beverly would like to give a special thanks to three vegan writers and thinkers whose works have had a profound effect on her development as a vegan, a chef, and a woman: Carol J. Adams, Joanne Stepaniak, and Nava Atlas. Thank you for the endless inspiration.

Special Thanks to the Technical Reviewer

The Complete Idiot's Guide to Vegan Living, Second Edition, was reviewed by an expert who double-checked the accuracy of what you'll learn here, to help us ensure that this book gives you everything you need to know about understanding how to live a vegan life. Special thanks are extended to Trish Sebben-Krupka, a New Jersey–based vegan chef, culinary educator, and food writer.

Trademarks

All terms mentioned in this book that are known to be or are suspected of being trademarks or service marks have been appropriately capitalized. Alpha Books and Penguin Group (USA) Inc. cannot attest to the accuracy of this information. Use of a term in this book should not be regarded as affecting the validity of any trademark or service mark.

Venturing into Veganism

Compassion for all—this sounds like some sort of pledge taken by the Three Musketeers or something you might find in the Hippocratic oath. In a way, it is a little like a pledge or an oath. Vegans base many of their life choices on compassion and consider the well-being of others whenever possible.

So you think you want to be a vegan? Well then, read on about the roots, history, and benefits of veganism, and prepare to begin your journey into a cruelty-free lifestyle!

Why Be Vegan?

In This Chapter

- Understanding the role of compassion in veganism
- Is vegan the right choice for you?
- Thinking about animal issues
- Growing as a vegan at your own speed
- Making choices and staying the vegan course

What are vegans? A tofu-eating race of extraterrestrial beings from the planet Vega who have come to Earth to surprise, confuse, befuddle, and conquer unsuspecting Earthlings? Well, they might as well be, considering the confusion some people seem to have about vegans and their approach to life.

In actuality, vegans are just plain ol' humans who have made a conscious decision to live their lives with a compassion directed toward all living creatures.

Compassion in Action

The definition of compassion, in simple terms, involves being sympathetic to the suffering or distress of others—but it doesn't stop there. It also includes a desire to help alleviate or eliminate that suffering. According to the definition of compassion, without the desire to make things better, compassion can't really exist. This concept actually forms the basis of what being *vegan* is all about: being aware that there is suffering, feeling a responsibility to do something about it, and acting on that feeling. Veganism is compassion in action.

DEFINITION

A **vegan** is one who avoids causing harm or exploiting other living beings as much as humanly possible. This involves excluding all animal foods and animal-based items from their lives.

Compassion is purely an emotional response. Most people feel compassion toward something or someone on some basic level. Living and showing compassion to all creatures big and small as much as possible is at the heart of being and living as a vegan.

It's common that many of us feel disconnected from the fellow creatures we share this planet with. We, as a species, seem to forget that other creatures are actually our distant relatives, forever linked to us by either evolution or a divine creator.

For many, it's hard to take the time to ponder this and other great truths of the universe while trying to meet all the daily commitments of a job, school, friends, family, and so on. But for those who do make it a point to try to understand who we are as a species, where we came from, and where we're going, it can be the start of a lifetime of increasing awareness and a positive struggle for internal and external change. As Gandhi said, "We must become the change we want to see."

Putting Forth Positive Energy

When you become aware that there's much needless animal suffering going on in the world and you become determined you'll no longer contribute to it, you've already taken the first step in bringing your compassion to the next level.

You and every other living creature on the planet only get one shot at this life you're living right now, and it only seems logical to make the most positive impact possible. Putting positive energy out into the universe brings more back to you. Doing your best to help effect positive change can cause a chain reaction of good things, the ripples of which can reach out into places previously unimagined.

Searching Your Soul

As the saying goes, a mind is a terrible thing to waste, and as humans, we have very developed brains that often are not used to their full potential. We really owe it to ourselves to be the best we can be on all levels: physical, mental, emotional, and spiritual. Doing a little soul searching can be a catalyst for good things, particularly when you think about how you view yourself and your role in society, as well as how you fit within the bigger scheme of things.

VEGAN VOICES

Man did not weave the web of life, he is merely a strand in it. Whatever he does to the web, he does to himself.

—Chief Seattle, leader of the Suquamish people, in a letter to the American government, 1854

It's okay to take some time to invest in yourself and your own growth. It's good to question things. The world around you is in a constant state of change, and it makes sense that you should be as well, particularly in developing who you are and the kind of person you want to be.

Looking around and really analyzing your life and the world around you can make you aware of pleasant and happy things, along with those that are more harsh and brutal. Some of what you see and experience will upset and concern you, and how, and to what extent you react, will be up to you. Some people prefer to follow a safe and steady course and not question things too much or get too involved, while others try to do whatever they can to help when they become aware of injustices. How you react is entirely up to you!

Is Vegan Living for You?

If you're wondering if living a vegan lifestyle might be for you, ask yourself the following questions:

- Do you love animals?
- Do you oppose the use of animals in entertainment?
- Do you feel sad seeing animals in pet-store windows?
- Do you sometimes find eating meat or dairy unappetizing?
- Do you find yourself gravitating toward the veggie side dishes on your plate first?
- Do you ever stop to ponder where the fur trim on your coat came from?
- Do you have any health concerns that may be diet related?

- Do you suffer from any food allergies or sensitivities?
- Does the knowledge that your lotion or mascara was tested on an animal make you think twice about using it?

If you answered "yes" to any of these questions, you could be a potential vegan in the making, and this book is certainly for you. We hope to educate, inform, and guide you through all the phases necessary to becoming, being, and living as a vegan.

These questions reflect some of the issues you may encounter as you begin to ponder the issues surrounding veganism and living compassionately. They should also spark more questions, whet your curiosity, and drive you to expand your knowledge base and thought processes. As you arrive at the answers to your questions, you may or may not be faced with making some major life choices to reconcile your feelings.

If you are compassionate and empowered to begin making decisions based on compassionate living, the vegan way of life could be for you. But only you know what is best for you.

Decisions, Decisions

By now you probably realize that transitioning to a vegan lifestyle is all about making decisions and choices. Being a vegan is about deciding to live as compassionately as possible and applying this to all the choices you make in your life, whether it's what to wear, what to buy, what to put in and on your body, and most importantly, how you choose to treat your fellow creatures on Earth.

If or when you feel you're ready to try to reduce the negative impact your life has on the animals we share this world with, do it in your own way and at your own pace. Begin by taking small steps and making decisions on basic issues first.

IN A NUTSHELL

Start your transition into a vegan lifestyle at your own speed and level. Keep in mind that sometimes an accumulation of small steps makes for a profound journey. As the Chinese proverb goes, a journey of 1,000 miles begins with the first step!

Never forget that with all your small yet positive changes, you are making a difference in the lives of other creatures. You may never know the results of the ripples of compassion you're causing to spread or how far they'll eventually reach.

As you move toward a vegan lifestyle, you'll have to make your own individual choices about what you will and will not feel comfortable doing in your life. For instance, will you continue to go to the zoo or circuses or support other forms of entertainment that use animals or keep them in confined areas? It might not bother you much in your first stages of becoming vegan, but you'll probably feel much different later on. Perceptions often change over time and when the time is right.

Benefits for You and Your Health

We all strive to live a long, healthy, and happy life, and although we can't control when we die, we can take control over the quality of our existence while we're alive. Choosing to go vegan is a huge step in the right direction for helping you achieve a healthier—and hopefully longer—life, as you will see in Chapter 3.

The latest research into optimal dietary needs, proper nutrition, and preventive approaches to fighting and treating disease seems to keep circling back to the garden plot, not the feedlot. The plant kingdom is where it's at in terms of proper nutrition, and our mothers, grandmothers, and Popeye the Sailor really did know best when they told us to finish our broccoli or eat our spinach if we want to grow up healthy and strong.

Leafy green veggies, fruits, and other plant-based foods contain multiple vitamins, minerals, and antioxidants our bodies need to function properly, and many of these nutrients are often lacking or totally absent in animal-based foods. Plant-based foods also tend to be lower in sodium, calories, and fats (especially harmful saturated fats that clog your arteries); contain beneficial dietary fiber; and are totally cholesterol-free, in contrast to their animal counterparts.

The standard American diet (SAD) relies heavily on animal-based foods, and many health experts believe that overconsumption of these types of foods is the cause of many chronic diseases and illnesses. As a result, larger numbers of people are transitioning to a more plant-based diet for their health.

Vegans have significantly lower incidences of cancer, stroke, heart disease, kidney disease, diabetes, and arthritis than those who eat meat, along with lower blood pressure and cholesterol levels. They tend to be more physically active and fit overall, with lower incidences of obesity. On average, vegans live 5 to 10 years longer than meat-eaters.

Spiritual Connection

For many of us, our personal ethics define our spirituality. Compassion, reverence for life, and passion for doing the right thing are central tenets of many of the great religions of the world—and of veganism, too. For vegans, these things often lay the foundation for the decisions made in life.

Albert Schweitzer spoke freely of his views on the reverence for life, which became a guiding force in his life as well as the inspiration for a group of writings on the subject. His writings were inspired by those of vegans or vegetarians before him, and the cycle continues, as his writings have inspired and will continue to inspire future generations of plant-based eaters.

> **VEGAN VOICES**
>
> By having a reverence for life, we enter into a spiritual relation with the world. By practicing reverence for life, we become good, deep, and alive.
>
> —Albert Schweitzer; humanitarian, theologian, musician, philosopher, physician, and 1952 Nobel Peace Prize recipient for his "Reverence for Life" philosophy

Throughout history, many different cultures and religions have been supportive of veganism and vegetarianism (see Chapter 2 for more information on vegetarianism). Most vegans try to live by the Golden Rule and treat others the way they themselves wish to be treated.

Cruelty-Free Living

As vegans, we choose to do no harm and live as much of a cruelty-free lifestyle as possible. That is, we make a conscious effort to ensure no animal had to suffer in the creation of the products we use and the foods we consume. We believe we can better sustain ourselves and the planet by using renewable, plant-based resources and by doing no harm to animals.

Vegans take consumerism very personally and are very careful about the products and services we support with our money. From a vegan perspective, it isn't right to put another creature through something we ourselves wouldn't be willing to go through. There are almost always alternatives to anything that has its roots in cruelty, and if not, there may be ways to avoid the product or practice altogether.

IN A NUTSHELL

When purchasing personal or household items, look for the V logo, or the words *vegan, certified vegan,* and *no animal testing.* These and other similar phrases are often accompanied by a drawing of a bunny on the product packaging. These types of designations signify that the product is free of animal-based ingredients or that it was produced using cruelty-free means.

Knowingly or not, vegans often practice *ahimsa*, which is an ancient Sanskrit word meaning "nonviolence," or more specifically, "to cause no harm or injury to another living creature." It is at the heart of cruelty-free living and forms much of the foundation veganism is built upon. (See Chapter 2 for more on ahimsa.)

Vegans: Square Pegs in Round Holes?

When you first decide to go vegan, you might feel at odds with the world and people around you. But just like anything in life, you can figure out things for yourself if you remain patient and persevere.

It helps to know that you as a vegan are not alone. Millions of other people in the world think very much like you do. You may not know any of them at first, but you eventually will. You will run into vegans in unexpected places—often when you least expect it!

We Come in All Shapes and Sizes

Vegans, like all the other creatures in the animal kingdom, come in all shapes and sizes. Big, tall, short, fat, petite, long-lived, or gone in a blink of an eye—like any subculture or religion, it's impossible to stereotype vegans into one boilerplate form. Vegans are hippies, yuppies, Republicans and Democrats (and even former U.S. presidents!), celebrities and entertainers, CEOs and business moguls, medical professionals, athletes, grandparents, and regular Janes and Joes.

People arrive at their chosen compassionate lifestyle for their own personal reasons, often in their own roundabout way. Some start out by being concerned with animal issues, while others come to a vegan lifestyle after first exploring seemingly unconnected issues. Sometimes dietary or medical concerns, including food allergies and weight-loss issues, start a person down a road that eventually leads him to veganism.

Then there are the raw foodists, the religious-minded, and those who view their bodies as temples and discover that eating vegan is the healthiest way to worship at that temple. Some just stumble into it out of pure curiosity while pursuing any one of the various issues surrounding the lifestyle or maybe due to peer or celebrity influence. We're all unique, and the paths we take to get here are equally unique!

Finding the Perfect Fit

Making contact with other vegans can really help you achieve a sense of vegan camaraderie and remind you that you belong to a larger community of people who share your ideals. This can help you stay the course and empower you as a vegan.

It might take time for you to find your perfect fit or just the right place in the world as a vegan, but be patient. The search for your own perfect place, which may be a physical or mental state, or even simply one or more supportive friends, can take some time. The internet can be a great way to connect with other vegans, through social networking websites, discussion forums, and even blogs.

If you don't find that your present physical location is supportive of your vegan lifestyle, you can always seek out a more veg-friendly place. Again, the internet can help you search for and discover new and wonderful places—just like we did when we discovered the very vegan-friendly city of Eugene, Oregon!

Wherever you live, and whatever your number of vegan friends, you can still always try to do all you can to improve things for animals, people, and environment in your current locale. Try volunteering at an animal shelter or joining (or founding!) a local pro-vegan group. This can really help make a difference in your area and further your commitment to the causes you care the most about.

The Least You Need to Know

- Compassion is a combination of being aware of the distress or suffering of others and wanting to help alleviate it.
- Many religions have compassion at the root of their beliefs, and veganism is similar in this regard.
- Finding support for your beliefs can be important in helping you stay the course.

Planting the Seeds of Veganism

In This Chapter

- The difference between vegans and vegetarians
- Illustrious veg-heads through history
- The birth of the Vegan and Vegetarian societies
- The spread of the vegan movement

The transition to a vegan lifestyle often involves a gradual progression, although for some, it happens almost overnight. As they learn more and more about the positive impact of a cruelty-free lifestyle and the wonderful health benefits gained from a plant-based diet, many people feel compelled to move further toward a complete vegan lifestyle. Enter, the veg-heads.

Veg-Heads

When a person decides to become a "veg-head"—a vegetarian, vegan, or someone who avoids animal-based products or foods to varying degrees—it's usually at his or her own speed and comfort level. Let's begin by taking a look at the similarities and differences between vegans and vegetarians, two of the main types of veg-heads.

The Vegetarians

Vegetarians choose not to eat animal flesh (meat, poultry, fish, and seafood), but they do often consume other animal-based products, such as milk, cheese, butter, eggs, gelatin, and honey.

There are several subcategories of vegetarians:

- Lacto-vegetarians eat dairy (lacto) but not eggs.
- Ovo-vegetarians eat eggs (ovo) but not dairy.
- Lacto-ovo vegetarians eat both eggs and dairy.
- Flexitarians eat mostly a vegetarian or heavily plant-based diet but still occasionally eat meat, poultry, fish, or seafood.

Most vegetarians fall into the lacto-ovo category. Although they don't eat animal flesh, some vegetarians do wear leather shoes or clothing and also use animal-based beauty products, like beeswax-based lip gloss or mascara or lotions made with lanolin from wool.

Flexitarians, who label themselves vegetarian while still eating meat, are often a source of controversy and discussion among vegans and vegetarians alike. Many see them as a contradiction in terms, similar to that of being a war-supporting pacifist or a polluting environmentalist. Others feel that an increase in people trying to be "mostly vegetarian" is ultimately better for animals, as well as for individual and planetary health, than if they had remained unrestrained meat-eaters.

The Vegans

Veganism takes the dietary compassion of vegetarianism to the next level, concerning itself with all aspects of a living creature's existence. Vegans eat a strictly plant-based diet and do not use or consume anything that comes from an animal, like meat, poultry, fish, eggs, dairy products, and honey or beeswax. They also avoid wearing things like leather, wool, silk, or feathers. If something came from an animal source—insects included—or involved something from an animal source used in the production of a product, vegans don't use or consume it. Basically, if it had a face, fins, wings, or feet, a vegan won't use it, eat it, or wear it.

Vegans are faced with many daily choices based on whether or not animal suffering or exploitation is present or involved. As much as possible, vegans abstain from any activity, food, business, or product that involves causing harm in any way to any living, feeling, and sentient creatures. This applies to human as well as nonhuman beings.

So Close, and Yet So Far

Both vegans and vegetarians agree that we should consume more of a plant-based, rather than animal-based, diet. But they disagree fundamentally when it comes to consuming and using animal-based foods at all. Much of being vegetarian centers on the dietary realm and does not spill over into other areas of life as much as being vegan does.

HOT POTATO

By continuing to consume dairy products and eggs, vegetarians are, even if unwittingly, still supporting the factory farm system and the corporations that profit from them. Vegans tend to vote with their dollars by not giving their money to industries that conflict with their cruelty-free focus.

Using and wearing products that come from animal-based sources is often not considered inconsistent with the vegetarian lifestyle. From a vegan perspective, much of this use is based on a lack of information and understanding of the underlying factors involved in the production of those items. It's wrongly assumed that just because the animal isn't killed (or at least directly killed) in the production of any given thing, the story ends there.

Some vegetarians think that moving toward a vegan lifestyle is difficult or inconvenient, and often they aren't quite sure how they would go about replacing the animal products in their lives. How can you find good nonleather shoes or get enough calcium and protein in your diet if you don't consume dairy products? Have no fear. It's actually quite simple if you're armed with the right information. These are the types of issues and life factors we address in this book.

Veg-Heads Through the Ages

Many influential people throughout history were either vegetarian or vegan. Veg-heads abound throughout all phases of history.

Evidence exists that some of the earliest humans were mostly vegetarians who ate meat only during extreme circumstances or while in hostile climates. Instead of the "hunter-gatherer" image we learned of in elementary school and beyond, our early ancestors were far more likely to be primarily gatherers.

In addition to the many gifts the ancient Greeks gave the world, they also did quite a bit to develop and spread the concept of vegetarianism. Among the influential Greek vegetarians was the philosopher and father of mathematics Pythagoras of Samos (580 B.C.E.), who is remembered most for his Pythagorean Theorem, which has helped and/or frustrated first-year geometry students for centuries. Other notable ancient Greek vegetarians include Plato, Porphyry, Epicurus, Plutarch, and Diogenes.

Major Eastern religions such as Buddhism and Jainism have, at their core, a strong advocacy of vegetarian and vegan values. Siddhartha Gautama, who later became the Buddha and founder of Buddhism, was a vegetarian. Through many spiritual writings, he mandated a vegetarian diet rooted in compassion. Mahavira, founder of the Jain religion in the sixth century B.C.E., advocated nonviolence toward human and nonhumans alike and mandated a strict veganism for all followers.

VEGAN VOICES

He who harms animals has not understood or renounced deeds of sin. ... Those whose minds are at peace and who are free from passions do not desire to live at the expense of others.

—Mahavira (599–527 B.C.E.), Hindu teacher and founder of Jainism

The quintessential Renaissance Man himself, Leonardo da Vinci, was also a vegetarian. He wrote in his journal that "I have from an early age adjured the use of meat, and the time will come when men such as I will look upon the murder of animals as they now look upon the murder of men." While the man who gave the world so many inventions and great works of art was busy painting, discovering, and writing, he was fueling his body and mind with a vegetarian diet.

Many famous writers have also led meatless lives. Through their writings, vegetarian poets Percy Bysshe Shelley, Ralph Waldo Emerson, and Lord Byron influenced others, including playwright George Bernard Shaw, to "go veggie." Percy's wife, Mary Shelley, herself a vegetarian, weaved vegetarian and anti–animal experimentation themes throughout her novel *Frankenstein*. Renowned Russian writer Leo Tolstoy was also a strong vegetarian advocate, as were Franz Kafka and H. G. Wells.

The complete list of other illustrious vegetarians and vegans throughout history is much too long to include here, but consider this small sampling:

- Albert Einstein, scientist

- Charlotte Brontë, novelist

- Harriet Beecher Stowe, writer

- Henry David Thoreau, writer

- Isaac Bashevis Singer, writer

- Mohandas Gandhi, humanitarian

- Sir Isaac Newton, scientist and mathematician

- Susan B. Anthony, women's suffrage pioneer

- Thomas Edison, inventor

- Vincent van Gogh, painter

The British Invasion: The Vegetarian Society

During the 1800s, more and more people who shared some of the same ideals started organizing meetings and publishing writings about their views and feelings toward animals. A monumental meeting took place on September 30, 1847, in London, when 140 people gathered to voice their feelings regarding the consumption of animals. This was the beginning of the Vegetarian Society of the United Kingdom. Members chose to call themselves "vegetarians" based on the Latin word *vegetus*, meaning "whole," "sound," "fresh," and "lively." (It wasn't based on the word *vegetable*, as many people think!)

The Vegetarian Society started the *Vegetarian Messenger* as a way to publish its writings that supported its positions and challenged the status quo. This publication helped further expand vegetarians' influence throughout the world as well as bring people together.

Members of the Vegetarian Society came from all walks of life. Some held political, religious, and esteemed positions within society. As members traversed the globe, their influences helped shape public opinions throughout the world. Many Christian religious leaders embraced the natural hygiene and vegetarian movements, helping further spread the good message of compassionate living.

IN A NUTSHELL

The natural hygiene movement's principles date back centuries, but the 1800s saw the most advances in this new area of emerging medicine. The approach suggested many "revolutionary" concepts for the time, such as consuming whole, natural foods; getting sufficient rest, sleep, fresh air, and sunshine; and bathing regularly.

Reverend William Metcalfe was one of the first religious leaders to help the British vegetarian message spread to the Americas when he emigrated to the United States in 1817. He influenced many people, including Bronson Alcott, father of the famous American writer and herself vegetarian Louisa May Alcott, who established one of the first vegan communities in America.

Metcalfe also influenced Sylvester Graham, who preached the "good book" as well as natural hygiene, raw and whole foods, and vegetarianism. He was also the creator of the graham cracker, made from graham flour, both of which are named after him. As the vegetarian movement grew in the United States, the America Vegetarian Society and the numbers of other such groups also grew.

The Vegan Society Emerges

A diverse group of people made up the Vegetarian Society. As members' consciousness raised and eyes opened to the suffering of animals, further questions and quandaries arose. Many began to question the practices they had once supported, including eating animal-based foods such as dairy products and eggs, and to examine the many moral issues tied to the raising and using of animals for various facets of life.

Donald Watson: Vegan Revolutionary

Articles that addressed these new issues and concerns began appearing in the *Vegetarian Messenger*. Many members opposed these "radical new views," which caused dissension in the ranks of the Vegetarian Society. In December 1943, Donald Watson spoke freely about his views in a lecture titled "Should Vegetarians Eat Dairy Products?" This lecture sparked questioning and contemplation for some of the members of the society, but for the most part, it was met with opposition.

In November 1944, Watson and several others gathered to discuss the formation of a society that supported their ideals of compassion for all creatures. From that gathering came the Vegan Society.

Members first referred to themselves as "total vegetarians" and then later shortened it to "vegans." In fact, Donald Watson was the first to coin the word *vegan*. He took the first three letters and the last two letters of the word *vegetarian* because, as he plainly put it, "veganism starts with vegetarianism and carries it through to its logical conclusion."

The Aims of the Vegan Society

Members of the Vegan Society believed in living as humanely and compassionately as possible, thus eliminating practices and products from their lives that lead to the exploitation or cruelty of animals. The aims of the Vegan Society were and continue to be as follows:

- To advocate that man's food should be derived from fruits, nuts, vegetables, grains, and other wholesome nonanimal products, and that it should exclude flesh; fowl; eggs; honey; and animal's milk, butter, and cheese

- To encourage the manufacture and use of alternatives to animal commodities

Donald Watson's and the Vegan Society's first newsletter was titled the *Vegan News*. Starting with only 30 subscribers, it soon became known as simply *The Vegan*, and thousands worldwide read the quarterly magazine.

In 2012, the Vegan Society is still doing its part to spread the vegan message by providing educational material on veganism to schools, organizations, and individuals. It also publishes the *Animal Free Shopper* and various books and videos on animal issues, lifestyle choices, cooking, and nutrition.

The Grassroots Spreading of Veganism

The Vegan Society's work eventually helped spread the concept of veganism to other shores as well, influencing people in Asia, India, Australia, New Zealand, and the Americas. Little did the founding Vegan Society members know how far-reaching their message would eventually be!

IN A NUTSHELL

In 1994, on the fiftieth anniversary of their first meeting, the Vegan Society declared November 1 World Vegan Day. It's celebrated every year with worldwide events to promote veganism.

Coming to America

Just a few years after the creation of the Vegan Society, Dr. Catherine Nimmo and Rubin Abramowitz started a branch in California. Their work caused a snowballing effect for veganism on North American shores.

In 1960, Jay Dinshah began the American Vegan Society, better known as AVS, and fittingly, its first member was Catherine Nimmo, who remained a member until her passing in 1985. The writings of Jay and many others were featured in *Ahimsa* (defined by AVS as "dynamic harmlessness"), the organization's magazine from 1960 to 2000. (In 2001, it became the quarterly magazine *American Vegan*.)

The AVS spells out ahimsa as an acronym, creating a moral code that can help guide a vegan through life. It is made up of "six pillars of the compassionate way." They are as follows:

- **A**bstinence from animal products
- **H**armlessness with reverence for life
- **I**ntegrity of thought, word, and deed
- **M**astery over oneself
- **S**ervice to humanity, nature, and creation
- **A**dvancement of understanding and truth

When Jay died in 2000, he was still working to spread the message of veganism and compassion. He was posthumously awarded the Mankar Memorial Award at the thirty-fourth World Vegetarian Congress in Toronto. At each congress, this award is given to those who have made a significant contribution to the cause of vegetarianism. Jay was honored for his work with the AVS, NAVS, American Natural Hygiene Society (known as the National Health Association since 1998), International Vegetarian Union (IVU), and Vegetarian Union of North America (VUNA). Jay's wife and children continue his work, as well as their own, of spreading the message of dynamic harmlessness.

IN A NUTSHELL

In 2011, a Harris Interactive telephone poll sponsored by the Vegetarian Resource Group (VRG) estimated that 2.5 percent of the U.S. population identifies as being vegan. This translates to roughly 7.7 million people, which is over double the number estimated in a 2000 Zogby poll.

Oh, Canada!

The first records of organized vegetarianism in Canada are the formation of the Toronto Vegetarian Association (TVA). In 1945, a small group of 20 or so vegetarians gathered at the home of Esther Greenburg to discuss their views. They came away with the basis of their organization, as well as a president, J. Don Scott. Within a year, their numbers had grown to 150, and they helped send surplus soy grits and vegetable-based oils to those in need in the throes of war in Europe. A few years later, members organized the Vegetarian Fund for India to help fight famine in the region.

The TVA is, to date, Canada's largest vegetarian organization. Its work has inspired other grassroots organizations, including Vegan Canada. This organization is dedicated to working with individuals and other vegan and vegetarian groups to educate, inform, and encourage a vegan lifestyle.

For more information, or to find addresses and websites for the organizations discussed in this chapter, see Appendix B.

The Least You Need to Know

- Vegetarianism is mainly concerned with diet, while veganism focuses on all aspects relating to animal cruelty and usage.
- Many influential people throughout history were either vegetarian or vegan.
- Donald Watson founded the Vegan Society in 1944 as an offshoot of the Vegetarian Society due to differences of opinion surrounding the use of animals in the diet and beyond.
- Watson coined the term *vegan* from the first three and last two letters of *vegetarian*.
- Through the work of Catherine Nimmo, Jay Dinshah, and others, the Vegan Society's message spread to the Americas and beyond.
- The Toronto Vegetarian Association (TVA) is Canada's largest and oldest established vegetarian organization.

On the Road to Good Health

In This Chapter

- Health concerns surrounding animal-based diets
- Healthful benefits of plant-based diets
- Preventive medicine and its proponents
- Reducing your risk of heart disease

Many new vegans, as well as their friends and family, are sometimes concerned that their new way of eating, free of animal products, won't be as healthy as their previous diet. Although you should always be conscious of whether or not your nutritional intake is adequately meeting your needs, eating a well-balanced vegan diet is actually *more* healthful than eating one that includes animal products.

All you need is a little information to help guide you along the way, and soon you'll be thriving on a vegan diet!

Meat Mayhem

Consuming food from animal sources has many pitfalls, and serious health concerns are certainly among them. We've discussed the spiritual and emotional reasons behind being vegan and the history of the veggie movement. Now we come to perhaps the strongest argument for a vegan lifestyle: the health disadvantages of eating meat and the health benefits you can gain by eating a plant-based vegan diet.

Food-Borne Illness Concerns

Food-borne illnesses are of serious concern to all of us, whether we eat meat or not. People often think they have the "24-hour flu" or the stomach flu, when in actuality they are having an intestinal reaction to food-borne or water-borne bacteria that has invaded their body and taken up residence. The most commonly known food- or water-borne bacteria are E. coli, salmonella, campylobacter, and listeria. Each takes varying lengths of time to rear its ugly and painful head, but the most common symptoms are abdominal pain and cramps, vomiting, and diarrhea often accompanied by blood.

According to U.S. government statistics, E. coli is present in about half of all cattle, which is 10 times higher than previously thought. Campylobacter infects more than 70 percent of chickens and 90 percent of turkeys, and between 20 to 80 percent of all chickens are also infected with salmonella.

Improper food handling can be blamed for the spreading of bacteria, but the most numerous and serious of incidents can all be traced back to animal-based contamination. Much of the meat, eggs, and dairy products Americans consume is infected with some sort of food-borne bacteria, which is then passed on to the humans when the food is consumed. Even when plant foods appear to be the source of an outbreak, the true source is often traced back to water that was contaminated by infected livestock or to improper handling of tainted meat.

What's Mad Cow Disease?

You may have heard of mad cow disease, but many people aren't really sure what it is. Mad cow disease is a transmissible spongiform encephalopathy (TSE) found in several species. In humans, it's called Creutzfeld-Jacob Disease (CJD); in sheep it's called scrapies; in elk and deer herds, it's referred to as chronic wasting; and in cattle, it's called bovine spongiform encephalopathy (BSE), or more commonly, mad cow disease.

Whatever you label it, TSE affects the central nervous system, causing disintegration of the brain, and it is fatal. Consuming infected meat and other parts—specifically brain and other organ meat—and spinal cord material most commonly transmits TSE. Problems occur when contaminated animals go undetected and get into the "food chain" of modern farming. The infected meat contains prions, small infected proteins that transmit the disease, which can pass from animal to animal and even species to species.

Mad cow crosses over to our species when humans eat the infected beef. Symptoms of the human version, CJD, can lie dormant for 20 years before making themselves apparent. Because the symptoms of CJD mimic those of other brain-wasting conditions such as Alzheimer's, CJD usually goes undiagnosed. At the time of this writing, the only way to positively test for the presence of the CJD prion is to take a tissue sample from the brain.

> **IN A NUTSHELL**
>
> In 1996, Texas cattle ranchers sued Oprah Winfrey and Howard Lyman, author of *Mad Cowboy*, for remarks they made involving mad cow disease and not eating hamburgers anymore. The ranchers said the two defendants slandered beef's good name. Oprah and Howard won against the ranchers. The pair were the first defendants sued under the then-new Texas Food Disparagement Act.

The Connection Between Diet and Disease

Heredity determines if you have a genetic predisposition for a particular illness or disease, but many other factors help determine the quality of your health. Getting adequate rest and plenty of fresh air and sunshine; drinking pure, filtered water; exercising regularly; and most importantly, consuming a well-balanced vegan diet rich in plant-based foods is necessary to your physical and emotional well-being.

Many health organizations, such as the American Cancer Society, the American Dietetic Association, the American Heart Association, the American Diabetic Association, and even the Senate Select Committee on Nutrition have stated that diet and lifestyle play a major role in developing certain illnesses and diseases. Studies have shown that many chronic diseases—including cancer, diabetes, hypertension, heart disease, kidney and liver disease, strokes, obesity, arthritis, gastrointestinal disorders, and osteoporosis—are indeed diet related.

The medical community is doing more research than ever before into the links between health and diet. They are most concerned about diets that are high in cholesterol and saturated fat, low in dietary fiber and complex carbohydrates, and lacking in adequate vitamins and minerals. Animal-based diets are high in saturated fat and very low in dietary fiber. In contrast, plant-based diets contain large amounts of dietary fiber and vital nutrients, have low levels of saturated fats, and are cholesterol free. Eating vegan can actually *decrease* your risk of disease.

> **VEGAN VOICES**
>
> Overconsumption of certain dietary components is now a major concern for Americans. While many foods are involved, chief among them is the disproportionate consumption of foods high in fats, often at the expense of foods high in complex carbohydrates and fiber that may be more conducive to health.
>
> —Surgeon General C. Everett Koop, in his 1994 report *Nutrition and Health in the United States*

Dietary Links to Cancer

The amount of cancer research has greatly increased in the last few decades, with much of it focusing on the ties between diet and the disease. In fact, the World Health Organization concedes that dietary factors account for approximately 30 percent of all cancers in Western countries, and up to 20 percent in developing countries. The American Cancer Society agrees and has determined that one third of all cancer deaths in the United States are attributable to nutritional factors.

Studies done in England, Germany, Canada, Japan, and the United States have all shown that eating large quantities of fruits and vegetables helps reduce your risks of getting cancer because such diets tend to be high in dietary fiber; low in fat; and contain many beneficial phytochemicals, antioxidants, and other anticancer compounds.

In contrast, meat and other animal-based products, as well as high-fat foods, have been found to increase your cancer risks because they increase your production of hormones (like estrogen and testosterone), which in turn promotes growth of cancer cells in hormone-sensitive organs such as the breasts, ovaries, and prostate. In addition, nearly 80 percent of all livestock in the United States are fed some sort of hormones, including synthetic growth hormones, to increase and extend production. When humans eat the hormone-fed meat, the hormones are also passed on and wreak havoc on our systems.

Animal-based foods are low in fiber, contain high concentrations of saturated fat, and as the result of cooking may also contain carcinogenic compounds (like heterocyclic amines), which greatly increase your chances of developing various kinds of cancer. Therefore, many health professionals have proclaimed that plant-eaters are at the lowest risk for cancer and have a significantly reduced risk compared to meat-eaters. According to the Physicians Committee for Responsible Medicine, "vegetarians are about 40 percent less likely to get cancer than nonvegetarians, regardless of other risks such as smoking, body size, and socioeconomic status."

Obesity on the Rise

The United States has the highest obesity rate in the world. Obesity has reached epidemic proportions, with more than two out of every three Americans being classified as overweight or obese. While more and more people go on diets to lose weight, 25 percent of the world's population is malnourished. High-fat fast-food diets, sedentary lifestyles, and plain old lack of energy all contribute to ever-expanding waistlines and rising numbers on the scale.

So how do you know if you are overweight or obese? Well, if you weigh 10 percent or more of what's considered the average recommended weight for someone your height and age, you are overweight. To be considered obese, you have to be 20 percent above the average weight.

Body mass index (BMI) is a simple index of weight and height commonly used by health professionals to classify weight for adults. BMI is defined as a person's weight in kilograms divided by the square of his height in meters (kg/m^2). Having a BMI over 25 is considered being overweight and over 30 is obese. As your weight increases, you also increase your chances of developing diabetes, cancer, heart disease, kidney disease, high blood pressure, high cholesterol, and breathing and sleep disorders.

If you are overweight, it's because you are taking in more fuel (food) than you expend as energy, and your body stores the excess as fat. Making serious dietary and lifestyle changes are the only nonsurgical ways to win the battle of the bulge. It isn't just sugars and other carbohydrates, as some diet books would have you believe; overindulge on fatty foods on a regular basis, and surprise, surprise, you'll probably gain weight.

Most animal-based foods contain several kinds of fats, but most troubling are the high concentrations of saturated fats. Saturated fats clog your arteries and add a layer of fat to your outsides as well. What you put in your body really does affect how it looks on the outside, so be sure to eat the best nature has to offer: luscious healthful veggies, whole grains, and succulent fruits!

Veg-Head Vitality

After many years of speculation, it has finally become widely accepted that a well-balanced vegan diet provides adequate nutrition and helps in the prevention and treatment of illness.

The idea of diet and health being tied together isn't new. Hippocrates, the Greek vegetarian man of wonder, saw the connection centuries ago. The father of modern medicine even reportedly cured many illnesses with fasting and raw foods.

Plant-Based Benefits

Across the board, vegans have lower incidences of cancer, stroke, heart disease, kidney disease, diabetes, and arthritis and lower blood pressure and cholesterol levels, just to name a few.

In the last few decades, much research has been conducted on the ties between various diseases and our diets, both in the United States and abroad. In study after study, the benefits of plant-based foods outweighed those of animal-based selections. This knowledge has empowered people to take the prevention or treatment of disease into their own hands by nourishing their bodies with a diet high in the kinds of vitamins, minerals, and other important nutrients that only come from fresh fruits, veggies, whole grains, and other plant-based foods.

In addition to the many vital nutrients fruits and veggies are loaded with, including vitamins and much-needed fiber, phytochemicals are included in the plant-based foods we eat. These chemical compounds are produced naturally by plants and are extremely beneficial in keeping the body happy and healthy. They provide our bodies with an arsenal of natural weapons we need to fight off cancer and other diseases.

Consider these examples of phytochemicals, along with the foods they are found in and the benefits they give us:

- Sulforphane, found in broccoli, helps fight cancer.
- Limonoids, found in citrus fruits, increase the activity of enzymes that eliminate carcinogens.
- Indoles, found in cruciferous vegetables like cauliflower, cabbages, and greens, lower the risk of cancer, especially breast cancer.
- Carotenoids, including lycopene, beta-carotene, and lutein, found in carrots, tomatoes, fruits, and greens, lower the risk of cancer, heart disease, premature aging, and degenerative eye disease.
- Flavonoids, found in cranberries and other berries, grapes, nuts, seeds, and olives, lower the risk of cancer and heart disease and also lower cholesterol levels.
- Isoflavones, found in beans, especially in soybeans, lower the risk of cancers, attack free radicals, and balance estrogen and hormone levels.

Longer and Healthier Lives

On average, vegans and vegetarians live 6 to 10 years longer than meat-eaters. That's primarily due to the many health benefits of eating a plant-based diet. They tend to have lower cholesterol and blood pressure levels, consume less saturated fat and more fiber, and get lots of good disease-fighting plant compounds. As a result, on average, vegans also tend to be more fit.

They tend to be more conscious of and concerned with what they put into their bodies, whether it be clean air, clean water, or good foods from organic sources whenever possible. They also tend to be more active, which helps keep their bones stronger for longer throughout their lives, and their joints and muscles moving as they should.

We're all familiar with how fat and cholesterol affect our health, but so do excess amounts of protein and calcium, especially where our internal organs are concerned. By not consuming excess amounts of meat and dairy, vegans have a better shot at avoiding those pitfalls. (We touch more on this in Chapters 5 and 6, where we discuss the body's protein and calcium requirements and take a look at some good sources from food.)

An Ounce of Prevention: Preventive Medicine

The medical community is finally starting to alert the public to the preventative aspects of a plant-based diet. Some physicians have taken it a step further and have become leaders in a field of medicine known as *preventive medicine*, with various clinics, organizations, and literature to support it.

> **DEFINITION**
>
> **Preventive medicine** is primarily concerned with helping healthy people *stay* healthy and providing the tools and information needed to keep disease at bay. It explores the environmental and dietary effects on disease and health and works to determine the root causes instead of reaching for quick fixes.

Preventive medicine is not really a new concept, but it has been winning over many within the medical community. Most doctors entered the medical profession out of a desire to help others, and giving patients the information and guidance needed for them to stay healthy in the first place is certainly one of the best ways to help them.

A number of doctors are on the forefront of this exciting field and advocate plant-based diets in their disease prevention techniques. Let's meet a few.

Heart-Healthy Eating with Dr. Esselstyn

Dr. Caldwell B. Esselstyn Jr. is a former surgeon, researcher, and clinician at the Cleveland Clinic. Through his 20-year nutritional study of patients who were diagnosed with advanced coronary artery disease, he achieved remarkable results through a treatment of dietary changes alone. With his help, they were able to dramatically lose weight, lower cholesterol levels, reduce angina symptoms, and even improve their artery blood flow—and all of this was done without having to resort to surgery.

Simply by placing these patients on a plant-based, oil-free diet, Dr. Esselstyn has helped them not only stop the progression of their heart disease, but in many cases, also reversed their diagnosis. It's his belief that heart disease can actually be prevented through dietary changes. To learn more about Dr. Esselstyn and his groundbreaking research and work, check out his book *Prevent and Reverse Heart Disease*.

Lifestyle Changes with Dr. McDougall

Dr. John McDougall, along with his wife, Mary, developed *The McDougall Program*, which guides people through making changes in their diet and lifestyle to achieve healthful living. Among the many positive lifestyle changes they recommend to their patients and their readers, the McDougalls' various health and advanced study programs advocate a diet free of animal foods. They have devoted their lives to helping people improve their health, diet, and overall well-being, without the use of medications or surgeries.

At the McDougall Health Center in Santa Rosa, California, patients can be part of a 10-day live-in program as they make transitional changes to their lifestyle and dietary habits. The center's program is vegan, and Dr. McDougall even offers a line of packaged vegan foods to make it convenient to eat healthful, vegan foods on the go; as part of school lunches; or at the office.

IN A NUTSHELL

John and Mary McDougall are the authors of several best-selling books, including *The McDougall Program: 12 Days to Dynamic Health*, *The McDougall Program for Maximum Weight Loss*, *The McDougall Program for Women*, and *The McDougall Program for a Healthy Heart*.

The Raw Cure for Diabetes with Dr. Cousens

Dr. Gabriel Cousens is a holistic physician and the founder and director of the Tree of Life Rejuvenation Center and Tree of Life Foundation in Patagonia, Arizona, a holistic medical spa and lifestyle educational campus that focuses on preventing and reversing illnesses and disease through a raw foods diet. He is the author of several books, including *Conscious Eating, Rainbow Green Live Food Cuisine,* and *There Is a Cure for Diabetes.*

Dr. Cousens and his Tree of Life Rejuvenation Center were featured in the movie *Simply Raw: Reversing Diabetes in 30 Days,* which followed several diabetic patients through their lifestyle changes and raw foods nutritional treatment at the center. With the aid of this program, Dr. Cousens helped them not only lose weight, but also reduce or eliminate their need for insulin and other medications and improve their blood sugar levels so significantly that they are no longer considered diabetic.

The Physicians Committee for Responsible Medicine and Dr. Barnard

The Physicians Committee for Responsible Medicine (PCRM) is a nonprofit organization comprised of well-known physicians, laypersons, and grassroots individuals. Founded in 1985, it promotes preventive medicine, conducts clinical research, and encourages higher standards for ethics and effectiveness in research.

The big deal about PCRM is that it focuses on preventive medicine and advocates taking conscious steps and making lifestyle changes, if necessary, to prevent a health crisis from settling on your shoulders. It employs these preventive techniques first, instead of gravitating toward medications or surgeries for quick fixes. The group also provides free informational brochures such as its *Vegetarian Starter Kit, Vegetarian Starter Kit for Restaurants,* and *Replacing Animals in Research* for use as educational tools.

Dr. Neal Barnard is the president of PCRM and author of *Turn Off the Fat Genes; Foods That Fight Pain; Eat Right, Live Longer; Food for Life;* and other books on preventive medicine. In all his books, he tries to show how following a plant-based diet, exercising, and taking direct control of your own health ensures that your life and health are all they should be.

PCRM's advisory board includes 19 well-known health-care professionals from a broad range of specialties. Here are a few of our favorites:

- T. Colin Campbell, PhD, Cornell University
- Caldwell B. Esselstyn Jr., MD, Cleveland Clinic
- Suzanne Havala Hobbs, PhD, MS, RD, LDN, FADA, Vegetarian Resource Group
- Henry J. Heimlich, MD, ScD, Heimlich Institute
- Lawrence Kushi, ScD, Division of Research, Kaiser Permanente
- Virginia Messina, MPH, RD, Nutrition Matters, Inc.
- John McDougall, MD, McDougall Program, St. Helena Hospital
- Milton Mills, MD, Gilead Medical Group
- Myriam Parham, RD, LD, CDE, East Pasco Medical Center
- Andrew Weil, MD, University of Arizona

IN A NUTSHELL

For more information on PCRM and its informative website, see Appendix B or pcrm.org.

The China Study and Dr. Campbell

Dr. T. Colin Campbell of Cornell University and Dr. Richard Peto of Oxford University have conducted a research project studying thousands of patients in China. The China-Oxford-Cornell Diet and Health Project, or the China Study, as it's more commonly referred to, is one of the most comprehensive studies done to date on the correlation between diet and disease.

Dr. Campbell and Dr. Peto chose to study the Chinese because in comparison to other cultural or ethnic groups throughout the world, a majority of Chinese people tend to remain in one area for many decades, even generations. They also tend to consume certain types of foods, regionally and routinely, that have sustained them and formed the basis of their diets for centuries.

Chinese diets generally contain only about 0 to 20 percent animal-based foods, compared to 60 to 80 percent for the standard American diet. The study has shown that the more westernized their diet becomes and the farther they stray from their former mostly plant-based diet, the more they experience an increase of heart disease, cancer, obesity, diabetes, and so on.

The study also found that the Chinese have fewer incidences of breast and ovarian cancer than people in Western countries. This may have a tie to soy, which is quite prevalent in the average Chinese diet and contains beneficial cancer-fighting *phytoestrogens.*

DEFINITION

Phytoestrogens are naturally occurring plant compounds similar to estradiol, the most potent form of human estrogen. The effects of phytoestrogens are not as strong as most estrogens and are very easily broken down and eliminated. They help regulate the estrogen levels in the body.

In addition, the study showed that a diet high in animal protein affects the rate at which young people grow and mature sexually. It found that hormones contained in animal foods, including bovine growth hormone, make humans grow taller and larger in disproportional and increased rates.

The many findings of the study discovered that chronic degenerative diseases, such as diabetes, cancers, and heart disease, occur most in areas where diets are higher in animal products and fat, such as in industrialized and urbanized Chinese locales. It also found that even adding small amounts of animal foods to an otherwise all-plant-based diet significantly raises cholesterol levels, as well as the risk for related diseases.

Lactose and Lactose Intolerance

Some people find their way to a plant-based diet because of allergies or intolerances to foods. Milk, dairy, eggs, shellfish, and even certain fruits, vegetables, and nuts are common allergens and negatively impact millions of people each year in the United States alone.

One of the most predominant food intolerances is to dairy products. If a person is lactose intolerant, his or her body is unable to break down lactose into glucose, which the body uses to provide energy and fuel.

All mammals breast-feed until a certain age and then, when they are weaned, their bodies no longer need to produce lactase, the protein enzyme needed to break down the lactose into glucose. For humans, this begins happening around age 2. So when we consume dairy products beyond that age, our bodies may no longer be able to digest the lactose they contain, thus causing some people symptoms of lactose intolerance.

Lactose intolerance is a common concern throughout a modern world that sustains itself on a diet of dairy-rich foods. In fact, only a small part of the world population can even digest cow's lactose throughout their entire lives, and it's mostly those of Eastern European descent. For the rest—nearly 75 percent of the population worldwide—consuming dairy products may start out as a harmless act but soon ends in pain and discomfort.

Symptoms of lactose intolerance include gas, bloating, cramping, nausea, and diarrhea and are experienced by many who consume dairy products in the form of milk, cheese, yogurt, ice cream, and so on. Left unchecked, it could lead to extreme weight loss and malnutrition.

Protecting Your Heart from Disease

Heart disease is becoming the number-one killer of men and women throughout the world. It was once thought that the only options when diagnosed with this disease were either to wait and see, take costly medications, or face a series of risky surgeries. Now doctors and laypersons know that by simply making changes in diet and lifestyle, you can greatly reduce your risks of having a heart attack and facing a lifelong battle with heart disease.

Begin by getting enough rest, reducing your stress levels, and enjoying some form of regular exercise—hopefully outdoors so you can breathe in fresh air. Check your weight, blood pressure, and cholesterol levels; heart disease is affected by all those factors.

Then analyze your diet and whenever you can, try to limit your consumption of excess sugar and sweeteners, fat and oils, and salt. Fortunately, whole foods that are part of a vegan diet tend to be high in fiber and low in fat, especially saturated fats, which will help you maintain a proper weight. As an added bonus, plant-based foods are also cholesterol free.

The average cholesterol level for someone who follows the standard American diet (SAD) is around 210. Your chances of having a heart attack decrease as your cholesterol levels dip below 150. So if you don't increase your cholesterol levels with your food intake and you combine that with eating cholesterol-fighting plant foods like oats, you'll be on your way to lowering your cholesterol naturally. Also as a vegan, unless you have a strong genetic predisposition for having high cholesterol, your levels should be around 125 and below. Your chances of having a heart attack at those levels are virtually nil. Consult with your doctor for other advice on helping keep heart disease at bay.

IN A NUTSHELL

The director of the nonprofit Institute of Nutrition Education and Research, Dr. Michael Klaper, believes that animal fats clog our arteries and make us fat, and that we have no nutritional requirements for animal protein or products. Because plant-based foods help lower our cholesterol levels, which helps us fight heart disease, he and other doctors are instructing heart patients to adopt a heart-healthy, low-fat, vegan diet.

The Least You Need to Know

- A diet high in animal fats, proteins, and cholesterol can lead to a plethora of health problems.
- A completely plant-based diet gives your body all the nutrition it needs to fight disease.
- Preventive medicine works at helping healthy people stay healthy and solving potential health problems before they arise.
- The China-Oxford-Cornell Diet and Health Project was a comprehensive study that showed a correlation between consumption of animal products and disease.
- Many people find their way to a plant-based diet due to food allergies or intolerances.
- You can lower your chances of getting heart disease and your cholesterol levels by modifying your lifestyle and switching to a vegan, plant-based diet.

Starting Your Vegan Transition

In This Chapter

- Beginning your journey to a vegan lifestyle
- Transitioning tips
- Out with the old and in with the new
- Being kind to yourself

Transitioning is a necessary part of your personal evolution to veganism. You're changing and adapting your sense of awareness of the world around you and your place within it. The rate and level at which you evolve is personal to you and you alone and should come naturally to you. Some people might be able to transition to a vegan lifestyle in one fell swoop, but for others, it might take many months, and many even have a few stumbles along the way.

It's best to be like the turtle (another illustrious plant-eater)—slow and steady to win the race. And for you, winning the race is reaping all the benefits of a vegan lifestyle. Go at your own pace and with what makes you feel comfortable. This chapter helps you transition from a meat-eating or vegetarian diet to a vegan lifestyle.

Taking Small Steps

For many, making life changes can seem intimidating; others embrace change and become energized by the process. However you approach your transition into veganism, think of it as taking small steps in making a positive change for yourself, the animals, and the planet. We discuss many of the health, physical, environmental, and social benefits of adopting a vegan lifestyle throughout the pages of this book. Take and absorb the information; then make changes in your diet and lifestyle as you see fit, at your own speed.

You decide which part of your life to change first, what goes into your body, onto it, or surrounding it. Having patience with yourself can really help empower you during the times you may stumble or falter in your transitioning process. But be confident and stay the course. No one is perfect; we all make mistakes and go astray along the way on our journey into veganism.

You also might have a problem sticking to your new dietary choices or vegan standards 100 percent of the time as you transition into the vegan way of approaching the various aspects of your life. Just try to do your best, and take slow and steady steps. If you slip, don't beat up on yourself. Remind yourself that you are making a difference, however small it may seem. Every time you live up to a vegan ideal, you are helping limit suffering and hopefully save an innocent life. It's hard for anyone to be 100 percent vegan when you start to scrutinize every aspect of your life. Remember, you can only do the best you can with the things you have control over.

Getting Your Diet in Order

One of the first transitional changes the vegan-curious make is to their diet. They often give up added cheese or butter toppings or avoid eating a burger and opt instead for a salad at lunch. These are positive steps in the right direction to changing your diet to a vegan one.

Transitioning Out Certain Foods

While increasing your consumption of fruits and veggies, you could start eliminating animal-based foods from your diet. Start by avoiding the foods you don't particularly care for or enjoy eating. Then begin making other small changes, like leaving the sour cream and butter off your baked potato and using a little nonhydrogenated margarine or olive oil instead. Or buy a carton of soy milk for use on your morning cereal instead of using cow's milk.

By approaching it one item at a time, before you know it, you've eliminated animal-based foods entirely from one meal and then another. If you find you don't miss the eliminated foods, keep going and try other eliminations or substitutions (see Part 5 for more on substitutions). Don't beat yourself up if you stumble and give in to a craving for a cheeseburger or pizza at first. Keep at it, and soon you'll find yourself choosing vegan selections naturally and eating all your meals vegan.

> **HOT POTATO**
>
> Don't let your food cravings derail your new vegan diet. Keep your freezer stocked with vegan convenience foods like frozen veggie burgers, veggie dogs, and dairy-free pizzas. When a craving hits for one of your former favorite nonvegan foods, you'll be prepared with a vegan alternative.

Eating Lots of Raw Goodness

As you switch your diet to being more plant-based, try to increase your consumption of raw fruits and vegetables. Even after washing and cutting, the vitamins and nutrients in these raw foods are left more intact—especially more of the beneficial digestive enzymes—than their cooked food counterparts.

A relatively easy (and delicious!) way to get more servings of fruits and veggies into your daily diet is by drinking fresh juices and smoothies. Try blending a variety of raw fruits and vegetables in your liquid libations, like leafy greens and cucumber with berries or bananas. This increases your consumption of beneficial phytochemicals and gets you one step closer to not relying on animal-based foods.

Getting Your House in Order

When making the decision to become a vegan, you have to analyze many of your past and present choices about how you eat, what you wear, and what products you use. Often this means getting rid of the old and buying all new. We offer some suggestions in the following sections, but ultimately, what you do with those no-longer-accepted vegan items is a personal decision.

Sorting Your Pantry

What should you do with those nonvegan food items? Your choices are basically consuming them one last time, giving them away, or discarding them altogether. We have often been faced with this choice when we've been given or inadvertently purchased nonvegan foods. Depending on how "unhealthy" or "wrong" the item is, we either pass them along to nonvegan friends, food banks, or as a last resort, the landfill.

We choose to throw things away as a last resort because it's wasteful. We acknowledge that the item has already been prepared, thus the wrong has already been done to the animal and we can't change it. We may be showing the animal further disrespect for the suffering it had to endure by just discarding the item when someone could receive a benefit from it. This is one of the many tough personal calls you will have to make for yourself.

> **IN A NUTSHELL**
>
> There's a Native American line of reasoning that you should pay homage to the life that has given its own to sustain yours. You should not show it disrespect in the giving of its gift, which would be an injustice and not in balance with nature.

Cleaning Out Your Closet

When it comes to clothing and accessories, you can apply the same type of reasoning as with foods. If the items are worn out, discard or recycle them. If they still have some use, pass them along to others who can put them to use. If you don't know someone who could use the items, donate them to charity. We feel best passing on these nonvegan items to those who can use them.

As you rid your closet and drawers of any leather, fur, wool, or other animal ingredients, you can seek out vegan-friendly substitutes. That means shopping! You can find many natural and plant-based fabrics used in clothing, coats, and accessories in most retailers and department stores.

Man-made materials are also used in these same types of clothing and in footwear, from sandals to dress shoes to boots. Begin by reading labels when you're in doubt of their origin. You can also go online for sources of vegan clothing and footwear. We offer some sources in Appendix B.

Cleaning Out Your Cabinets

Check your local health-food store and retailers for cruelty-free beauty and personal products. Most offer a selection of shampoos, conditioners, lotions, perfumes, and makeup that are free of animal ingredients and not tested on animals. These items tend to cost a bit more because they're often made with organic and better-quality ingredients. So begin by replacing one item at a time, and don't put a crimp on your pocketbook!

Many health-food stores offer shampoos, conditioners, and lotions for sale in bulk quantities, which makes these products even more affordable. You can even make your own natural household cleaners by mixing water with a little vinegar or lemon juice. This mixture can clean your windows, bathrooms, countertops—you name it—all natural and very inexpensive!

Staying the Course

Lifelong journeys begin with short, sure, and steady steps. Start with small changes at first, in your diet for instance, by giving up one animal food or group at a time. If it's something you aren't sure you can live without, search out substitutes to help fill the void so you won't feel deprived or like you're on a "fad diet." The internet and your local library can help you find a wide variety of information, as well as recipes and cookbooks to inspire you.

IN A NUTSHELL

Check out www.veganchef.com for some of Chef Beverly's vegan recipes and menu ideas—from vegan soups to vegan desserts! You'll also find some of her tasty vegan recipes in *The Complete Idiot's Guide to Vegan Cooking; The Complete Idiot's Guide to Gluten-Free Vegan Cooking,* which she co-authored with Julieanna Hever; and *The Complete Idiot's Guide to Vegan Slow Cooking.*

You'll likely have times when a craving hits you so hard you think you'll just have to go get some nonvegan food. Most everyone has experienced this at one time or another. During these rough moments, remind yourself that you're making the right choice by going vegan and that it's good for you and the rest of the planet. And if you need more help, you've got it right now, in your hands. We provide you with further encouragement throughout the book. Keep turning pages, and know you're doing something great for yourself and for the world!

The Least You Need to Know

- Transitioning to a vegan lifestyle in your own way and at your own pace helps keep you from feeling overwhelmed by all the changes.

- When transitioning to a vegan lifestyle, you'll face many decisions. Just do the best you can, at your own pace.

- Eliminating one nonvegan aspect of your life at a time is often a gentle way of transitioning. For extra help, find alternatives for those nonvegan foods at the top of your craving list.

- Replace animal-based ingredients with similar plant-based substitutes, and increase your consumption of raw fruits and vegetables.

- You'll feel more empowered as a vegan after you clean out your pantry, closets, and cabinets and rid them of animal-based food, clothing, and personal products.

Myths and Misconceptions About Veganism

Part

2

There's a lot of confusion about what it means to be vegan, including how we can possibly survive without animal foods. If vegans had a dollar for every time we were asked questions such as "How can you get enough protein if you don't eat meat?" or "How can you get enough calcium if you don't drink milk?" quite a few wealthy vegans would be roaming the streets.

The chapters in Part 2 provide the answers to those questions—and a whole lot more—for your own knowledge and to help you handle your next veg-curious encounter.

No Meat? What About Protein?

In This Chapter

- Getting enough protein in your diet
- The importance of fiber
- All about beans, grains, and greens
- The many faces of soy
- A look at meat substitutes

How will you ever get enough protein without eating meat?

Without a doubt, when you're transitioning to a vegan diet, this is one of the most commonly asked questions you'll hear. The veg-curious in your inner circle of friends and family and even complete strangers will ask you this question again and again. As you begin your journey toward eating vegan, you might even find this is an issue that's often on your own mind.

Where *will* you get your protein, and are you sure you'll get enough of it without eating animal-based foods? You have no need to worry. The plant kingdom is full of protein-rich foods!

Plants: Powerful Protein

Plants provide us with so much, nutrition-wise: proteins, carbohydrates, natural sugars, heart-healthy fats, phytochemicals, vitamins, minerals, and more, and we discuss all these in this book. But first, let's talk about protein.

How much protein does your body really need? It's recommended that 1 out of every 10 calories you take in should come from protein, and exactly how much that amounts to depends on your weight. The Recommended Daily Allowance (RDA) for protein for healthy adults 19 and older is .8 grams per kilogram of body weight, and daily intake should be about 45 grams for a woman and 55 grams for a man; pregnant or lactating women and children need at least 1 gram per kilogram of body weight. Athletes also have increased protein needs, and the National Strength and Conditioning Association recommends that athletes consume 1.5 to 2 grams per kilogram of body weight, depending on the intensity of their training.

Interestingly, most Americans consume 4 to 8 times their daily requirement of protein, which translates to 15 to 20 percent of their caloric intake. For vegans, roughly 10 to 12 percent of our calories come from protein, and the World Health Organization only recommends getting 5 or 6 percent of your total calories from protein to replace what you utilize every day. So you see, getting enough protein on a plant-based diet is actually pretty easy!

HOT POTATO

Being on a high-protein diet has consequences. For one thing, taking in too much protein messes with your calcium absorption, which in turn increases your risk of kidney disease and osteoporosis. (We touch more on the body's calcium requirements and absorption capabilities in Chapter 6.)

The Benefits of Plant Proteins

Proteins help your body build and maintain muscles, bones, hormones, enzymes, and many other body tissues. Proteins are made of building blocks—22 amino acids, to be exact—and combinations of these amino acids form the proteins that exist in all living creatures. Your body makes 13 of the amino acids; the other 9, referred to as *essential amino acids*, must be supplied by dietary sources. Your body uses these essential amino acids to aid in synthesizing your own amino acids.

DEFINITION

Essential amino acids (EAAs)—histidine, isoleucine, leucine, lysine, methionine, phenylalanine, threonine, tryptophan, and valine—are your body's key protein-building blocks. They must come from dietary sources.

It's a myth that animal protein is naturally packed with essential amino acids, and therefore superior to the protein found in plant foods. In reality, all the amino acids in animal foods derive from the vegetation the particular animal consumed, whether it be the grain fed to cows and chickens or the plankton, algae, or kelp the swordfish swallowed. Plant-based foods are the source of all the essential amino acids, and they also have significant amounts of protein. For instance, asparagus, broccoli, and tofu are all around 40 percent protein as a percentage of calories. Watercress weighs in at a whopping 83 percent!

It's also a common misconception that you need to combine plant proteins at each meal or in each dish to make them form "complete proteins," or proteins that contain all the essential amino acids. This is not necessary. Even the American Dietetic Association agrees that eating a diet rich in a wide variety of fruits, vegetables, and whole grains provides *all* your amino acids and protein needs, *and* vitamins and minerals to boot! Plus, plant-based foods are cholesterol free and low in calories and fats, unlike their animal-based equivalents.

Soybeans contain all nine essential amino acids, making them a perfect food. Soy-based products include tofu, tempeh, mock meats, nondairy ice creams, soy milk, and a vast assortment of vegan cheeses, yogurts, sour creams, and other dairy-free alternatives.

Hemp seeds are also a good source of all nine essential amino acids and contain an ideal ratio of essential fatty acids as well. A plethora of vegan hemp seed–based products are becoming increasingly available, including hulled seeds, seed meal, milk, seed butter, ice cream, and hemp protein powder.

Moving Through the Works

Your body can better and more easily utilize plant-based protein sources than meat-based sources because it's built for the plant version. Human saliva contains a carbohydrate-digesting enzyme, called salivary amylase, that's responsible for the digestion of starches. Animal-based protein sources contain very small amounts of carbs and little to no fiber, so if you consume as much meat and dairy as the average American, your colon and elimination time can become a lot like a game of *Tetris*. You keep consuming large quantities of food, which keep getting compacted down, but you only eliminate a small part of it at a time. You may feel bloated or gassy, develop indigestion or digestive problems, and even put on weight.

The amount of fiber in foods affects digestion time and efficiency. Because proteins are generally not digested until they're in the small intestine, sometimes having the slow digestion of plant material is beneficial. Your body can draw out more of the nutrients and put them to use.

When you begin to shift toward an all-vegan diet, you may experience a few digestion problems at first, especially when consuming beans or cruciferous vegetables like cabbages or cauliflower. This will greatly improve as you consume these types of foods more often, because your body begins to produce enzymes that help you process them. Cooking your vegetables and beans thoroughly may also improve digestibility. Try eating any bothersome foods in small quantities at first, and vary your selections. Also, be sure to chew your food thoroughly because chewing really kick-starts the whole digestive process into action.

Down with Fat, Up with Fiber

The medical community has widely accepted that if you want to reduce your risk of chronic disease, you should consume a diet low in fat, high in fiber, and full of fruits and vegetables. Plant-based foods are excellent sources of low-fat protein and are high in fiber, so they meet all the criteria.

Depending on your level of health, your daily diet should include no more than 10 to 20 percent fat. If you need to make major alterations to your cholesterol levels, it's best to consume an even lower-fat diet of between 5 to 10 percent fat for several weeks or more or until your cholesterol levels take a serious nosedive.

Pay attention to your consumption of tropical oils like palm and coconut because they're very high in saturated fat. Stick with olive, flax, hemp, pumpkin, sunflower, and sesame oils for flavor with added health benefits.

You need 25 to 30 grams fiber in your diet per day for proper colon function. Fiber comes from cellulose, which makes up the cell structure of plants. Dietary fiber is best described as the parts of vegetation that can't be broken down by digestive enzymes. Animal products contain no dietary fiber, so they tend to accumulate in the colon, stubbornly refusing to be moved along.

In contrast, all the fiber in fruits, veggies, and other plant-based foods cleans your pipes. It acts just like a brush and keeps things moving as it should. As an added benefit, a diet low in fat and high in fiber will have you shedding extra pounds and looking good!

Not all fiber is created equal. Fiber can be broken up into two categories: soluble and insoluble. When mixed with water or other liquid, soluble fiber turns into a gel that contains fatty acids and other nutrients your body can easily absorb and utilize. In contrast, insoluble fiber, which doesn't easily dissolve in water, passes through your digestive tract mostly intact.

Soluble fiber, found in flaxseeds, barley, oats, beans, apples, oranges, and carrots, helps lower cholesterol levels and helps diabetics regulate blood sugar levels. Insoluble fiber found in corn, wheat, cruciferous vegetables, green beans, and the skins of many fruits and vegetables aids in digestion, elimination regularity, toxin removal, and system balancing. Each type of fiber has its own benefits, so be sure to include sources of each in your daily diet.

Keeping Things Regular

The fiber in plant foods, often known as roughage, helps keep your bowels moving regularly like they should and helps prevent painful constipation. Fiber provides bulk and binds with fats and toxins in your system, which are quickly eliminated by fiber's cleansing action. Most importantly, fiber keeps bile from recirculating in your system. Bile is formed from the cholesterol in your body, so you want to eliminate it instead of having it absorb into your bloodstream and affect your cholesterol levels.

High-fiber diets help with your natural elimination process. In addition, because they're quite filling, high-fiber foods help you maintain a proper weight. They also require more chewing, which gets the digestion process off to a good head-start. Adding water into the mix gives you a feeling of fullness and satisfies your hunger even faster.

IN A NUTSHELL

Drinking a lot of filtered water—8 to 10 glasses per day—is highly recommended when you're increasing your fiber intake. It prevents constipation as fiber absorbs water, toxins, and bile from your system and flushes them away.

It's best to include as many sources of fresh raw fruits and veggies in your daily diet as possible, and be sure to include some protein-rich leafy greens. The RDA is at least five servings a day, but vegans often consume more servings than that in one meal alone. Foods in their raw state are easily broken down on a nutrient level, hastening their utilization and processing. (We discuss the benefits of eating foods in their simple, raw state in greater detail in Chapter 12.)

Protein-Packed Plant-Based Foods

Where will you get your protein as a vegan? If you look to the plant kingdom for sources of protein, you'll be amazed at what you'll find. Protein is abundant in plant foods. Beans have it; grains do, too. And you can find lots of protein in most nuts, seeds, and veggies—especially green leafy ones.

Veggies are such powerhouses that even if you ate only one of these types of foods as the majority of your daily diet, you would easily meet and exceed your RDA for protein. But it's recommended and much more exciting to eat a variety of plant foods to have a well-balanced diet. They don't say variety is the spice of life for nothing!

Know Beans About It

It's recommended that you get 3 or 4 grams protein for every 100 calories you consume. Legumes such as beans, lentils, and peas deliver those numbers very easily. Most provide 12 to 15 grams protein per 1-cup serving, which is easy for a vegan to consume in a bowl of bean-and-veggie chili or split-pea soup.

Legumes are also excellent sources of iron, zinc, calcium, phosphorus, potassium, vitamins A and B, and trace minerals. In addition, most are complex carbohydrates, low in fat and calories and high in fiber. Soybeans are one of the most commonly consumed forms of bean proteins for vegans (we discuss them a little later in the chapter), but certainly not the only ones. Get creative!

The following table lists some other beans you might want to try, along with their amount of protein in grams per 1-cup serving.

Legume	Protein	Legume	Protein
Black beans	15 g	Peas (fresh)	9 g
Chickpeas	14.5 g	Soybeans	28.5 g
Lentils	18 g	Split peas	16.5 g
Navy beans	16 g		

The fiber in beans helps you feel full faster, so they help control your appetite, which comes in handy if you're trying to drop a few pounds.

Some people experience digestion problems, like gas or stomach pain, when they start adding large amounts of beans to their diets for the first time. If this happens to you, don't drop beans altogether; just cut back a bit. If using dried beans, you can greatly improve their digestibility by presoaking them before cooking, or by cooking them with a piece of kombu (a sea vegetable) or a bay leaf. Also, try eating a smaller portion at one meal until your system adjusts. Then as your symptoms subside, increase your serving size, and feel free to include them at more than one meal.

A Grain of Truth

What are grains exactly? It's easiest to describe them as the seed heads of grasslike plants. Sometimes they're also referred to as "cereal crops." Foods such as brown rice, corn, wheat, spelt, quinoa, amaranth, barley, bulgur, couscous, millet, pastas, and even those rice blends you find in bulk bins or boxes on your local store shelves qualify as grains.

Humankind has used and cultivated grains throughout the centuries, and some of these grains have become more popular and widely used than others. Cultural and regional conditions often determine a particular grain's predominance in the daily diet. Mediterranean diets favor pastas, corn, and wheat, while Eastern European diets center on spelt, wheat, and barley, which all add heartiness to the dishes they're cooked in. Most Asian diets are predominantly rice based, whether it be in whole-grain or noodle form.

Whole grains are amazing. They contain complex carbohydrates, protein, vitamins B and E, phosphorus, potassium, and more—all of which are good sources of fuel to provide long-lasting energy for your body. With all the delicious whole-grain options available, it's really easy to incorporate several servings of protein-packed grains into your daily diet. For example, you can find 4 to 8 grams protein in 2 slices of whole-grain bread or 1 cup cooked grains. You can find up to 10 grams protein in 2 ounces cooked pasta (that's before you add your favorite sauce or topping).

For optimal nutrition and health benefits, it's best to consume whole grains. These are your best choice for getting the most vitamins and fiber benefits. Whole grains have all the germ and bran intact, which provide your body with vital fiber. Germ and bran are usually stripped away during the bleaching process, resulting in a whiter-looking (and less-nutritious) flour.

When selecting grains, avoid products with words like *bleached, white, enriched*, or *bromated* in the ingredient list. These words mean that vital fiber has been removed from the grains. Instead, look for terms like *whole grain, sprouted grain*, and *whole wheat* to ensure you get all the grainy goodness nature intended.

Lean, Mean, and Green

Leafy green veggies such as lettuce, spinach, Swiss chard, collards, kale, and cabbage contain so many good-for-you things, including calcium, protein, iodine, magnesium, iron, plenty of fiber, complex carbohydrates, and vitamins A, B, C, E, and K. To get 3 or 4 grams protein, you would need to consume 3 or 4 cups raw spinach, kale, or lettuce, or 1 cup cooked collards, cabbage, or spinach.

All these veggies are delicious eaten raw, steamed, or sautéed; cooked into soups or stews; used to encase fillings; or added to your favorite dishes. If you munch on them as a salad or enjoy them in a green smoothie, your saliva's digestive enzymes immediately start breaking down the nutrient-dense leaves, which will give you an instant energy boost. Plus, all the fiber in leafy greens gives you a feeling of fullness faster and satisfies your appetite. So dig into a fresh, crisp salad full of a variety of greens, veggies, and even some beans, whether you want to eat well or just drop a few pounds!

To preserve as much dietary fiber and nutrients as possible when cooking leafy green veggies, it is best to quickly sauté or stir-fry them until crisp-tender or just wilted. Or cook them into soups, stews, or with a lot of water and aromatic herbs until they reach the desired tenderness, and fully enjoy the vitamin-rich liquid they produce.

IN A NUTSHELL

In the South, many people love the "pot liquor" that results from cooking greens. They use this vitamin-rich broth in sauces, for cooking grains, or for making soups. Some people like to drink it, but it's especially good if you soak it up by dipping bits of cornbread or other bread into it!

Soy—Oh Boy!

Ah, the magnificent soybean! We have the great Benjamin Franklin and a few other agriculture pioneers to thank for soy reaching the shores of America when it did. After learning about the amazing "cheese" made from soybeans on a visit to Paris, Franklin had several soybean plants sent to Pennsylvania farmers. Franklin himself was a vegetarian (for at least part of his life) as well as a writer, inventor, and states-man. He convinced farmers to grow soybeans as crops, which were then used to make the soybean cheese, better known to us as tofu, in addition to soy sauce and vermicelli-like soy noodles.

Asian cultures are the true masters of the soybean, though. They have been enjoying it for centuries in everything from beverages to main dishes to desserts. They soak and grind soybeans into a refreshing soy milk and eat green soybeans, better known as edamame, as a snack. *Miso*, which is a fermented soybean paste, is a popular condiment used in Asian cuisine to flavor sauces and soups. Pieces of tofu or tempeh often find their way into appetizers like spring rolls, which are sometimes rolled in yuba, the dried skin removed during the process of making soy milk. Tofu and tempeh are also used to make an array of interesting alternatives to meat and dairy products (see the following sections for more on tofu and tempeh).

> **DEFINITION**
>
> **Miso** is a thick, pastelike condiment made from fermenting soybeans with salt and koji (a beneficial type of mold), often in combination with other beans or grains like chickpeas, barley, or rice. Miso ranges from sweet, mild, and mellow with a light beige color, to strong and rich with earthy dark brown or red tones.

Soy and Your Health

The medical community has conducted numerous studies to analyze soy's nutrient content and its many positive effects on our health and well-being. For one, it's a great source of phytosterols, which reduce blood cholesterol levels.

Soybeans also contain phytoestrogens, which are plant-based compounds that act in a similar manner as the estrogen (female sex hormone) that's found naturally coursing through a woman's body via her bloodstream. These phytoestrogen allies, although weaker than our own, have been found to beneficially help women regulate their estrogen levels. And don't worry, men, research has shown that phytoestrogens don't adversely affect your manly testosterone, so they won't make your breasts start to grow or have a negative impact on your virility or fertility. Actually, studies have shown that consuming soy products reduces the risks of estrogen-related cancers, prostate cancer, osteoporosis, menstrual and menopausal symptoms, and cardiovascular disease.

To reap the most medical benefits from soy, you should consume more minimally processed forms of soy products, like edamame or cooked soybeans, soy milk, tofu, tempeh, and miso. Some vegan packaged foods, like meat analogue products and protein bars, contain ambiguous forms of soy, like soy protein isolates. While these foods are great for transitioning vegans and occasional use, they aren't as good for you from a nutritional standpoint as less-processed forms, and they may even have some drawbacks. Also, try to only consume organic soy products or those not made with genetically modified soy, as much controversy surrounds the safety of consuming genetically modified foods.

> **HOT POTATO**
>
> *GMO* is the abbreviation for "genetically modified organism," a term used to describe foods whose genetic makeup has been scientifically altered to produce qualities like pesticide resistance (so more can be applied) or toxicity to natural pests. Among other crops, soybean and corn are often genetically modified. Many people are concerned about the potential health risks of GMO foods. To avoid them, look for products labeled "non-GMO" or "GMO-free," or even better, opt for certified organic foods, as organic certification standards don't allow GMOs.

However, for many unfortunate people who are allergic, soy is off limits. Symptoms of a soy allergy vary from individual to individual. Some are mild, like hives, but in some rare cases, consumption can cause a life-threatening allergic reaction (anaphylaxis). Many people allergic to soy are also allergic to other legumes such as chickpeas, lentils, peas, and peanuts. If you have a soy allergy, you need to become a diligent label reader, as soy products are becoming widely used in all sorts of foods, beverages, and snacks. To help in this task, the Food Allergen Labeling Consumer Protection Act (FALCPA) of 2004 requires that all packaged foods declare if they contain common allergens like milk, wheat, soy, peanuts, and tree nuts.

Tofu to Ya!

You may have stumbled across tofu in your grocery store. You know, those white blocks submerged in liquid, in plastic or aseptic containers. It does look a little curious, floating there in that liquid, but don't be put off by tofu's appearance.

We have Asia to thank for this miracle food. More than 2,000 years ago, Chinese culinary masters figured out how to process the simple soybean in such a way as to increase its digestibility and nearly double its protein content. This process is very similar to that of cheese-making, but instead of starting with cow's milk, it starts with soaked and cooked soybeans that are then ground to make soy milk. A coagulant is added to the soy milk and then the magic happens, turning this noble bean into a custardlike mass.

There are basically two types of tofu, regular and silken. Regular tofu is made very much like cheese. After the coagulant is added, the solids or curds are separated from the liquid or whey. The accumulated curds are then packed into molds, pressed, and left to drain to the desired consistency and texture. This separating of the curds and whey could explain why tofu is also referred to as *bean curd*. Depending on how much water is removed, the tofu is labeled as either soft, firm, extra-firm, or super-firm. You'll find most varieties of regular tofu packaged and immersed in water, but super-firm often is not, and you'll find them in the refrigerated case of most grocery and natural foods stores, as well as Asian specialty markets. Silken tofu, on the other hand, is made a lot like yogurt, and the solids and whey are not separated.

Silken tofu is also available in soft, firm, and extra-firm varieties. It has a softer, creamier texture, making it better suited for puréeing for use in sauces, soups, smoothies, and dairy-free desserts like vegan cheesecake. You'll also find many brands of silken tofu packaged in water in the refrigerated case. However, some manufacturers, like Mori-Nu, pour the soy milk and coagulant directly into aseptic packaging. This type of silken tofu firms inside the packaging and does not require refrigeration until the package is opened.

In China, tofu has been nicknamed "the meat without bones" because of its versatility in creating so many meatlike replacement products. Tofu has a spongelike texture that puts off some people at first. But keep in mind that, like a sponge, it can take on a lot of flavor from whatever surrounds it, and it has an endless array of uses in your vegan kitchen. (Need some ideas? We discuss substitutions and recipe ideas in Parts 5 and 6, respectively.)

Tempting Tempeh

Tempeh is a vegan delicacy that originated in Indonesia. There, folks developed and introduced a fermentation technique to the tofu-making process that resulted in something totally different, texture- and flavor-wise.

Tempeh is made with soybeans alone or in combination with other beans or grains such as lentils, rice, millet, quinoa, or barley. In a procedure similar to that of making blue-veined dairy cheeses like Roquefort, a special mold (or fermenting culture starter) is injected into the soybean mixture and left to ferment. The mold binds together the mixture, and the result is a thick slab with veins running through it. The veins are mostly white, but sometimes you'll see gray, brown, and black veins, too. The fermentation process gives the tempeh a richer, almost mushroomlike flavor.

For those of you who think you'll miss beef when eating vegan, give tempeh a try. It can be fried, sautéed, or baked or added to sauces, stews, or stir-fried dishes. Steaming it makes it swell in size and soak in additional flavorings, like its spongelike cousin tofu does.

IN A NUTSHELL

Many people who have a problem digesting soy products such as tofu and soy milk don't experience the same symptoms with tempeh. This is mainly the result of increased digestibility arising from the fermentation process.

TVP: Textured Vegetable Protein

TVP, a.k.a. textured vegetable protein or textured soy protein, is considered a "second-generation" form of soy protein. It's made from defatted soybean meal that's cut into chunks or small flakes and then dried.

Cooks use TVP to extend meat dishes in many schools and government-funded institutions because it is economical and high in protein. It's often used as a substitute for ground hamburger in burgers, chilies, sauces, and veggie loafs. You can find it in packages and in the bulk section of your local grocery or natural foods store.

Soy Many Choices

A popular snack trend in the United States is edamame, or fresh, immature, and still-green soybeans. You can find them fresh for a limited time and in the freezer section of your grocery store almost any time of the year. You can boil them in their pods, season them with salt, and then pop them out of their pods directly into your mouth. Soy nuts made from split soybeans that are then roasted and often seasoned are also available in most snack aisles. These goodies pack a whopping 34 grams protein in a ½-cup serving.

You can purchase the fully matured soybeans in the regular beige variety, as well as the black ones that come canned or dried. The black bean paste commonly used to flavor many Asian dishes is made from fermented black soybeans and seasonings.

You can also find many mock meat products in the refrigerator and freezer sections of your local grocery and natural foods stores. You will be amazed by the wide selection of products, ranging from veggie hot dogs, sliced luncheon meats, sausages, and ground-meat replacements to the ever-popular mock turkey products used during the winter holiday season. Many grocery stores carry soy protein powders; soy-based nondairy ice creams, cheeses, and cream cheese; and soy-based beverages, yogurts, and, if you're lucky, luscious desserts.

It might take a bit of experimenting to discover which products you like best because they all vary in terms of flavor, consistency, and nutrition. If you don't care for a particular brand, don't be put off; just try another until you find one that suits your taste. (In Parts 5 and 6, respectively, we discuss substitutions and give you some recipe ideas.)

Other Meatless Options

We have the Buddhist monks—with their strict vegetarian, nearly vegan lifestyle—to thank for developing so many mock meat products. Not only did they come up with some amazing soy-based substitutes, but their culinary expertise and wisdom also helped develop even more amazing foods from what some would consider nothing.

They developed techniques for turning grains into everything from beverages to savory items to desserts. They transformed little morsels of humble nuts, seeds, and mushrooms that many just passed by or overlooked into culinary creations that produced intricate layers of flavor and texture while providing a hearty and filling meal that satisfied the palate.

Seitan: The Wheat Meat

One of the most amazing culinary developments the monks made is definitely the development of seitan. Somehow, these wise disciples figured out how to rinse the starch out of wheat flour and leave only the gluten part, which they then sent on an amazing transformation.

In an elaborate and timely process, they mixed together wheat flour and water, kneaded it to develop the gluten structure in the flour, and rinsed it. They repeated this procedure until all the starch and bran had rinsed away and all that remained was the gluten part of the flour. They then simmered it in either water or a flavorful broth so the grain swelled in size and became infused with flavor.

The traditional method for making seitan is quite labor-intensive and can take hours to prepare. However, for an easier and faster way to make a batch of seitan, other alternatives are available, and many people opt to use *vital wheat gluten* instead of whole-wheat flour. Vital wheat gluten is available in the baking and bulk bin aisles of most grocery and health-food stores. Boxed products are also available, such as Seitan Quick Mix, which often only require a little water and a few minutes to make a batch of homemade seitan.

> **DEFINITION**
>
> **Vital wheat gluten** (also known as instant gluten flour) is a powdered form of dehydrated pure wheat gluten. It's often mixed with liquids and seasonings and used to make seitan and its many meat analogue variations. Find it in bulk bins or packaged in most grocery and natural foods stores.

From this point, your seitan can be adapted to make many products that resemble the taste and texture of beef, chicken, and seafood. For example, you can simmer small morsels in soups, sauces, or stocks. Or you can develop its chewy texture by baking or steaming it in loaves, sausages, or small pieces.

Not only is the versatile seitan delicious, but it's also quite nutritious. A 2½-ounce serving contains no cholesterol or fat, has only 70 calories, and delivers 12 grams protein. That's not bad for a little flour! Seitan does have one drawback: because it's made from pure wheat gluten, it's not suitable for those who suffer from celiac disease or wheat or gluten allergies.

Some Chinese restaurants, particularly vegetarian ones, use mock meats, many of which are soy and gluten based, in their menu items. If you see some of these faux meats on the menu, be a little adventurous and try one. This can be a great way to introduce yourself to gluten before attempting your own such concoctions at home.

The all-vegan Lotus Garden restaurant in vegan-friendly Eugene, Oregon, features many soy- and gluten-based mock meats in their many menu selections. They even make terrific batter-dipped and fried pieces of seitan that resemble those infamous fast-food chicken nuggets—only lighter in taste and crispier!

The Fungus Among Us

Many cultures throughout history have used mushrooms for food, medicine, and spiritual purposes. Actually fungi, mushrooms grow on organic material, preferring nutrient-rich soils and decaying tree limbs for their host homes. They grow wild as they see fit, even if we have managed to cultivate a few varieties, and their earthy aroma and flavor tantalize the senses.

Mushrooms come in thousands of varieties, but most of us only have access to a few types all year around, the most common being white button, shiitake, crimini, and portobello. Some areas have better access to mushrooms with more exotic varieties like porcini, morel, chanterelle, truffle, oyster, lobster, enoki, and wood ear, just to name a few.

Mushrooms contain 70 to 90 percent digestible vegetable protein, a substantial amount of B vitamins, selenium, copper, and some other trace minerals. They are low in calories (1 cup raw mushrooms has about 20 calories), low in fat, high in dietary fiber, and cholesterol free. Moreover, researchers have discovered that some mushrooms contain antibacterial and other medicinal qualities, including antitumor compounds called triterpenoids.

You can purchase mushrooms fresh, frozen, canned, dried, and even in the supplement form. Their rich, almost "beefy" flavor and chewy texture work well as a meat substitute. You can marinate and grill whole portobello caps and enjoy them as burgers or mushroom "steaks." You can also slice or chop mushrooms and add them to veggie chilies, tomato sauces, or stews. The flavor and texture fools your palate into thinking it's meat, which is perfect for those who may be new to the vegan way of eating.

HOT POTATO

Unless you're an expert on wild mushrooms, you shouldn't just pick and eat any ol' mushroom you find growing in your yard or in the woods. Some of them can be extremely poisonous!

Just Nuts About It

Nuts and seeds are one of the earliest and simplest protein sources available. Many species enjoy these savory morsels as they grow abundantly in thousands of varieties and hang from trees within easy grasp. Just like a piece of ripe fruit, there's nothing like picking a handful of nuts fresh from a tree, cracking them open, and enjoying them in their natural, raw state. It's best to eat nuts and seeds raw to get the most of their many benefits, but many people enjoy the more developed flavors of dry-roasted nuts.

Nuts and seeds are important protein sources for raw foodists, vegans, and vegetarians alike. They are high in protein; most contain 3 to 8 grams protein in a small, ¼-cup serving. They also contain calcium, zinc, selenium, vitamin E, and other antioxidants and provide phytochemicals that help with mineral absorption.

Nuts and seeds do contain high amounts of fat and calories because they are such nutrient-dense foods, but fortunately, most of the fats are unsaturated and thereby considered healthier sources of dietary fat. In addition, many nuts and seeds contain significant amounts of *essential fatty acids* (*EFAs*) that help reduce blood cholesterol levels and prevent and fight disease. These EFAs are also found in dark-green leafy vegetables, grains, soybeans, broccoli, and sea vegetables.

You can chomp on a handful of nuts for a quick and easy snack that will provide you with concentrated energy and help get you over the hump until your next meal. They are also often ground into nut and seed butters, such as peanut, almond, or cashew butters and sesame-based tahini. They are available freshly ground, salted, unsalted, raw, and in roasted varieties to suit all tastes.

DEFINITION

Essential fatty acids (**EFAs**) are made of alpha-linoleic acid and linoleic acid, necessary for the formation and maintenance of cells. These fatty acids are commonly referred to as omega-3 and omega-6 fatty acids, respectively, and they compete for dominance within your body. Having a greater proportion of omega-6 can increase your risk for chronic diseases, as it cancels out the beneficial effects of omega-3 acids.

Surely you must have had your share of peanut butter and jelly sandwiches, but have you ever tried a cashew or almond butter sandwich topped with raisins, chopped fruit, or seeds? Delicious! Ground nuts and seeds can even add protein, texture, flavor, and binding qualities to veggie burgers, loaves, cutlets, and baked goods.

The vital oils found in nuts and seeds require a bit of special treatment to preserve them and prevent rancidity, so be sure to refrigerate or freeze nuts and seeds you have at home. Also keep nut butters in your refrigerator to preserve their freshness.

The Least You Need to Know

- It's easy to get enough protein on a vegan diet. Many plant foods are loaded with it.
- Fiber is essential for keeping your system moving and working efficiently. Be sure to regularly consume sources of both soluble and insoluble fiber.
- Legumes, green leafy vegetables, and whole grains are fundamental parts of a good vegan diet.
- The soybean is a versatile and nutritious food that can be prepared in a wide variety of ways.
- Vegans and others who want to move toward a plant-based diet can easily find many healthful and nutritious meat substitutes.

No Dairy? What About Calcium?

In This Chapter

- Eliminating calcium concerns
- The advantages of avoiding cow's milk
- Plant-based milk substitutes
- The truth about dairy cheese
- The wonderful world of nondairy cheeses

Where will you get your calcium if you're not eating cheese and drinking milk?

In addition to the often-asked questions regarding protein, you'll most likely hear this question, as well as other versions of it, as people learn you're going vegan and wonder how you'll ever survive without dairy products.

What many people don't realize, however, is that it's relatively easy to meet your calcium requirements while consuming a completely plant-based diet.

What the Other Animals Do

Calcium is one of Earth's most common minerals. It's also the one most abundant in your body. How does it get there? Plants absorb calcium into their cells, and you then access the plants' calcium when you eat calcium-rich foods or ingest them as either human or animal breast milk that has become fortified with the mother's dietary calcium. Consuming plant-based dietary sources of calcium is much easier and supplies much larger amounts of absorbable calcium.

Not Past the Age of 2

In general, most creatures who nurse their young do not breast-feed beyond the age of 2; therefore, the need for milk no longer exists past that age. This is the case for humans as well, and by the time we reach age 4, most of us have lost the ability to digest lactose.

Lactose, which we touched on briefly in Chapter 3, is a type of sugar present in all animal breast milks, including human. As you age, your gastrointestinal tract matures and reduces your need for lactose as weaning is completed. When lactose isn't digested properly, it reaches the intestines, where bacteria attack it and try to break it down. During the "attack," acids and gases are produced; these are what cause the many painful symptoms associated with lactose intolerance.

Not Your Mama's Milk

It makes sense for our young to consume their mother's breast milk—after all, that's why it's produced in the first place. Most breast milk contains colostrum, which supplies newborns with all the vitamins, nutrients, and antibodies they need for the early developmental stages of life. It seems only logical that if you're going to consume any milk, it should be early in life and it should be human milk because it contains the right kind of colostrum specific for your body.

Humans are the only species on the planet who consume the milk of another species and who continue to drink milk after weaning. So what's wrong with cow's milk and its colostrum for humans? Cow's milk's main function is to take a young calf and "beef it up" to several hundred pounds in its first year of life. If you consume cow's milk instead of breast milk as an infant, it can definitely affect your size and development, which can also explain the increased obesity of toddlers in this country.

HOT POTATO

Cow's milk can contain growth hormones and antibiotics that are given to dairy cows to increase their milk production and alleviate conditions like infected udders. All these substances are then passed on to those who consume dairy products. Some have been linked to various forms of cancer and disease, food allergies, growth abnormalities, and birth defects.

It's interesting to note that mature cows don't need to consume milk to produce lots of calcium-rich milk. In their natural habitat, they would eat a diet based on grasses and vegetation. Similarly, humans don't need to drink cow's milk to get calcium or produce milk for their own babies, either. Consuming plant-based forms of calcium to stay healthy and help produce our own milk, as the cows do, is the ideal way of getting it straight from the source instead of secondhand.

Calcium Concerns

Your body uses calcium to maintain strong bones and teeth, send nerve impulses, metabolize iron, regulate your heartbeat and other muscle contractions, and reduce the risk of chronic diseases. Yes, you should be concerned about whether or not you're getting enough calcium from dietary sources, but you should also be aware of your body's ability to absorb and utilize the calcium from those sources.

It's also important to hold on to the natural calcium already present in your bones and also take in dietary sources of calcium to make up for the losses that occur naturally as you age. What you eat directly affects your calcium loss and the strength of your skeleton, so be sure to choose low-fat forms of plant-based protein, watch your salt intake, limit your caffeine to 2 cups of coffee a day, quit smoking, and get plenty of exercise outdoors. It's believed that if you avoid the calcium depleters while consuming an average level of calcium in your diet, you can maintain strong, healthy bones.

The people of India and their cultural diet are a great example of the pitfalls of following a dairy-rich diet. There they follow a mostly vegetarian diet, but most of their native dishes contain large amounts of yogurt, milk, cheese, and ghee (clarified butter). As a result, Indians have high incidences of diseases associated with high-cholesterol and high-fat diets such as cancer, especially prostate and breast cancer, and heart disease. According to projections made by both the Indian Council of Medical Research (ICMR) and the World Health Organization (WHO), by 2020, the population of India will top the charts worldwide with the highest numbers of heart attacks, hypertension, and diabetes.

Sources and Absorbability

What are some calcium-rich foods, and how much of their calcium are you capable of absorbing and holding on to? For proper calcium absorption, you need to consume food sources that contain types of calcium that are easily digested, assimilated, and absorbed. Keep a watchful eye on your protein, sodium, and other mineral intakes, as they all affect this process.

Especially important to note is the special relationship between magnesium and calcium. These close buddies rely on each other, and both need to be present for proper absorption. Usually it's in a 2:1 ratio, with 2 parts calcium to 1 part magnesium. Because of the calcium-magnesium ratio in dairy products, your body does not properly absorb the calcium they contain. Excess stores of animal-based calcium accumulate in your blood and urine and can cause kidney problems, like kidney stones and gallstones, or worse yet, kidney failure.

The presence of vitamin D also affects calcium's absorption capabilities. The body easily absorbs vitamin D with just 15 minutes of sun exposure per day. Vitamin D is produced within the body when the sun hits your skin. The sun triggers ergosterol, which is transformed into vitamin D, which is stored in your liver and helps you absorb calcium from the foods you consume directly into your bloodstream. Many believe that vitamin D you get from sun exposure during an average summer can be stored within your body and used throughout the winter. The liver is capable of storing up to a 3-year supply of vitamin D at one time.

So what about your body's ability to absorb plant-based sources of calcium? You can find plenty of calcium in leafy greens and cruciferous vegetables, and 40 to 60 percent of their calcium content is absorbable by your body. Unfortunately, some of these same foods are also high in *oxalates*, which can impact calcium absorption and have been blamed for causing kidney stones, among other problems.

DEFINITION

Oxalates are organic acids that occur naturally in leafy greens, berries, nuts, black tea, and other foods. They can significantly reduce your body's absorption of iron, magnesium, and calcium, and an accumulation of oxalates in the body could lead to kidney stones.

The good news is that you can greatly reduce the oxalate content of these foods simply by cooking them. Boiling them, for example, reduces the oxalates by 80 percent. If you're susceptible to kidney stones and gallstones, you might want to limit your consumption of leafy greens to several times a week. Also, drinking plenty of water can help prevent the formation of stones by diluting the concentration of oxalic acid and dissolved minerals in the urine.

Today, many foods are fortified with calcium, magnesium, and vitamin D. As a matter of fact, most of the vitamin D present in cow's milk is actually added later as a supplement, which is also the case with fortified nondairy milks. Check your grocery and natural foods store shelves for fortified soy-based products, cereals and grain products, boxed mixes and food items, and orange juices and other beverages.

You'll absorb more calcium if you spread out your food choices throughout your meals and throughout the day. With all the delicious plant-based choices available, it's virtually impossible to have a calcium deficiency if you consume a well-balanced vegan diet.

Comparing Food Sources

The U.S. RDA for calcium for men and women between the ages of 19 to 50 is 1,000 milligrams, and after age 50, it increases to 1,200 milligrams, depending on your protein intake. But many feel that number is too high. The WHO recommends between 400 and 500 milligrams calcium daily—half of the U.S. RDA. As we've discussed, plant-based sources of calcium are generally more absorbable than animal sources because we can digest the plant-based foods easier and break them down and utilize the nutrients better.

Proteins also have a negative effect on calcium stores because amino acids contain sulfur, which in turn affects the body's pH balance. Plant-based proteins tend to have lower concentrations of sulfur-based amino acids and are more alkaline in nature. Meat, on the other hand, is very acidic, and the body reacts to rebalance itself by leaching alkaline calcium out of the bones to neutralize the acid. For every 1 gram protein in your diet, you can expect 1 milligram calcium to be lost or eliminated in your urine.

Through his research, Dr. T. Colin Campbell, author of the China Study (see Chapter 3), has determined that even though most Chinese consume no dairy products in their daily diets, *osteoporosis* is uncommon in China. The Chinese consume only half the amount of calcium consumed by Americans; instead, they obtain all their dietary calcium from plant-based sources.

DEFINITION

Osteoporosis is a bone-thinning disease that can rob you of 30 to 40 percent of bone tissue. Calcium passes from the bones, filters through the kidneys, and is eliminated in the urine. Factors like excess salt, animal protein, and high-protein dairy products in your diet cause rapid calcium losses and increase your chances of developing osteoporosis. Women in the United States take note, as osteoporosis affects one in four women in North America.

Ironically, osteoporosis is highest in those countries that consume the highest amount of calcium from animal-based sources. Because the high concentration of acidic protein in animal-based sources causes the body to lose more calcium than it consumes, a vegan diet actually reduces your chances of developing osteoporosis.

Plant-Based Possibilities

Many plant-based foods are rich in calcium (and many are also excellent sources of protein; see Chapter 5). In the leafy green vegetable category, you have many choices, including spinach, collards, kale, Swiss chard, lettuces, rhubarb, mustard and turnip greens, and even broccoli.

Soy foods have naturally occurring calcium and are also often enriched to further increase the calcium amount. Calcium-rich soy products include soy milk, nondairy cheeses, edamame, tofu, tempeh, and veggie burgers and other mock meats, just to name a few. In cereals and grains, calcium can be found in quinoa, amaranth, corn, wheat, and brown rice. And you might be surprised to learn that many sea vegetables, nuts, seeds, dried fruits, oranges, and even blackstrap molasses all contain significant amounts of calcium.

Here's a small sampling of vegan foods high in calcium:

1 cup hijiki	648 milligrams
1 cup tofu	516 milligrams
1 cup cooked collard greens	358 milligrams
1½ cups calcium-fortified oatmeal	326 milligrams
1 cup calcium-fortified orange juice	270 milligrams
10 medium figs	270 milligrams
1 cup cooked spinach	244 milligrams
1 cup cooked white beans	160 milligrams

The Disadvantages of Cow's Milk

Even though cows eat a low-fat plant-based diet naturally, their bodies transform the polyunsaturated fatty acids they consume into saturated fats contained in their milk to help their young grow quickly. As a result, cow's milk and most dairy products in general are high in fat, especially high concentrations of saturated fat and trans-fatty acids. These types of fats are associated with increased risks of chronic disease and obesity and higher mortality rates.

High-fat dairy products, such as whole cow's milk, butter, and cheese, also contain larger amounts of pesticide residues and other environmental contaminants than their low-fat vegan counterparts.

Allergen Alert

Around 75 percent of people throughout the world develop some degree of lactose intolerance after weaning, and this leads to problems digesting dairy products. Besides being allergic to lactose, many find themselves allergic to casein, one of the types of proteins found in cow's milk. Many further suffer from colic, which has been linked to consumption of cow's milk.

IN A NUTSHELL

In 2005, the Dairy Council dropped its popular slogan, "Milk: it does a body good" after a lawsuit brought by the Physicians Committee for Responsible Medicine (PCRM; see Chapter 3) alleged that milk actually contributes to disease and in fact does *not* do a body good.

An allergic reaction to dairy can cause a wide variety of symptoms, including diarrhea, constipation, respiratory problems, muscle and abdominal pain, colitis, depression and irritability, skin rashes, and chronic fatigue. Diligent label-reading is your best defense. If you suffer from such allergies, avoid products with the following words on the ingredient label: *whey, milk solids, calcium caseinate, sodium caseinate, sodium lactylate,* and *lactalbumin.* As a vegan, you'll naturally avoid these substances anyway. You should always take food allergies very seriously because, in some instances, they can be life-threatening.

Kick Your Cold

Dairy products also produce excess mucus in your system. This leads to such problems as sinusitis, nasal stuffiness, and runny nose, which in turn can lead to colds and increased ear infections, asthma, and sinus infections.

Plant-based substitutes for cow's milk, such as those made from a soy or rice base, are associated with fewer allergies. Those who suffer from chronic colds or dairy allergies should explore dropping dairy products from their diet to relieve their symptoms. Many see positive results within a few weeks after making dietary changes.

Finding Plant-Based Milk Substitutes

Our bodies don't have a physical need for milk after a certain age, but there's no doubt the use of dairy products has had an impact on our cuisine. We have acquired tastes for rich and flavorful foods and creamy textures.

But just because you shun dairy doesn't mean you have to give up creaminess and satisfaction. Many plant-based substitutes to cow's milk exist, and each has its own distinct and unique flavor and consistency or texture. Creamy, milklike beverages are made from soybeans, rice, grains, coconut, nuts, and even seeds, and these are also low in fat and excellent sources of complex carbohydrates. And not only are plant-based milks suitable for drinking or on your bowl of cereal, they can also be used in your favorite recipes measure for measure as a replacement for their dairy-based counterparts. (See Part 5 for more information on using substitutions. Then if you like, turn to Part 6 for recipe ideas!)

If you look around your local grocery or natural foods store, you'll easily find several varieties of nondairy milks, in aseptic packaging, making them shelf-stable; in the cereal and juice aisles; or in cartons in the refrigerated sections next to their dairy-based counterparts. They're sold in a wide assortment of sizes, like the convenient juice boxes and quart or half-gallon sizes, as well as in unsweetened or lightly sweetened varieties and fantastic flavors such as plain, vanilla, chocolate, chocolate mint, carob, coffee, and even holiday varieties like eggnog.

Soy Milk

Soy milk is made from cooked ground soybeans and is rich in iron, calcium, and phosphorus. You can easily make it at home or purchase it premade in assorted sizes and flavors.

Soy milk is delicious and nutritious, and in a 1-cup serving, you get 9 grams protein, 2 grams fiber, 4½ grams fat, and only ½ gram saturated fat. Soy milk is also high in soy isoflavones, the beneficial phytoestrogens that have so many positive effects on your body. Some brands are also fortified with extra calcium and vitamin D, making soy milk even more nutritious.

Rice Milk

Rice milk can also be homemade or purchased commercially in assorted sizes and flavors, and it's usually made from fermented rice alone or in combination with soy milk or other grains. It has a slightly thinner consistency and sweeter flavor than soy milk, and is a great alternative for those with food allergies.

Rice milk is a high-quality source of carbohydrates and B vitamins, and each 1-cup serving contains 1 gram protein, 2 grams fat, and no saturated fat.

Other Nondairy Milks

If you love the taste of nuts and seeds, look for luscious-tasting and protein-rich almond, cashew, hazelnut, hemp, and sunflower milks.

One of the most popular plant-based beverage options these days is coconut milk, and its rich and creamy flavor and consistency is winning people over from coast to coast, especially those who suffer from soy allergies. Not only is it available as a drinkable beverage, but you can also purchase pint-size cartons of coconut nondairy liquid creamer (soy versions, too!) for use in your cup of coffee or tea, and of course, your favorite recipes.

You will also find other grain-based milky beverages, like oat milk and multigrain milk (made from a mixture of amaranth, barley, brown rice, oats, soybeans, and triticale). Per serving, these grain-based milks deliver between 4 to 7 grams protein, around 2½ grams fat, and no saturated fat.

Cheese: Melting Through the Layers

Cheese is, hands down, the most popular of all dairy products. And it comes in so many varieties, from cow's milk, goat's milk, and sheep's milk, to the ever-popular buffalo mozzarella made from—you guessed it—water buffalo milk.

In the 1970s, the average American consumed close to 11 pounds of cheese per year, and now that figure is more than 30 pounds per year—per person! Cheese is essentially concentrated milk, so it also comes with higher concentrations of fat, calories, sodium, cholesterol, and agricultural contaminants like antibiotics and pesticides.

HOT POTATO

One pound of cheese contains 10 times the amounts of hormones and antibiotics (used in factory farming) as the milk from which it came.

It may seem difficult or daunting to give up dairy cheese at first, but no worries! Just check out the refrigerated case at your local grocery or natural foods store, and you'll find a wide array of fabulous dairy-free alternatives. But before we get into the vegan cheese alternatives out there, let's delve deeper into the problems with consuming too much animal-based cheeses.

Cholesterol and Sodium Levels

Cholesterol, as previously mentioned, is produced by the body and also found in animal-based foods. One cup whole milk contains 10 milligrams of cholesterol, and cheese made from a high concentration of milk has a larger proportional amount of cholesterol.

Here's an example of the kind of cholesterol numbers you can expect to find in a 1-cup serving of some popular cheese products, according to the U.S. Department of Agriculture (USDA):

Cheddar cheese	240 milligrams
Ricotta cheese	125 milligrams
Parmesan cheese	64 milligrams
Cottage cheese	32 milligrams

Salt is used in cheese-making to add flavor, to ripen, and to cure the cheese. The exact amount of sodium in cheese depends on the variety and processing methods, but as with cholesterol and fat, there's also a higher sodium content in cheese compared to other dairy products. Processed cheeses, cheese foods, and cheese spreads contain more sodium than naturally aged cheeses; cottage cheese's sodium content falls somewhere between the two types.

More Fat Than Protein

The current RDAs for dairy products recommend two or three servings a day. Most Americans don't follow the recommended serving sizes when it comes to eating cheese. An average serving constitutes about 1 ounce, which could be 1 slice hard cheese (like mozzarella or cheddar), 1½ slices American cheese, or ⅓ cup shredded cheese. These cheezy servings come with 6 grams artery-clogging saturated fat, and your average slice of cheese-laden lasagna or cheese-lover's pizza could have 20 to 25 grams saturated fat!

Cheese is also a very concentrated source of protein, and about 80 percent of milk and cheese is made up of the protein casein. Casein plays a major role in cheese-making, where it's used to bind the other milk proteins together, giving the cheese structure and a stretchy, gooey quality when melted.

Cheese-making also uses coagulants to bind or give structure to the cheese. These coagulants can come from plant- or animal-based sources, and rennet is the most commonly used. What's wrong with rennet? For one thing, it comes from the digestive systems of pigs and other mammals. Ponder that for a moment the next time you get a craving for a hunk of havarti!

The Pains of Lactose Intolerance

Many lactose intolerant have fewer problems digesting cheese and yogurt because of the friendly bacteria and enzymes added during their production processes. However, the lactose that's still present may cause some to experience constipation, abdominal pain, digestion problems, and migraine headaches.

Over time, continuing to suffer the lactose-related irritation to your system weakens your immunity and digestion processes.

HOT POTATO

Whether or not you started out lactose intolerant, as you transition to a vegan diet, you might become so rather quickly after giving up the dairy products. Read product labels carefully and thoroughly to avoid dairy-based ingredients. Watch out for words such as *rennet, casein, whey, calcium caseinate, sodium caseinate, sodium lactylate,* and *lactalbumin* on ingredient labels.

Dairy-Free Substitutes

In the last decade, the demand for more nondairy and animal-free food products has grown dramatically, and this has not gone unnoticed by the retail industry. In response, a plethora of vegan alternative products have flooded the markets. On the shelves of most grocery and natural foods stores, you can find some astounding dairy-free substitutes, right there alongside their animal-based counterparts.

Plant-based milks of all sorts are available, and the ones sold in shelf-stable, aseptic packages enable you to keep your pantry stocked with vegan options to be opened when needed—and they're also great for traveling. Most nondairy milks come in juice-box, quart, and half-gallon sizes to suit all needs and family sizes.

You can also find many products in the refrigerated case. Among them are soy- and coconut-based liquid creamers, which can be used in coffee and other beverages, or in recipes as desired. You'll also find nondairy milks in quart and half-gallon sizes in various flavors from plain to chocolate, and specialty options, like eggnog and other holiday or seasonal selections. Several cultured options are available as well, like vegan yogurts, kefir, sour cream, cream cheese, and even fluffy vegan whipped toppings for embellishing your piece of pie. Or if you want it à la mode, check the freezer for nondairy ice creams and other frozen novelties made with a soy, rice, coconut, hemp, or nut milk base.

For some, cheese is one of the hardest things to give up when going vegan, but it doesn't have to be. You can make or buy your own dairy-free substitutes, and you'll also find a wide array of vegan soft and spreadable cheeses, hard blocks of cheese, slices and shreds, and even shredded Parmesan-style cheese alternatives, ready and waiting for you in the refrigerated case at your local grocery or natural foods store.

Most people like melted cheese on their pizza, and vegan versions of nondairy cheeses, found at most stores, can do the job. You can also make and drizzle a vegan cheese sauce on your pizza for a different change of pace. (See Chapter 22 for Vegan Cheezy Sauce, a versatile sauce to help those suffering from cheese cravings.)

Not all prepackaged brands of vegan cheese are the same, and each has its own unique flavors and textures. Do a little experimenting to see which ones you like best. Some are strongly flavored, and others are mild. Some have softer or firmer textures than others, making some more suitable for slicing and shredding. Types, flavors, and availability vary depending on where you live, and some natural foods stores even make their own homemade vegan cheeses.

IN A NUTSHELL

Not all packaged vegan cheeses are equal, especially when it comes to meltability (some do and some don't). One of the most popular brands of meltable vegan cheese is Daiya. Made with all plant-based ingredients, it's suitable for those with food allergies because it contains no dairy, gluten, eggs, soy, peanuts, and/or tree nuts (excluding coconut). Other notable brands of vegan cheese are Vegan Gourmet Cheese Alternative by Follow Your Heart, Teese by Chicago Soydairy, and Dr. Cow.

Cheezy Nutritional Yeast

Nutty and cheezy-tasting nutritional yeast is a great ingredient vegans can use to enhance the flavor and cheesiness factor of their foods. Nutritional yeast is an inactive type of yeast grown on a molasses medium, not to be confused with the kind of yeast used to make beer or bread. Nutritional yeast is high in supplemented B_{12} and is also gluten-free.

Look for the readily available Red Star vegetarian formula in small and large flakes as well as in a fine powder, packaged and in bulk bins at most grocery and natural foods stores. You can use it as a condiment, add it to boost the flavor of a recipe, and as you'll soon learn, it's often used to make nondairy cheese recipes because of its nutty, slightly salty flavor. There's really nothing quite like it!

The Least You Need to Know

- Thanks in part to the many plant foods high in calcium, it's easy to get enough calcium in a well-balanced vegan diet.
- By avoiding dairy products, you're also avoiding a lot of fat, agricultural adulterants, inferior calcium, and lactose intolerance.
- Soy milk, rice milk, coconut milk, hemp milk, and nut milks are all delicious and healthful alternatives to cow's milk.
- Dairy cheese is a concentrated form of dairy milk and contains concentrated forms of cholesterol and fat as well.
- You can find many nondairy products and cheese alternatives available in most grocery and natural foods stores.

Don't Carbohydrates Make You Fat?

In This Chapter

- A look at the carb craze
- The differences among carbs
- Eating whole-grain goodness
- The dangers of a low-carb diet

During the past few decades, there has been a dramatic increase in the popularity of diets that espouse a low-carb, high-protein approach to weight loss. Most of them claim that by dramatically decreasing your carbohydrate intake, while increasing your protein consumption and not worrying much about your fat intake, you can lose weight.

Unfortunately for many people, these trendy, low-carb diets all seem to boil down to eating lots of meat and dairy and not getting enough fiber, fruits, and veggies. Is this a reasonable and healthy road to weight loss, or just another dead end on the road to good health and fitness?

The Highs and Lows of Carbs

People following these low-carb, high-protein diet plans have to obsess over their intake of carbs, and a good recollection of high school math really comes in handy with all the calculating and figuring required. What's more, most people really aren't even sure what carbohydrates are or what they do.

Carbohydrates provide the basic energy needed to fuel your body. Plants make carbohydrates from the carbon, hydrogen, and oxygen they take in during their cycle of life. Carbohydrates usually come in the form of starches and sugars and are found in fruits, vegetables, nuts, seeds, and grains.

Carbohydrates are essential for providing energy to every part of your body, from your cells to your muscles, so they're certainly an important part of your diet. If you limit your carbs without being aware of what they are and why you need them, you could be doing your brain and body wrong—big time. Carbohydrates are an absolute necessity for brain function, so if you like your brain activity to be quick and responsive, you'll find carbs quite useful.

VEGAN VOICES

The American Heart Association doesn't recommend high-protein diets for weight loss. Some of these diets restrict healthful foods that provide essential nutrients and don't provide the variety of foods needed to adequately meet nutritional needs. People who stay on these diets very long may not get enough vitamins and minerals and face other potential health risks.

—American Heart Association Recommendation, 2002

The slamming of carbohydrates has caused a lot of confusion regarding the differences among the three types of carbs: complex, simple, and refined carbohydrates. (More on these in the next section.) Consuming more complex carbohydrates, limiting your simple carbohydrates, and restricting or eliminating refined carbohydrates should make up the basis of a well-balanced diet for anyone—veg-heads and meat-heads alike—especially those who suffer from chronic diseases.

Of note to diabetics, modern medicine is siding with the veg-heads because it turns out that excess meat-based proteins seem to affect insulin levels more than complex carbohydrates do. Studies have also shown that following low-carb diets should not become lifestyle choices, as these diets open the door to numerous health problems that may not be reversible without expensive surgeries, medications, and drastic changes. Not coincidentally, heart disease and various forms of cancer do seem to be plaguing some of the more vocal supporters of these types of diets.

Carbs: Complex, Simple, and Refined

Complex, simple, and refined carbohydrates really are miles apart, and it's quite easy to distinguish the good from the bad. They each have a role in your life, and how big a role each plays in your daily diet seems to be the key to the size of your waistline.

Carbohydrates are made of sugars and starches. Complex carbohydrates are starches in their whole forms, such as in whole grains and flours, beans, and fresh and frozen vegetables. They provide your body with dietary fiber to aid in digestion, keep you regular, and lower your risk of chronic disease. Whole grains and seeds like brown rice and quinoa, unrefined flours, corn, pasta, beans, root vegetables, and green leafy vegetables all provide high concentrations of complex carbohydrates. You benefit greatly from centering your daily diet around foods like these.

Simple carbohydrates are found in fresh, frozen, and dried fruits like berries, citrus fruits, apples, cherries, dates, melons, peaches, and plums, and commonly used sweeteners like agave, sugar cane, brown rice syrup, and maple syrup. They provide you with quick energy and help satisfy your sweet tooth with a better choice than a piece of candy. Enjoy these carbs more sparingly than the complex variety, but enjoy them nevertheless, especially fruits, because they're loaded with vitamins, enzymes, fiber, and lots of other good stuff!

Refined carbohydrates are abundant in highly processed and packaged foods such as snacks, candies and confections, cookies, cakes, and other baked goods made with ingredients like white sugar, white flour, high-fructose corn syrup, hydrogenated oils, and lots of artificial colorings and flavorings. Consume these foods only occasionally—or better yet, not at all!—because they're empty calories that can lead to weight gain, cause fluctuations in blood-sugar levels, and provide very little on a nutritional level, as many vitamins, minerals, phytochemicals, fiber, protein, and beneficial essential fatty acids are removed during the refining and manufacturing process.

Low-Carb: Diet Craze, or Just Crazy?

The Atkins, Zone, South Beach, and other low-carb diets push high-protein portions mostly in the form of meat, eggs, and dairy—and along with them come artery-clogging fats. Conversely, carbohydrates are practically demonized and avoided at all costs.

These diets call for limiting the intake of sugar (itself a type of carbohydrate), which in actuality is not a bad thing, but they take it a step further by limiting one's choice of fruits and veggies because they contain sugars. In the process, all the beneficial vitamins, minerals, enzymes, and essential fiber that those fruits and veggies contain are also limited.

All this, they believe, will make you a shining example of good health and cause you to lose tremendous amounts of weight without ever having to exercise. It's all the foods' fault you're fat, they say, not that you possibly made bad food choices when going back for that third piece of fatty meat or cheese—both of which these diets encourage you to keep enjoying to your heart's (dis)content, by the way.

VEGAN VOICES

Dr. Atkins advocated substituting simple carbohydrates with high-fat, high animal-protein foods such as bacon, sausage, butter, steak, pork rinds and brie. I would love to be able to tell you that these are healthy foods, but they are not. Telling people what they want to believe is part of the reason that the Atkins diet has become so popular.

—Dr. Dean Ornish, *Journal of the American Dietetic Association,* April 2004

As we discussed in Chapter 5, too much protein in your diet can lead to numerous health problems, the most life-threatening being heart disease and various forms of cancer—but that's not the only problem with these diets. Proponents want you to believe that if you base your diet around lots of animal protein and dairy products, with seemingly unlimited intake of fats, you'll actually lose weight as long as you give up all your breads and pasta. What they usually don't tell you, at least not in the many TV ads or articles, is *why* you'll lose weight by eating this way.

The reason for your weight loss is because your body is sent into ketosis, which is the physical state where your system is fooled into burning stored fats instead of sugars. Carbohydrates and fats are the body's two main forms of energy, and when you extremely limit your carbohydrate intake, your body then switches to burning deposited fats. Carbohydrates are usually burned and put to use immediately, while fats are usually stored in deposits for later use.

In ketosis, everything is turned topsy-turvy. When your body burns fat as its main source of energy, toxic ketones are released into your system. Ketones are strong acids that are harmful to your body; they build up in your blood and urine. In high levels, ketones are poisonous to body tissue. Ketones also are the reason why some people on these types of diets have such foul-smelling breath.

Tipping the Scales in Your Favor

If you want to lose a few pounds, begin by increasing your intake of plant-based foods. The produce section of your grocery or natural foods store is the best place to start when you're looking for good sources of carbohydrates.

The biggest and smallest animals all chomp down on a little raw vegetation from time to time, often for the fiber benefits alone, and they're definitely more tuned in to their proper natural processes than we humans are. Eating a big carrot or leafy green salad definitely fills you up faster, whether it be from the digestive enzymes released or the high fiber content. This means less food passing by your lips, and ultimately, less ending up on your hips.

Refining Our Way of Life

After the world wars, the powers-that-be got it in their heads that everything had to be pristine white to instill a sense of cleanliness in the minds and hearts of those in the United States. Whitewash covered every part of society, from uniforms and clothing, to architectural structures, to modern conveniences and appliances, right down to the foods we eat. Across the board, white was right, and brown caused a frown.

Manufacturers of grains and sugars also began bleaching and polishing their foods to make them appear better and healthier to consumers, in addition to giving them a slightly longer shelf life. In the process, they stripped items such as flour, rice, and sugar of their vital nutrients, fiber, and bran—all of which made these foods beneficial in some way to our diet. No real nutritional benefits (although some brands add back in some synthetic vitamins) were added during all this bleaching and refining, only negatives.

HOT POTATO

During the bleaching process that turns beige-colored, unrefined cane sugar into white sugar, all the good nutritional components are stripped away. Among them are the molasses, vitamins, and minerals that were present. The only things left are refined carbohydrates and empty calories. Even more disturbing, from a vegan standpoint, is that often during the bleaching process, cane sugar is filtered through bone char (animal-based charcoal; for more about this, see Chapter 18).

You *need* bran, fiber, and other naturally present nutrients. Your insides are color-blind and don't care if a product is white or brown in color, just that it's wholesome and gives you the fuel you need to stay up and running like a well-oiled machine.

When you're choosing dry goods for your pantry, pick those that appear in shades of brown, not white. Select brown rice instead of white, whole-wheat or oat flour instead of bleached and bromated, and evaporated or unbleached cane juice instead of bleached white sugar. Buy whole grains such as whole-wheat couscous, quinoa, millet, brown rice, and so on.

When purchasing grain or rice blends, be sure the words *brown rice* or another whole grain appears on the label either instead of or before *white rice*. Whole-grain pastas, for example, are made from whole-wheat flour, and sometimes even brown rice, corn, quinoa, and vegetables. You can find them next to their white-flour counterparts on grocery shelves. You might even be able to find them at a savings in the bulk section of many stores as well. For some good recommendations of delicious and nutritious vegan food items to help stock your pantry, refrigerator, and freezer, turn to Part 3.

The Least You Need to Know

- Eating a low-carb, high-fat, and high-protein diet can be detrimental to your health, especially when the diet becomes a way of life.
- Complex carbs should be the basis of a well-rounded vegan diet. Simple carbs should be enjoyed more sparingly, and refined carbs should be rarely used or avoided altogether.
- When choosing carbohydrates like grains and sugars, always look for whole or unrefined varieties.

Aren't All Vegans Weak and Sickly?

In This Chapter

- Getting fit and trim, the vegan way
- A look at vegan athletes
- Fueling your body with the right stuff
- The slow burn of carbs

For some reason, people sometimes have the impression that vegans and other plant-based eaters are frail, too thin, weak, or sickly. This couldn't be further from the truth, although vegans are much more likely to be fitter and trimmer than their nonvegan counterparts. Vegan athletes abound and excel in the sports world, and some of our greatest athletes have followed a completely plant-based diet.

Be confident knowing that being vegan does do a body good, and your physique won't suffer from your new way of eating. In fact, it will almost certainly improve. Remember, small steps taken in the right direction can have a positive impact on your journey to good health and happiness. Each of the changes you're making in your lifestyle has an effect on your quality of life now and down the road.

Veganism: It Does a Body Good

The American Dietetics Association and the Dietitians of Canada have stated many times that a well-balanced vegan diet is appropriate for all stages of life, from pregnancy, through the early stages of infancy on into childhood, through the growth spurts of adolescence, and on into adulthood. Vegan diets provide nutritional benefits in abundance. This translates into a body that is a lean, mean, vegan machine.

VEGAN VOICES

My best year of track competition was the first year I ate a vegan diet. Moreover, by continuing to eat a vegan diet, my weight is under control, I like the way I look … I enjoy eating more, and I feel great.

—Carl Lewis, winner of nine Olympic gold medals

As you know, vegan diets are lower in fat than other kinds of vegetarian and animal-based diets. Plant foods are fiber rich and often lower in calories, which assists in weight loss. Evidence exists that, due to their low-fat and high-carbohydrate diet, vegans have higher metabolic rates than people who consume animal-based foods.

A higher metabolic rate means you're burning calories faster, which is good for weight loss. As you age, your basal metabolic rate (BMR) steadily decreases. When you're young and strong, your BMR is very high. Then as you get older, you lose lean body mass, which in turn slows down your BMR. The more lean body tissue you have, the higher your BMR. The more "fatty" body tissue you possess, the lower your BMR. You can raise your metabolic rate by getting regular vigorous exercise and consuming a healthy vegan diet.

Worth the Weight?

On average, vegans have lower incidences of obesity and tend to be leaner and trimmer. Most people who try a vegan diet for any length of time generally experience some weight loss, whether it be just water weight initially or some serious poundage. When going vegan full throttle, it's not uncommon to lose a significant amount of weight, especially as you rid your system of excess fat stores and cholesterol you may have accumulated. Vegans are also well equipped for avoiding yo-yo weight fluctuations and usually consistently maintain their ideal weight.

Carbohydrates and simple sugars are the main sources of fuel for our bodies, and these are not found in meat. Providing your body with the proper fuel gives you endless amounts of energy and causes you to burn more calories. As a rule, plant-based foods are usually low in salt, saturated fats, and calories, which makes them perfect for those crunching their dietary intake numbers. Also, if you only consume foods that are low in fat and high in fiber, you are off to a good start for supplying your body with the optimal fuel it needs.

VEGAN VOICES

Since becoming vegan, my running has improved considerably. Vegan food is ideal: high carbohydrate, low fat and plenty of vitamins and iron. I'm proud that I run without exploiting animals in any way.

—Sally Eastall, marathon runner

The Skinny

A vegan diet can help you reach and maintain your optimum weight. A plant-based diet is full of fiber from plant vegetation and whole-grain sources that help flush out toxins, keep foods digesting properly, and make elimination time faster and more efficient.

Veggies are also low in calories. Beans and green and yellow vegetables, like zucchini and summer squashes, celery, greens, peppers, onions, and carrots, all are perfect low-calorie munching foods. If you want to drop a few pounds, stick with your vegan diet. You can easily expect to have double the weight loss than someone following a low-fat animal-based diet.

Eating well is important when it comes to weight loss, but physical activity and vigorous exercise are also a must. Exercise boosts your metabolism and controls your appetite. Putting your body into a fast-paced mode during exercise triggers your body's "fight or flight" response. As a result, your digestion processes and appetite go into a holding pattern for a while to help your body handle the increased workload. Exercising an hour before eating helps you satisfy your hunger with much less food— and burns more calories, to boot.

The Buff

Vegans tend to have more lean muscle on their bodies and better overall muscle tone in general. You don't need to eat animal protein to put on muscle. Look at the elephant, one of the largest and strongest creatures in the animal kingdom. It eats an entirely plant-based diet full of roughage and fiber. It simply strips the leaves off the branches and chows down.

Some think we vegans survive on eating "leaves and twigs," as some foods, especially trail mix, appear this way to some. But maybe we *would* all eat more leaves and twigs if we thought it would help us grow to be as strong and healthy as elephants are!

Vegans Fit and Famous

It's a common misconception that you need animal-based protein to meet your protein needs and that you need extra amounts of protein if you're an athlete or lead a physically demanding lifestyle. Doctors have discovered that you really don't utilize proteins any more rapidly while at work or play than you do at rest.

Meat and dairy products are high-fat forms of protein, and although high-fat foods do provide you with energy, just as high-sugar foods do, they don't give you *sustained* energy. Rather, your uplifting feeling fades quickly, leaving you feeling sluggish and out of it. Instead, grab a carrot, a handful of nuts, or some broccoli. Plant-based proteins amply support muscle development and endurance during physical exertion and activity.

The *Yale Medical Journal* has concluded that strong evidence exists that a meatless diet is conducive to endurance. Similarly, Dr. Ioteyko of the Academie de Medicine of Paris has discovered that vegans and vegetarians averaged two to three times more stamina and recovered from exhaustion in one fifth of the time as meat-eaters.

This increased endurance and stamina comes from a high-carbohydrate vegan diet. Carbohydrates give a slow, steady burn and provide a constant energy source (fuel) for the body. That's why many athletes carb-load before a big race or competition. Lean sources of protein that are low in fat and high in fiber, like beans and other veggies, are like powder kegs for the body. And athletes know it!

Many well-known athletes know the benefits of a meatless diet. Here are a few fit and famous vegans:

- Brendan Brazier (pro Ironman triathlete, ultramarathoner, and author)

- Mac Danzig (pro mixed martial arts fighter and instructor)

- Sally Eastall (marathon runner)

- Ruth Heidrich (three-time Ironman finisher, marathoner, age-group record holder, and author)

- Jack LaLanne (fitness guru and author)

- Carl Lewis (winner of nine Olympic gold medals)

- Scott Jurek (ultramarathoner and 24-hour distance record holder)

- Martina Navratilova (champion tennis player)

- Robert Cheeke (bodybuilder and author)
- Kenneth Williams (bodybuilder and personal trainer)
- Christine Vardaros (pro cyclist)

IN A NUTSHELL

In a position paper on athletic performance and physical fitness, the American and Canadian Dietetic Association and Dietitians of Canada recommended that for most athletes, 60 to 65 percent of total energy should come from carbohydrates. Those who compete in prolonged endurance events, or who exercise intensely on consecutive days, should increase their carbohydrate-based energy to 65 to 70 percent.

Finding Balance

No matter how or what you do or do not eat, the most important thing you can do to ensure your good health is to eat a well-balanced diet, full of fruits, vegetables, grains, healthful fats, lean proteins, and complex carbohydrates, with plenty of water and other liquids. Fruits and veggies are the good stuff your body needs, so try to eat a wide variety in a rainbow of colors. This helps you easily get all your nutritional needs—and do it far better (and tastier, too!) than animal-based foods.

There's nothing like a little grain to fill out your meals and satisfy your appetite—especially whole grains, which provide protein, carbohydrates, fiber, and an endless supply of energy with their slow burn. What you put into your body, you do get out of it. Good, wholesome foods will result in your whole being—body, mind, and soul—functioning in a happy, healthy way.

Being a vegan is not about being on some trendy new diet; it's a lifestyle. It's a way to think about the world and your relationship to it, as well as a moral code to make life choices by. It's not only the most cruelty-free way to nourish ourselves, but it's also the healthiest. That's an indisputable fact. Veganism as a way of life and a way to approach eating is meant to sustain us for the long haul. Although it certainly is growing in popularity around the world, it is not just the latest fad diet or "in thing" to do. A vegan diet is sound nutrition for a lifetime.

The Least You Need to Know

- Eating a well-balanced vegan diet is appropriate for all stages of life.
- A plant-based vegan diet can help you shed excess pounds and maintain your optimum weight level.
- Many athletes have achieved fame and fortune by fueling their bodies with a completely plant-based diet.
- Fueling your body with plenty of fruits, veggies, whole grains, and lean, plant-based proteins provides the steady source of sustained energy needed for physical exertion.

A Vegan Survival Guide

On the ever-popular survival reality shows that grace our television screens, the contestants are left to their own resources to feed themselves, and they sometimes go hungry. What they need is an educated vegan, preferably a raw foodist, to show them all the wonderful plant-based foods that surround them!

Plants are definitely where it is, nutritionally. They give you a strong and healthy body, provide plenty of energy and endurance, and keep you mentally quick and alert. Eating vegan definitely gives you an advantage to help you win the game. After reading the following chapters, you'll have a leg up on the ins and outs of vegan nutrition, whether you're a child, young adult, pregnant, or in the prime of life. All you need to win at the game of life is right here!

Nourishing Yourself

In This Chapter

- The development of dietary guidelines
- The Four Food Groups versus the New Four Food Groups
- Reshaping the Food Guide Pyramid into MyPlate
- A look at the standard American diet
- The meatless Power Plate
- Meeting all your vegan nutritional needs

Many people are confused when it comes to what's actually needed by our bodies, in terms of fuel, to keep them moving and working as they should. A lot of this confusion stems from the fact that most of what we believe about eating properly and meeting our nutritional needs we learned in grade school. In this chapter, we discuss dietary guidelines and how to adequately meet all your nutritional needs with a vegan plant-based diet.

You may not have been much of a chef or short-order cook in your prevegan days, but if you truly want to embrace your new vegan lifestyle to the fullest, you're going to need to roll up your sleeves and get cooking. Check out your pantry, refrigerator, and freezer for supplies and inspiration. Sometimes wandering in the market or cleaning out your cabinets can really spark some culinary creativity that results in a fabulous vegan meal. To further assist you with this task, we also share some helpful advice and tips for planning vegan meals that are good for you and taste great!

Knowing how to properly fuel your body with good-for-you plant-based foods also comes in handy in later parts of this book, when we guide you through the process of stocking your pantry with vegan goods (Part 4) and provide you with suggestions on how to use some of the vegan alternatives you might not have used—or even heard of—before (Part 5). Then in Part 6, we provide you with some vegan recipes you can add to your repertoire to help you through your transition into eating vegan, as well as a few dishes to impress the veg-curious or veg-skeptical in your life.

The Formation of the Food Guidelines

The idea of using formal or semiformal dietary guidelines has been around for quite some time now, but it wasn't really widely used until the last century. Having recommended daily intake guidelines to follow for specific types of foods makes it easier for some people to be sure they're getting enough of what they need. Several dietary guidelines exist—from food groups to pyramids to plates—and are widely used by carnivores and vegans alike. We look at a few of them, and a bit of their histories, in this chapter.

Congress created the United States Department of Agriculture (USDA) in 1862, and right from the start, concerns existed over conflicts of interest. The USDA became the overseer of farmers' crops and the regulator of the nation's food-supply levels. It was also in charge of educating the public on all things agricultural, including instructing and advising on what they considered proper nutrition via their own recommended food guidelines. The combination of these two roles meant the USDA essentially controlled both the supply of and the demand for the nation's food.

The USDA soon found itself coming under the influence of heavy-hitting special interest groups like the meat and dairy industries. The first public food guidelines were published in 1916, and since their very beginning, their nutritional accuracy has come under scrutiny.

In the 1950s, the Basic Four Food Groups began their climb to fame and comprised the bulk of what most schoolchildren learned about proper nutrition for more than 30 years. The Basic Four Food Groups—which were made up of meat and other protein sources, milk and dairy products, grains, and fruits and vegetables—became the first of the food guidelines to give serving recommendations. We were told to eat in this manner every day:

> 2 servings milk and dairy products
>
> 2 servings meat, fish, poultry, eggs, dry beans, and nuts
>
> 4 servings fruits and vegetables
>
> 4 servings grain products

IN A NUTSHELL

Food-industry special-interest groups greatly influenced the Basic Four Food Groups serving suggestions. The National Dairy Council was one such influencer. It produced a vast amount of its own food-groups promotional literature, including posters and other "educational materials" that were used in classrooms.

The New Four Food Groups

Not everyone agreed with the USDA's recommendations. The Physicians Committee for Responsible Medicine (PCRM) strongly felt that the food guidelines should better reflect what had become widely considered as the most healthful way for people to eat: a diet low in fat and cholesterol and high in veggies and whole grains. In 1991, PCRM introduced a healthier and meatless alternative set of dietary guidelines, the New Four Food Groups, which recommended consuming the following each day:

5 or more servings whole grains

3 or more servings vegetables

3 or more servings fruit

2 or more servings legumes

The New Four Food Groups was intended to be a low-fat, zero-cholesterol, completely vegan way of meeting the daily nutritional requirements of the average adult. Several weeks before the USDA had planned to launch its Eating Right Pyramid, PCRM approached it about substituting the old Four Food Groups with its New Four Food Groups. Unfortunately, the USDA rejected the idea.

VEGAN VOICES

The old four food groups serve to misinform consumers about some aspects of nutrition. Two of the four food groups—meats and dairy products—are clearly not necessary for health and, in fact, may be detrimental to health. … Populations with the lowest rates of heart disease, colon and breast cancer, and obesity consume very little meat or no meat at all.

—From a 1991 PCRM report recommending the New Four Food Groups

Building a Pyramid

In 1977, the Senate Committee on Nutrition and Human Needs published dietary goals for the United States that totally supported a plant-based diet. In it, the committee recommended lowering cholesterol levels by limiting the amount of fats, especially saturated fats, in the diet and consuming generous amounts of fruits, vegetables, and whole grains. But after the meat and dairy industries complained and flexed their political muscle, the committee had to revise the report to be more accommodating to those industries.

In 1988, the USDA began to develop what it called the Eating Right Pyramid as a replacement for the old Basic Four Food Groups. This new food guide stressed the importance of plant-based foods by placing them at the foundation of the pyramid (the group with the largest number of servings per day) and relegating meat and dairy products to a small section at the top of the pyramid (with the least number of servings per day). For the first time in USDA history, meat and dairy would no longer take center stage in the recommended food guidelines.

Just weeks before the scheduled release date, the National Cattlemen's Association teamed up with the National Milk Producers Federation and other pro-industry groups to oppose the Eating Right Pyramid. A few weeks later, amidst protest from various health and medical groups, the USDA scrapped the Eating Right Pyramid, claiming children would find it "confusing." A year later, they released a new version of the Food Guide Pyramid, called MyPyramid, after it had undergone 33 changes, many of which were demanded by special-interest groups.

This "new and improved" version was made up of six categories of food groups—one minor and five major—that could provide all a person needed nutritionally on a daily basis. These six categories were arranged in pyramid shape and in ascending order according to the recommended servings for each. The plant-based food groups featured prominently in the food pyramid design, with the base layer of 6 to 11 servings of breads, cereals, rice, and pasta. Next were 2 to 4 servings of fruits and 3 to 5 servings of vegetables. Above these were the animal-based foods levels, or the milk and meat groups, which recommended 2 or 3 servings of each from legumes, nuts, eggs, fish, poultry, and meat for protein sources and various dairy products for the calcium requirement. Lastly, at the very top of the pyramid were fats, oils, and sweet indulgences, to be consumed sparingly.

IN A NUTSHELL

Want to shed a few pounds or eat a more heart-healthy diet in general? Choosing lean sources of protein such as beans instead of bacon and cholesterol-free soy milk instead of whole milk products is a step in the right direction.

Stepping Up to the Plate

In 2011, in an effort to make the dietary guidelines easier to understand, the USDA revised, reshaped, and renamed MyPyramid. This time, they chose the familiar image of a place setting for a meal and called it MyPlate, which illustrates how to build and fill your plate using five food groups: fruits, vegetables, grains, protein foods, and dairy. Specific daily need recommendations are broken down by age, sex, and level of physical activity.

Let's take a look at the arrangement of your MyPlate place setting.

Dividing Your Plate

Like most place settings, the USDA's MyPlate setup consists of a plate and a beverage. Let's start with your dinner plate. Divide it into four sections—one quarter section for each of the fruits, vegetables, grains, and protein food groups.

Two of the quarters, or one half of your plate, should contain fruits and vegetables. These can be fresh, frozen, canned, dried, whole, cut, mashed or puréed, or juiced.

The other half of your plate should be half grains and half protein. Opt for half of your grain servings to be whole grains like oats, quinoa, bulgur, and whole-wheat flour. The other half can be products made from refined grains, like white flour and white rice if you like.

For the protein food group, include plant-based foods like beans and peas, processed soy products, nuts, and seeds. (The USDA also recommends animal-derived foods here.)

The beverage part of the place setting is reserved for mainly dairy products, like milk, cheese, and yogurt, but the USDA also suggests calcium-enriched soy milk.

As part of the MyPlate dietary guidelines, you're encouraged to cut back on foods that are high in added fats, sugars, and sodium. Many packaged foods are made with overly processed ingredients and contain excessive amounts of fat, sodium, and calories, so only consume them on an occasional basis. Compare brands to make the wisest choice, and also check the Nutrition Facts label for the fiber, saturated fat, trans fat, caloric, and sodium content.

What's a Serving, Anyway?

So let's put this in perspective. In terms of fruit, 1 cup cut fruit or 100 percent fruit juice, a whole apple or banana, or ½ cup dried fruit is 1 serving of fruit. A big carrot, ½ cup chopped vegetables, or 1 cup leafy greens are all you need to get 1 serving of veggies. A slice of bread, 1 cup cold cereal, or ½ cup cooked rice or pasta is considered a 1-ounce serving of grains.

In the protein group, the USDA breaks down portions into 1-ounce sizes, such as a 1-ounce serving of fish, poultry, or meat; 1 egg; ¼ cup cooked beans; 1 tablespoon peanut butter; or ½ ounce nuts or seeds. A cup of milk, soy milk, or yogurt; 1½ ounces natural or 2 ounces processed cheese; or 1½ cups ice cream constitute a serving from the dairy group. As you can see, keeping the amount of dietary fat and cholesterol under control can be difficult following the USDA guidelines.

IN A NUTSHELL

Many nutritionists, dietitians, and doctors recommend you consume several small meals throughout the day instead of only 3 large meals a day every 5 or 6 hours. They believe this helps better regulate your blood sugar levels, thereby helping prevent mood swings and fatigue. Ever notice that depriving yourself of your afternoon snack sometimes results in a cranky or sleepy you? That could be the result of a mood swing stemming from low blood sugar.

There's no one-size-fits-all answer when it comes to the exact number of servings you need from each of these five food groups every day. It depends on your age, sex, and level of physical activity. On average, children require the least amount of servings, women require fewer servings than men, and athletes or people who are more active require more servings than those with sedentary lifestyles.

As a general guide for making your daily food choices, based on a 2,000-calorie diet, the USDA recommends the following:

>   2 cups fruits
>
>   2½ cups vegetables
>
>   6 ounces grains (mostly whole grains)
>
>   5½ ounces protein
>
>   3 cups dairy

For more specific information on the MyPlate guidelines, check out choosemyplate.gov.

The Vegan Power Plate

The USDA does offer some suggestions for adapting the MyPlate dietary guidelines for vegetarians. Following their lead, PCRM has taken its New Four Food Groups concept to the next level, creating what they call the Power Plate, which is geared toward vegans, with recommendations from only plant-based sources. The Power Plate skips the beverage part of the USDA's MyPlate place setting model. Instead, it focuses entirely on dividing your dinner plate into quarters and suggests filling your plate with a wide variety of whole grains, legumes, and plenty of colorful fruits and veggies for a powerful healthy and optimal vegan diet.

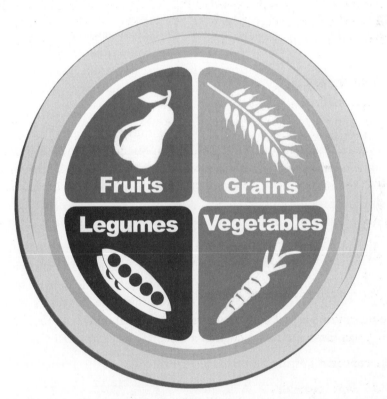

The PCRM Power Plate illustrates how to easily fill your plate with plant-based options at each meal to satisfy all your vegan dietary needs.
(Courtesy of PCRM)

PCRM's position is that there's no need for animal-derived products in your diet, and you're actually much better off without them. It also believes that by eating only plant-based foods, you can fulfill all your nutritional needs, achieve good health, and prevent and reverse many chronic illnesses and diseases. Be sure to include a reliable source of vitamin B_{12}, such as a multiple-vitamin supplement or fortified foods, with your Power Plate diet.

For additional information on the vegan PCRM Power Plate, check out pcrm.org or thepowerplate.org.

The Standard American Diet: SAD

The United States leads the world in the amount and quality of its food supply, but many people don't fully appreciate it or use it to their best health advantage. Instead of being a nation of healthy and well-nourished individuals in great physical shape, a growing number of Americans are actually overweight or obese, deficient in nutrients, and prone to disease—often all at the same time. When you list the dietary factors that increase the risks of cancer, heart disease, stroke, diabetes, gastrointestinal and digestive disorders, and other chronic and degenerative diseases, the standard American diet (SAD) includes them all.

Over time, the SAD has evolved from meaning nutritious homemade meals prepared with love, to nutritionally inferior meals of convenience designed to fit hectic lives and schedules. As a result, most Americans have to rely on quick fixes and fast foods for many of their daily meals, and those types of menus usually don't feature the wisest and most nutritious options.

The SAD tends to be made of overly processed foods very high in fat, calories, cholesterol, and animal-based ingredients. At the same time, they're also low in crucial dietary fiber, complex carbohydrates, and sources of vitamin and nutrient-rich fruits and vegetables. Often, a slice of tomato or lettuce leaf are the only fresh vegetables some people get in their fast-food diet, and even then, the vegetables are usually buried under a fried all-beef patty, gobs of cheese, and oil-laden sauces. It's not easy for the body to find nutrients hidden in all the fat and empty calories.

In 1990, chances of getting cancer were 1 in 33; today, it's estimated that 1 in 2 men and 1 in 3 women in the United States will develop cancer during their lifetime. The American Heart Association claims that 82 million Americans suffer from one or more forms of cardiovascular disease, including arteriosclerosis, strokes, and high blood pressure.

VEGAN VOICES

There are 4,000 heart attacks every single day in this country. The traditional four food groups and the eating patterns they prescribed have led to cancer and heart disease in epidemic numbers, and have killed more people than any other factor in America. More than automobile accidents, more than tobacco, more than all the wars of this century combined.

—Neal Barnard, MD, *Food for Life*

Furthermore, according to the U.S. Census Bureau's Statistical Abstract (2009) on the American diet, the average consumption of major food commodities per person, per year, included the following:

607 pounds dairy products

135 pounds wheat

106 pounds red meat

79 pounds fats and oils

63 pounds sugar

24 pounds ice cream and other frozen dairy products

23 gallons coffee

In the course of the past 50 years or so, American mealtime went from elaborate homemade spreads that included tossed green salads, entrées accompanied by two or more side dishes, freshly baked bread, and even a dessert, to the total epicurean opposite of so-called "fun meals" and meals in a box. One major contributing factor is a little thing called advertising, which shapes minds and targets all ages with whatever message the major food manufacturers or fast-food restaurants want to spread. Many people give in to these messages, buy their products, learn to love them and feel they need them, and don't see the harmful dietary drawbacks.

To truly see if products or foods are good for you and provide actual sound nutrition often requires taking a step back, analyzing products, and reading labels. Often, fast-food businesses don't have the nutritional information available for you to easily access, and food companies use slick advertising and double-talk to mislead you about the nutritional content of their products. Using common sense when making food choices for yourself and your family helps guide you through the quagmire of advertising mumbo jumbo.

A Look at Other Cultural Diets

Cultures that eat the reverse of the standard American diet—diets that are low in fat, high in complex carbohydrates and fiber, and more plant based—have lower incidences of cancer and coronary artery disease (CAD). What's even sadder is that countries whose populations can afford to eat the healthiest, disease-preventing foods often don't. The United States has spent more money on cancer research than any country in the world, yet the American diet contributes to the very diseases money is being spent to prevent.

Cultures that have adopted a more Westernized way of eating have all experienced elevations of many forms of chronic and degenerative diseases. Many countries are becoming aware of the connection between diet and disease. Thankfully, they're trying to establish healthier dietary guidelines to help turn around the health of their people before it's too late and epidemics take hold.

Many of the cultures that have the longest and oldest-recorded histories have traditional diets based on plant-based foods. Three significant geographical regions—Asia, Latin America, and the Mediterranean—are the focus of our discussion because a diverse world population enjoys their way of eating. The nutrient composition of the traditional rural Asian diet is very similar to both the Latin American and Mediterranean diets in that they're largely plant based and meat is consumed less frequently and in only very small amounts.

In these three traditional diets, fruits and vegetables are, for the most part, locally grown or gathered, seasonally fresh, and often consumed minimally processed or even raw. They also have heavily starch-based diets that feature beans, nuts, potatoes, rice, corn, wheat, and other grains that are all also locally cultivated, thus preserving more of their nutrients.

These cultures also avoid or limit their use of dairy-based products, yet they don't have the calcium deficiencies or problems with osteoporosis plaguing the United States. Those who follow their more traditional diets also experience better overall health and maintain proper body weights. When they adopt a more SAD way of eating, their health, figure, and well-being often go right up in a puff of smoke with their charbroiled burger.

IN A NUTSHELL

According to Dr. T. Colin Campbell, people eating plant-based and dairy-free Asian diets experience low rates of osteoporosis. Western nations that get most of their calcium from dairy products have much higher rates of osteoporosis.

The Vegan Diet Vantage

Overall, vegans have the best diet of all—full of vitamins, minerals, and essential amino acids—and they can easily fulfill all their dietary requirements. Eating plenty of fruits, vegetables, and grains from every color in the rainbow provides you with many phytochemical-rich foods and gives your body an arsenal of beneficial nutrients it needs for good health and to prevent and treat disease.

Most plant life contains many different phytochemicals that work in symbiotic relationships within foods. Cooking increases the availability of some phytochemicals, while it diminishes others. So be sure to enjoy both fresh, raw produce and cooked cuisine to get the most nutritional benefits you can.

A well-balanced vegan diet is generally lower in fat, cholesterol, and calories than the SAD and vegetarian diets. A diet that is lower in calories makes you more resistant to various forms of cancer, can reduce the signs of aging, and can lower your risk of developing diabetes. And by not eating an animal-based diet, you lower your risk for both high cholesterol and excess saturated fat, which can lead to many health woes from obesity to heart disease.

The key to it all is your body's ability to digest foods properly: how many vitamins and minerals you are able to utilize for various body parts and functions; how much energy you receive from carbohydrates, proteins, sugars, starches, and fats; and whether you burn them immediately or they go into reserves or fat storages.

Meeting Your Vegan Nutritional Needs

In the last few decades, research and modern medicine have acknowledged the nutritional soundness and advantages of a completely plant-based diet. Time and time again, the evidence has shown that a well-balanced vegan diet positively sustains people of all ages and backgrounds and greatly reduces risks of the major diseases plaguing our global village. Also, it has been shown that those who suffer from malnutrition, obesity, and disease can use a vegan diet to reverse, prevent, and reduce suffering associated with those ailments. In fact, both the American Dietetic Association and Dietitians of Canada take the position that appropriately planned vegan diets are healthful and nutritionally adequate and provide health benefits in the prevention and treatment of certain diseases.

Vegan plant-based foods can easily supply all your nutritional needs—and do it far better than animal-based foods. Start by eating a wide variety of foods from each of the vegan New Four Food Groups, as food sources are always the best choices for top-notch nutrition. However, most of us—vegans as well as those following the SAD—need to keep an eye on our intake of vitamins B_{12} and D. The easiest way to cover your bases with these two vitamins is by eating fortified foods or taking a multiple-vitamin supplement (see Chapter 10 for further information on supplements). You should also keep your consumption of sweets, fats, and overly refined foods to a minimum. They're usually just empty calories with no real nutrient value. These types of foods will fill you up but won't provide the sustained energy you need.

Physical activity and exercise are as important to your quality of health and body frame as proper diet, so you need the right fuel to keep you energized and moving as you should be. Also, get plenty of fresh air and sunshine, and stay properly hydrated as well. You should drink about $\frac{1}{2}$ gallon filtered water and other liquids per day.

IN A NUTSHELL

Limit your consumption of alcohol and caffeine products such as coffee, soda, and black tea to occasional use only. Instead, drink water and other liquids such as fruit or vegetable juices and green and herbal teas to help flush your system; keep you hydrated; and provide you with phytochemicals, vitamins, and minerals.

Fantastic Fruits and Veggies

As previously mentioned, eating a daily abundance of fruits and veggies provides plenty of the good stuff your body needs. All fruits and vegetables contain antioxidants, and generally, the more vivid the color a fruit or veggie is, the more phytochemicals it contains. To ensure you get as many beneficial antioxidants and phytochemicals as possible, try to eat a wide variety of foods from every color of the rainbow: reds, yellows, oranges, greens, blues, and purples.

The USDA's 2010 Dietary Guidelines for Americans recommends you consume about 3 cups vegetables per day. It breaks up the vegetable group into five subgroups and recommends you include the following in your diet each week:

> 2 cups dark-green or leafy vegetables
>
> 6 cups red- and orange-colored vegetables
>
> 2 cups beans and peas
>
> 6 cups starches
>
> 5 cups other vegetables

Vegans can easily meet those numbers because those types of veggies make up the majority of most well-rounded vegan diets.

Fruits are like nature's desserts and are excellent sources of natural sugar to satisfy the cravings of those of you with a sweet tooth. Reach for a piece of fruit instead of that next piece of candy; you'll get antioxidants, vitamins, minerals, and fiber instead of empty calories and mood swings after your blood sugar spikes and crashes from processing all the refined sugar.

Amazing Grains

There's nothing like a little grain to fill out your meals and satisfy your appetite. Whole-grain foods like barley, brown rice, amaranth, quinoa, bulgur, corn, millet, triticale, buckwheat groats, oats, and wheat are all smart choices for your body. They provide protein, carbohydrates, fiber, and an endless supply of energy with their slow burn.

You also receive a good deal of vital vitamins and minerals from whole grains, in addition to *lignans* and other phytoestrogens and antioxidants. These and other disease-preventing nutrients cannot be found in supplements and can only be found in actual food sources.

> **DEFINITION**
>
> **Lignans** are a variety of phytoestrogen, similar to isoflavones, that help regulate estrogen production in the human body. Lignans have been shown to have cancer-fighting properties that can help inhibit or prevent the growth of breast, colon, and prostate cancers.

A Well-Balanced Vegan Diet

Eating healthily as a vegan is actually pretty simple. Just approach it with a little common sense, and apply what you know about proper nutrition to your everyday food choices. If you focus on consuming a good variety of fruits, vegetables, and whole grains, along with legumes, nuts, or seeds throughout the day, you'll have no problem meeting or exceeding the recommended serving amounts, even without giving too much thought about serving sizes or quantities. As they say, variety is the spice of life, and it gets pretty boring eating the same foods day in and day out, so be sure to keep things interesting for your taste buds by eating a smorgasbord of delicious plant-based foods.

It's best to begin by basing your daily diet on a wide variety of fruits and vegetable food sources first, especially fresh veggies, which have more of their live enzymes intact. In a pinch, frozen and canned sources work, too. Also, strive to make whole grains, breads, and pastas a part of most of your meals. Grains and starches are nutrient-dense foods that provide slow-burning fuel for sustained energy. Consume whole grains and stone-ground grains instead of white, polished, or nutrient-stripped versions.

HOT POTATO

When whole grains are processed or refined, much of their nutrients are stripped away, and only a few of them are added back in during any subsequent fortification. As refined carbohydrates, they rapidly release sugars into your system, which raises your insulin and triglyceride levels and negatively impacts your health. Consume these refined and processed foods as secondary grain group selections or as only occasional food choices.

Fulfill your remaining calorie and nutrient requirements each day with protein-based food sources like beans and soy products, leafy greens, and other veggies. Many of these same foods also contain significant amounts of calcium, and vegans can easily fulfill their RDA for calcium by eating plenty of these options in addition to other calcium-rich foods (see Chapter 6 for a refresher).

Not only is eating a balanced vegan diet a wonderfully healthful and nutritionally complete way to eat, but it's also a good way to drop a few excess pounds. As you know, veggies are low in calories and high in fiber, and humble whole grains such as rice and quinoa are also low in calories and fat; high in fiber, calcium, and protein; and contain lots of other good stuff your body needs. Eating lots of whole grains and veggies can help make you feel full faster, which means you consume less food and maybe drop a few pounds, if that's what you're aiming to do. And think how healthy you'll become in the process!

Daily caloric requirements do differ from person to person and depend on various factors, but the average American takes in about 2,200 calories per day. If you want to lose some significant weight, you can start by making wise food choices and reducing your intake of processed foods and fats by limiting or eliminating fried or other fatty foods. Be sure, however, to include regular sources of good fats, such as the beneficial omega-3 and -6 essential fatty acids, which are found in some vegetable oils like safflower, sunflower, hemp, flax, and soybean as well as in seeds and nuts like pumpkin, hemp, chia, sesame, and walnuts.

The Least You Need to Know

- Following proper dietary guidelines can be a useful tool in being sure your diet isn't lacking in essential nutritional elements.

- Regularly partaking in a wide variety of foods from each of the vegan New Four Food Groups ensures that you meet all your nutritional needs.

- The standard American diet lacks many healthful components that are found in a vegan plant-based diet.

- Keep your consumption of sweets, fats, and refined foods to a minimum, and eat as many fruits, veggies, whole grains, and legumes as you like!

Seeking Supplementation

In This Chapter

- Food-supplied vitamins and minerals
- Keeping an eye on key nutrients
- Monitoring your need for supplements
- A look at the vitamin B_{12} issue
- Finding sources for vegan supplements

If you eat a well-balanced vegan diet, you should have no problems getting the vitamins, minerals, and other vital nutrients your body needs to be healthy and happy. Getting all those good things straight from food sources is the most beneficial way to get them, but at times you might want to take a supplement of one sort or another, be it a basic daily multivitamin or something more specialized, just to play it safe.

In this chapter, we look at some of the issues surrounding supplementation you should know about as you embark on your voyage into veganism.

Mining for Nutrients

Phytochemicals, which are found only in plant foods, help treat and prevent many health disorders, including cancer. When seeking beneficial sources of nutrients in your diet, look first to foods as the primary sources. Supplements should be used only in addition to, and not in place of, proper nutrition and a nutrient-rich diet. Many people rely too heavily on multivitamins and should really go straight to the food sources to get the best nutrients.

Vegan diets are abundant in vitamins, which are found in all the vegan food groups. Fruits and vegetables have vitamins A and C. Grains, veggies, legumes, and sea vegetables contain B vitamins. You can easily obtain vitamin D by spending a few minutes in the sunshine, but you can also get it from some herbs and fruits. Vitamins E, F, H, and K—yes, there are more letters in the vitamin alphabet than you may have known about—are found in many fruits, vegetables, grains, nuts, seeds, and plant-based oils.

Minerals abound in nearly all plant-based foods. Calcium, copper, chromium, iron, magnesium, potassium, *selenium*, iodine, and zinc appear in all colored vegetables, leafy green vegetables, grains, mushrooms, legumes, soy foods, nutritional yeast, and sea vegetables. Many fruit juices, breads, grains, and soy-based products are also fortified with various vitamins and minerals these days.

DEFINITION

Selenium is a rare mineral, closely related to sulfur, with a distinctive red-gray metallic appearance. It's an essential trace element that helps stimulate metabolism and protect against the oxidizing effects of free radicals. These days, most supplemental selenium is produced and obtained as a by-product of the copper refining process.

Many plant-based foods overlap in food group membership and contain multiple nutritional benefits. For instance, beans, grains, and greens are each full of protein, carbohydrates, calcium, B vitamins, and many other key nutrients your body puts to great use for many different functions. Nature does some amazing things, and combining many different types of nutritional benefits into a single food source is on that list. Consuming these types of foods as often as possible gives you a leg up on your quest for good health.

There's no reason your vegan diet shouldn't provide you with all your vitamin and mineral needs, as long as you try to keep it varied on a daily and weekly basis. And that's really the best way to approach your dietary needs, on a weekly basis, as it fits most people's lifestyles and gives you the opportunity to do a little home cookin'.

Think Outside the Bottle

Other animals don't need to take pills to meet their nutritional needs, and when we eat an optimal diet rich in all the good stuff we need, neither do we. The importance of eating a well-balanced diet simply can't be stressed enough, whether you're vegan or not. You only get one body, and although it will certainly go through many changes over time, it is strictly one per customer. You owe it to yourself to take the best care of your body, inside and out, you possibly can. Putting in good foods keeps you up and running at optimum capacity.

To satisfy your nutritional needs, it's best to start with natural and whole forms of foods. A vegan diet is rich in vital nutrients. In fact, a vegan diet contains higher amounts of vitamins A, C, E, and B, especially folate and biotin, and also copper, iron, magnesium, manganese, and potassium than most omnivorous and many vegetarian diets.

Specific nutritional needs can vary from person to person, however, and also from day to day, depending on how you feed yourself throughout the course of any given day. So if you think you'll fall short of fulfilling any of your daily requirements from food sources alone, you may want to think about taking a supplement like a multivitamin or a specific nutrient.

Keep in mind, though, that a healthy and fit body doesn't come from a bottle, at least not for the long haul. Don't be fooled by advertisers or so-called health experts who try to convince you to pop pills to achieve good health. Instead, take matters into your own hands nutritionally by making proper food choices. If you want health and vitality, you have to go for it and continue to work at it. Invest in your future by filling up your plate, not your medicine cabinet.

Foods: Your First and Best Sources

What should be your first line of defense in protecting your body and safeguarding your health against imbalances and ill health? Good clean living, as they say, with plenty of fresh air, clean water, and sunshine, vitalizes your spirit and body. Physical activity and exercise are necessary to keep your body moving and running properly, so don't skip out on it. Then be sure to nourish yourself properly and adequately. Begin by eating right in the first place and then turn to supplements as a backup.

IN A NUTSHELL

Often your body tells you what it needs if you learn to listen to it. If you get cravings for specific vegan foods, go with the cravings (within reason, of course).

Be sure to eat plenty of fruits and veggies every day, as well as a couple servings of whole grains as either breads, starches, or as part of your meal selections. Try to eat green leafy salads or obvious protein-rich foods like soy or other legumes to be sure you cover your calcium, iron, and protein needs.

Eating fruits and vegetables provides you with an array of phytochemicals. In fact, you get hundreds of them in a simple carrot—hundreds of different compounds, all arranged in a nice, neat sequence, just as nature intended, and usually in the correct form for another part of nature (your body) to utilize to its fullest potential. Certain compounds or substances seem to be present together because they work better that way, even if we don't always see the connection or correlation. That's why it's best to consume actual foods to try to obtain as many phytochemicals as you can, if solely for the antioxidant benefits alone.

Medical science has figured out how to isolate and identify certain vitamins, minerals, and nutrients, but it doesn't understand everything that's a part of our natural world yet. So it doesn't hurt to give yourself a little insurance and cover your bases in both areas. Eat right as often as you can and take a multivitamin, and any other supplements, sensibly and as you see fit, as a way of safeguarding your good health and ensuring the best life possible.

Key Nutrients to Watch

Nutrient deficiencies not only occur in third-world countries where there isn't enough food to eat, but also in the United States, where many follow a standard American diet (see Chapter 9). Many Americans live on a diet full of empty calories, fat, sugar, sodium, and cholesterol and get very little needed beneficial nutrients.

What key nutrients should you be concerned with? You know fruits and veggies contain tons of vitamins and minerals. You get essential amino acids and fatty acids from leafy green plants, legumes, nuts, and seeds. Then there's protein and calcium, which hopefully are no longer of concern to you now that you know good vegan food sources of both, like green leafy vegetables and beans.

But did you know that these same types of foods provide you with iron, zinc, and selenium as well? Even so, why do you need to be concerned about these nutrients?

Ironing Out Your Iron

You need to get plenty of iron for your blood. The level of iron in your blood plays an important function in the amount of oxygen that's fed to your cells, as well as the carbon dioxide that's released and eliminated from your body.

Iron is an essential part of hemoglobin, the oxygen-carrying component of your blood. A "precious" metal, iron is found in two forms: *heme iron*, which comes from animal-based sources, and *nonheme iron*, which comes from both plant- and animal-based sources. Athletes, pregnant and menstruating women, and children need to be the most concerned about the amount of iron in their diets and be sure to have iron-rich blood.

From nation to nation, across all corners of the globe, iron deficiencies are a major nutritional concern. How do iron deficiencies occur? The main causes are quite obvious:

- Blood loss from heavy menstruation or hemorrhaging
- Growth spurts, in the case of infants, children, and even pregnant women
- Strenuous exercising and excessive sweating, of concern to athletes
- Inadequate dietary intake

An iron deficiency that goes unchecked often results in iron deficiency anemia. You have little control over the other factors that effect iron, but you certainly can have control over your own diet, which you can directly and quickly impact.

HOT POTATO

Cooking your food in a cast-iron skillet supplies your body with some additional iron because your food absorbs some iron from the pan during the cooking process. Beware, though, because the same can be said of aluminum and aluminum cookware. Ingestion of aluminum has been linked to Alzheimer's disease, so avoid cooking in aluminum.

Vitamin C affects your absorption of iron. Eating vitamin C–rich foods with iron-rich foods increases your absorbability of iron several times over. So add a little colored pepper or orange, or have a little citrus vinaigrette on your next leafy green salad to increase the amount of iron your body receives.

Getting Your Zinc in Sync (Selenium, Too)

Your body and immune system need adequate levels of zinc and selenium to keep you on your toes and fighting off disease and infections. A few Brazil nuts, each containing around 70 micrograms selenium, can easily supply your daily needs.

Getting your zinc balance right can be a bit tricky. Getting daily doses less than 100 milligrams can enhance or boost your immune system, while doses more than 100 milligrams often depresses your immune system. Add to that the fact that phylates, a form of phosphorus found in whole grains and legumes, bind with zinc, which interferes with its absorption. The amount of calcium in your diet can affect your body's ability to absorb zinc, too. Supplements with high levels of calcium, iron, and copper can also interfere with zinc absorption and balance in your body.

But the culinary techniques you employ can help you increase the *bioavailability* of zinc. You can soak beans, grains, nuts, and seeds prior to cooking them or sprouting them for your own homemade sprouts, in addition to consuming fermented foods like tempeh or sauerkraut, to help increase your absorbability of zinc. Remember that the next time you're munching on a vegan tempeh Reuben sandwich!

DEFINITION

Bioavailability is the proportionate amount or level of a certain nutrient contained within a specific food that's actually used or utilized by your body.

Is B_{12} an Issue?

One vitamin seems to come into question time and time again for vegans and vegetarians, and that's vitamin B_{12}. Your body needs it in very small amounts for healthy blood cells and proper nerve functioning.

Vitamin B_{12} is actually made by bacteria and other microorganisms in nature. The bacteria attach themselves to a host and work their way into its system. B_{12} is not naturally produced by plants or animals directly, but plants and animals often find themselves as its hosts.

It's a good thing the human body can amply store vitamin B_{12}. You can store up to a 3- to 5-year supply in your liver, and the recommended daily allowance (RDA) for adults is a mere 2.4 micrograms per day. Keeping this in mind, you generally only need to worry about your intake of B_{12} on a weekly, rather than daily, basis.

B₁₂ Origins

Vitamin B$_{12}$ is prevalent in nature in the soil, which is how we once got all we needed naturally: by eating foods fresh from the soil with a little bit of dirt still on them and then perhaps licking our fingers clean. And before toothbrushes, dentists, and modern personal hygiene became a part of our daily lives, the B$_{12}$ bacteria would get stuck between our teeth and grow, as our mouths were warm and welcoming hosts.

Vitamin B$_{12}$ is present in many meat products, but how did the animals get it in the first place? Most of the animals that end up on American dinner plates consume a (mostly) plant-based diet themselves. When they graze on grasses or ingest traces of soil, manure, or other contaminants, the beneficial B$_{12}$ bacteria gets in their systems. The animals' livers then process the bacteria to absorb the vitamin B$_{12}$.

Much of the traces of B$_{12}$ found in meat products come from the gastrointestinal tracts of the animals and not exactly from within the cut of filet mignon itself. Without going into all the gory details, the slaughtering process is what really helps disperse the B$_{12}$ onto the meat. Fortunately for vegans, there are many better ways to get vitamin B$_{12}$!

Plant-Based Food Sources

Plant-based foods are far better sources of B$_{12}$, as they contain zero cholesterol and are lower in fat than animal-based sources. Because vitamin B$_{12}$ is from bacteria in the soil, you can easily get a reliable source from your own freshly and organically grown foods. Simply wipe off or give your foods a gentle rinsing in water, if needed, and you'll reap the benefits of clinging B$_{12}$. Eating foods in their raw state also preserves more of the naturally occurring B$_{12}$.

IN A NUTSHELL

Dr. Frey Ellis and Dr. T. A. B. Sanders, both British hematologists and natural hygiene pioneers, along with Dr. E. Lester Smith, the discoverer of vitamin B$_{12}$, showed in their studies in the 1960s that vegans have generous levels of vitamin B$_{12}$, even without supplementation.

But you don't need to rely on dirt particles alone for your B$_{12}$. Vitamin B$_{12}$ is fortified into so many vegan-friendly foods, including orange juice, grains, breads, nutritional yeast, cereals, sea vegetables, and many other soy-based products. A cup of fortified soy milk or orange juice can contain between 1 and 2 micrograms B_{12}—well meeting your daily needs. With an adequately planned, well-balanced vegan diet, you shouldn't have to worry about being deficient in B_{12}.

Stock up on these food sources of B_{12}:

- Fortified fruit juices

- Fortified soy milk and soy-based products

- Fermented soy-based products such as tempeh, miso, shoyu, and tamari

- Enriched grains, cereals, and starch-based products

- Nutritional yeast (1 tablespoon nutritional yeast supplies 4 micrograms— more than you need)

Just because it's easy to get enough vitamin B_{12} while being vegan, don't get careless about it. Deficiencies in vitamin B_{12} can cause serious problems, including increased risk of stroke, heart disease, and Alzheimer's. Stay on your toes, and be sure to regularly include good sources of B_{12} in your diet!

Supplemental Sources of B_{12}

There's much talk about how the processing of foods affects their B_{12} levels. As a result, some people feel you shouldn't count on foods as reliable sources, but that goes against the law and logic of nature. Foods are always the best way to feed your body and should be the first option you choose to achieve good health.

But there's nothing wrong with having a little insurance now and again, which is why supplements come in so handy. Including some sort of B_{12} supplement certainly won't hurt, and you only need to think about it a couple times a week. Follow the manufacturer's suggestion for dosage; most supplements come in 500 to 1,000 microgram doses, which makes it easy to meet your needs.

Vitamin B_{12} is naturally made of the mineral cobalt and nitrogen amines and is also commonly referred to as cobalamin. But on most fortified foods and supplements, you will see the words *methylcobalamin* or *cyanocobalamin*, which are the synthetic forms of B_{12}. When choosing supplementation, look for sublingual (absorbed beneath the tongue) form, which is the quickest and best-absorbed form. You can also purchase B_{12} tablets, but carefully check the ingredients when purchasing B_{12} supplements in pill form, as many supplements (particularly lower-quality brands) tend to have a nonvegan gelatin base.

Red Star vegetarian formula nutritional yeast is the most widely available form of nutritional yeast in the United States, and it's a deliciously convenient vegan source of vitamin B_{12}. A natural bacterial fermentation process not involving any animal products produces the B_{12} used in this nutritional yeast, and a supplemented B_{12} is added as well for good measure. Nutritional yeast also contains amino acids, important minerals, and folic acid.

Do You Need to Take Supplements?

Read labels to be sure you're receiving the proper dosages of nutrients and not falling under or over recommended dosages. Sometimes more is not better, especially when it comes to taking supplements. Taking too much of some nutrients can actually cause you harm and even do irreversible damage.

Taking excessive amounts of iron and vitamins A, B_6, D, and E can be toxic, so keep this in mind when choosing a multivitamin. You should choose the one that best suits your needs … but how do you know which one to pick? First, analyze your diet. You know it's important to eat well, but do you actually do it? How well you eat determines whether you need a multivitamin with megadoses of nutrients, or one with levels that provide you with part or all 100 percent of your RDAs for certain nutrients.

If your diet is generally full of lots of servings of fruits, veggies, and grains on a daily basis, maybe you only need a multivitamin with the basics—vitamins A, B, C, D, E, and so on—with levels that are below or bring you up to 100 percent of your RDAs. With an adequate diet, you also receive many nutrients, and you don't want to put your levels over the top or at a point where they actually start doing you harm instead of good.

If, on the other hand, you tend to not eat as well as you should more often than you would like to admit, think about taking a supplement with slightly higher doses. But remember, it isn't wise to rely on supplements as your main sources of needed nutrients, so you really should be getting your eating habits in order. You owe it to yourself!

There will be times when you may want to take a specialized or single nutrient–type supplement. For instance, if you're feeling a little sluggish, you may not be getting enough B vitamins. They are the real movers and shakers in your body, fueling many functions and adding luster to your hair, skin, and nails. During times of stress, your body can require even more B vitamins. If this applies to you, you may want to take a B vitamin complex supplement every once in awhile or at those times when you feel you're especially in need of them. You'll definitely feel a boost in your energy levels.

Most are familiar with taking a little extra vitamin C to build up your immune system and fight off colds. But be careful: taking too much vitamin C at one time can cause stomach upset, especially when taken on an empty stomach. If this is the case for you, look for "buffered vitamin C." It should be gentler on your system.

> **HOT POTATO**
>
> Excessive amounts of vitamin C can have a laxative effect. Some people even intentionally use vitamin C, in doses of 5,000 milligrams per day and more, as a natural laxative on an occasional basis to aid in regularity or to relieve constipation.

In recent years, it's come to be known that taking a little extra vitamins C and E can actually help reduce the signs of aging and fight off many chronic diseases and cancer. Especially significant are their effects on preventing and treating skin cancer. Topical applications have had some amazing results for basal cell carcinoma victims. As it turns out, vitamin C is toxic to melanoma and causes it to dry out, leading to scabbing and eventually scarring over.

One of the best and most inexpensive forms of supplemented vitamin C is the crystalline form of ascorbic acid, available at natural foods stores. A mere ¼ teaspoon mixed into a glass of water provides 1 gram (1,000 milligrams) pure vitamin C, and you don't have to worry about the fillers that accompany vitamin C in its pill form, whether you're a vegan or not.

Finding Vegan-Friendly Supplements

As a vegan, taking a supplement isn't as simple as running down to the corner drugstore. For one thing, *gelatin*—that gelling agent often used to make the outer coating of many supplements—is derived from animals. If you see the words *gel cap*, you'll have to do a bit of investigating to see if it's a gelatin- or veggie-based gel.

> **DEFINITION**
>
> **Gelatin** (or gelatine) is a gelling agent made from boiling the connective tissues and skins of animals. It's used in the manufacturing of many products, including foods, beverages, beauty products, pills, and even photographic film.

Some brands do say "vegi-cap" or "suitable for vegans or vegetarians" on their packaging if the gelling agent used is from plant sources. If it doesn't say what the capsule is made of, it's best to assume it's made of gelatin and avoid it, just to be on the safe side. If you have an option of buying the supplement in different pill forms, avoid capsules and look for tablets instead because they're usually gelatin free.

Also beware of supplements containing vitamin D_3. In pill form, most vitamin D_3 is derived from animal sources, so if you see vitamin D_3 among the vitamins listed on your multivitamin, perhaps as cholecalciferol, it probably isn't vegan. Recently, however, a few companies have started selling 100 percent plant-based D_3. Instead, look for a vitamin D_2 (ergocalciferaol) supplement, which is vegan, or simply be out in the sun for 15 minutes or less to get your D requirements.

You might be able to find some brands of vegan supplements in different drugstore and retail chains. But for the most part, you may have to search the shelves of your local natural foods store when first looking for vegan supplements.

A word of caution: supplements can be expensive, but you do usually get what you pay for. Look for those derived from natural sources whenever possible; supplements produced from food sources are much better in terms of bioavailability and safety.

Some popular vegan supplement manufacturers include Deva, Freeda, Garden of Life, Nature's Life, Nature's Plus, New Chapter, Rainbow Light, Solgar, and VegLife, just to name a few. After you find vegan brands you like, you can search for other sources and do a bit of shopping around and comparing prices. The internet is a great tool for purchasing vegan supplements at a savings. Check out Appendix B for some good websites where you can begin your search.

The Least You Need to Know

- Get as many nutrients as possible directly from their food sources primarily, and use supplementation only as a backup.
- In addition to the nutrients naturally present in fruits and vegetables, many packaged food items are also fortified with additional vitamins and minerals.
- Iron, zinc, and selenium are three very important dietary minerals, so watch your levels to be sure you're getting the right amount.
- It's a good idea to take a vitamin B_{12} supplement on at least a weekly basis.
- Finding good sources of vegan supplements isn't difficult, but it requires a little thought and research beforehand. The web can be a big help.

Healthy Vegan Mothers and Kids

In This Chapter

- Having a safe vegan pregnancy
- Looking at motherly nutritional needs
- Considering breast-feeding issues
- Raising and feeding vegan children
- Getting to the truth about vaccinations

Ah, the joys of motherhood! To bring a new life into the world is a wonderful and amazing thing. The experience brings with it a wide range of emotions as both mother and child develop and grow.

As a new vegan and a new mother, you'll naturally be concerned about the physical changes your body is—and will be—going through. Be confident in knowing that a good vegan diet can easily ensure you a healthy and happy pregnancy, and you and your baby will grow and develop as you should.

Handling a Vegan Pregnancy

Being sure your nutritional needs are met is a concern all expectant mothers face, vegan or not. As a vegan, you can also expect friends, family members, and especially your own mother and mother-in-law to be concerned that your vegan diet may not be able to provide you and your growing baby with all the nutritional requirements during pregnancy.

Have no fear. A vegan diet can cover all the bases—and then some! Just arm yourself with some good information, read all you can about vegan nutrition during pregnancy (we share some good books in a bit), and apply what you learn to eating as healthily as you can during this important time. It will soon be apparent to everyone that your vegan diet is having wonderfully positive effects on both you and your growing child.

Many medical studies have backed up the positive effects of a vegan diet during pregnancy. One of the largest involved is The Farm, a vegan community in Summertown, Tennessee. In the study, researchers gathered information from more than 775 pregnancies. They discovered that a vegan diet had no impact on infant birth weights (all were normal or above); most had relatively easy labor; and only 1 in 100 women delivered their babies by cesarean section, which is only a fraction of the national average of 1 in 4. Also, in over 25 years, only one case of *preeclampsia* has been reported with the group participants.

> **DEFINITION**
>
> **Preeclampsia** is a condition involving hypertension, retention of fluids, protein loss, and excessive weight gain during pregnancy. It occurs in at least 2 percent of all pregnancies in the United States.

The women at The Farm sustain themselves and their families on an all-vegan diet, and they are living examples that it really is the optimal way for us to nourish ourselves, pregnant or not. So relax and know that if you eat a well-balanced vegan diet, you and your baby will be all the better for it.

Here's a short list of some of the great books out there for vegan mothers-to-be to help get you started:

- *Pregnancy, Children, and the Vegan Diet* by Dr. Michael Klaper (Gentle World, 1988)

- *Raising Vegetarian Children: A Guide to Good Health and Family Harmony* by Joannne Stepaniak and Vesanto Melina (McGraw-Hill, 2002)

- *The Vegetarian Mother and Baby Book* by Rose Elliot (Pantheon, 1996)

- *Vegan Pregnancy Survival Guide* by Sayward Rebhal (Herbivore Books, 2011)

If you're a vegan who eats all or mostly organic foods, you can also be confident in knowing that you and your baby will have less exposure to the antibiotics, hormones, pesticides, and other toxic chemicals commonly found in conventional produce and animal-based foods.

Mother-to-Be Nutritional Needs

When you discover you're pregnant, you need to be concerned about what you put into your body and what you expose yourself to, because the life growing inside you feels the effects secondhand. It is highly recommended that you quit smoking and stop drinking alcoholic or caffeinated beverages as soon as you discover you're pregnant because these can lead to pregnancy complications, birth defects, and health problems in newborns. Remember that everything you do or that affects you on a physical or emotional level also affects your baby. Keep this in mind when making lifestyle choices and decisions.

Now more than ever is a good time to analyze the way you eat and start making wise food choices. After all, as the saying goes, "you are eating for two." You need to be sure the foods you're eating provide you with a legitimate benefit instead of being just empty calories to satisfy one of the many cravings you might experience while pregnant.

Eat a wide variety of foods, in every color of the rainbow, to be sure you're getting all the vital phytochemicals you and your baby need. Plant foods can more than adequately meet many of your increased needs for B vitamins, calcium, iron, zinc, and protein. You need to increase your daily intake of protein and calcium because your baby is sharing in your intake as it grows and develops. Try adding additional servings of protein- and calcium-rich foods like leafy greens, whole grains, legumes, nuts, and seeds to each of your meals.

While you're pregnant and lactating, you should try to consume at least 2,500 calories per day. This shouldn't be difficult, as your appetite usually increases after morning sickness lessens and goes away completely. Increase your servings from each of the food groups, and be diligent to consume four or more servings of fruits, vegetables, and protein. More importantly, get six or more servings of whole grains and whole-grain–containing products. Such foods contain significant amounts of B vitamins, which help with proper fetus development; deficiencies can lead to birth defects.

In addition to eating right and getting some form of exercise, it's also recommended that pregnant women, vegan or otherwise, take proper supplements to be sure they're regularly meeting all their baby's needs as well as their own. As with all supplements, search out high-quality brands and be sure they have all-vegan ingredients. Remember, you get what you pay for, and you really want to do the best you can for your growing baby and give him or her all the advantages you can.

Whichever brand vegan supplement you choose, be sure it contains the following at least:

30 milligrams iron

10 to 15 milligrams zinc

500 to 600 milligrams calcium

400 to 600 micrograms folic acid (folate)

3 micrograms B_{12} (increase to 5 to 10 micrograms while breast-feeding)

10 micrograms vitamin D

Also, be sure to include in your diet adequate sources of omega-3 essential fatty acids, which are important for the development and growth of your baby's brain. Foods such as flaxseeds, pumpkin seeds, soybeans, whole grains, and green-leafy vegetables supply loads of omega-3s. Peruse the shelves of many natural foods stores and retailers, and you'll also find several good vegan brands of prenatal supplements such as Deva, Garden of Life, Rainbow Light, and Simply One.

Dietary Suggestions for Vegan Mothers

Yes, you are now eating for two, and your food intake requirement has increased, but that doesn't mean you should munch on any old thing—especially tons of junk food or fried foods full of added fats. These will put on the pounds needed to support the extra life growing inside you, but such foods do not provide the proper vitamins and minerals. You'll have less excess weight to take off after your pregnancy if you fill your plate with a lot of complex carbohydrates such as whole grains, pasta, legumes, soy-based foods, nuts, and seeds.

> **IN A NUTSHELL**
>
> Expect to gain between 20 and 35 pounds during a normal pregnancy. You may not gain a lot of weight at first, but you should expect to gain at least 1 pound per week during your second and third trimesters.

For breakfast, have a few pieces of fresh fruit or blend them into a smoothie with some leafy greens, nuts, and seeds. If you're feeling really hungry, have a bowl of oatmeal or granola with some soy milk and a little sprinkle of dried fruits, raisins, or nuts. Or perhaps try a tofu-and-veggie scramble with some hash brown potatoes and a few slices of whole-grain toast. Choosing any of these breakfast options helps start you off on the right foot and gives you enough energy and nutrition to meet your needs.

To hold you over between your meals, opt for healthy snacks for a nutritious energy boost, like some trail mix, a few carrot sticks with a glass of juice, or even some hummus with pita bread and veggies as dippers.

For lunch, you could have a taco salad made of assorted greens and veggies, as well as a bowl of soup or soy and bean–based chili topped with salsa or guacamole and a little nutritional yeast flakes. If you're hankering for a sandwich, opt for one made on whole-grain bread with some crisp raw veggies and slices of mock meat, or the beloved PB&J or other nut butter–and–fruit spread sandwich.

Your dinner should be filling but not too heavy; otherwise, it could cause heartburn and indigestion, which are already common occurrences for pregnant women. Try a nutritious and satisfying dinner of stir-fried veggies and cashews over rice, quinoa, or pasta, or maybe some marinated and baked tempeh or tofu (preferably organic and non-GMO) with sides of your favorite cooked whole grains, leafy greens, and roasted or steamed veggies.

If you get the urge for an after-dinner treat, be sure you limit your binges of high-fat and high-calorie foods. Just because some pregnant women eat tons of ice cream and pickles doesn't mean you have to. Although, here's a little food for thought: most nondairy ice creams are much lower in fat than traditional milk-based ice creams.

Bouncing Vegan Babies

If you're eating properly, there's absolutely no reason your vegan baby shouldn't be as healthy as any other young mother's child. Study after study has shown this to be true. Adequate nutrition is what's most important for good health, for both mother and baby.

How do vegan babies measure up in terms of weight and size? The birth weights and lengths of vegan babies are relatively the same as, if not slightly higher than, those born to meat-eaters. Healthy, strong vegan babies abound, while low birth weights and preterm births are on the rise in the United States and around the globe. Inadequate nutrition is most certainly to blame, but not so with the average baby born to a vegan mother!

> **IN A NUTSHELL**
>
> If an expectant mother's in tip-top physical shape, she'll have an easier time during labor. It's also been shown that well-rested mothers have an easier time during labor, fewer complications, shorter delivery times, and fewer incidences of cesarean sections. It's recommended that you get at least 8 or more hours sleep per night, especially as your due date draws nearer. Try relaxation techniques, soothing music, and massage to ease your discomforts and increase your hours of sleep.

The Logical Dr. Spock

One of the most respected pediatricians and child-rearing experts was Dr. Benjamin Spock. He was the author of *Baby and Child Care*, first published in 1946. (In December 2011, the ninth edition was released on the sixty-fifth anniversary of the original publication.) Dr. Spock's book is America's second-best-selling book after the Bible and has helped generations of parents address questions and concerns regarding pregnancy and child rearing.

Dr. Spock went vegan in the 1990s in an effort to improve his health, which it did, and he was so impressed that he began focusing his research on learning all he could about vegan nutrition. He caused quite a stir with the seventh edition of his book, issued in 1998 after his death at the age of 94. Why all the uproar? Because he advocated a vegan diet for kids!

Dr. Spock wanted to share with parents what he had learned himself while turning his own health around. He told parents that if their children were raised as vegans, they were less likely to be overweight and have fewer incidences of diabetes, heart disease, high blood pressure, and various forms of cancer. He felt compelled to share the information to help parents as he had always done throughout his illustrious career.

Breast-Feeding Benefits

Nature has provided mammals with the most convenient and wholesome means to adequately feed their babies: breast milk. It is the perfect food, full of the proteins, carbohydrates, and fats your baby needs to develop properly during the first stages of life.

During the first several weeks after giving birth, your breast milk is rich in colostrum, which contains immune-boosting antibodies that help reduce your child's risks of allergies and illnesses. Your milk adjusts to your baby's needs over time, as well as your own.

Because you share all your nutritional intake with your baby while breast-feeding, eating a vitamin-rich diet during this time is very important. Your body divides and sorts the nutrients from everything you consume and passes a portion of them along to your baby via your breast milk.

Sometimes, breast-feeding doesn't come easy at first or seems unnatural to new mothers. It takes a bit of practice to get things right. Correct angles for nursing, irritation, and supply-and-demand issues can cause concern and frustration. But keep at it and be patient. It's certainly well worth the effort in terms of the health benefits to your child.

Breast-feeding also helps you develop a bond with your child. Your baby begins to recognize you by the touch, smell, and sound of your breathing and voice. This bonding process is vital to helping you address needs, concerns, and problems throughout your baby's growth and development.

It's suggested that you exclusively breast-feed your baby up to at least 6 months of age. Experts generally recommend breast-feeding for the first 1 or 2 years of a child's life, but you and your child should know when the time is right. Check with your doctor for additional guidance as needed.

Fulfilling Your Baby's Nutritional Needs

When breast-feeding, the best way to be sure all your baby's nutritional bases are being covered is to concentrate on your own diet. Ultimately, what you eat and drink makes up your baby's diet as well, and in a more concentrated form. Be sure to eat well-balanced meals on a regular basis, as well as a few healthy snacks throughout the day, to not only keep you energized but to also boost the nutritional levels of your breast milk. Avoid empty calories and excessive amounts of fats and sugars. These will cause fluctuations in your blood sugar levels, energy levels, and overall mood, as well as affect your baby's digestion, energy, sleep cycle, and moods. Put good things into your body, and you and your baby will get all the right things out.

IN A NUTSHELL

Breast-feeding your baby in direct sunlight for 15 minutes is a great way for both you and baby to get your daily requirements of vitamin D, in addition to making you both feel rejuvenated and revitalized by the warmth of the sun's rays.

Breast-feeding is the cheapest, most natural, and optimal way to feed your baby. Unfortunately for some new mothers, it's not always an option. Some mothers may have low milk production levels or medical issues, or they may not want to breast-feed. If this is the case, you can feed your baby a fortified infant formula (not just a plant-based milk) for up to the first 2 years of age. Finding a 100 percent vegan fortified infant formula can be next to impossible because most are made with supplemented vitamin D_3 derived from animal sources such as lanolin. So compare brands to find the best fortified vegetarian formula you can, made with organic ingredients, including added vitamins and minerals like vitamin B_{12}, vitamin D, DHA, iron, zinc, calcium, and others.

The right time to begin adding supplemental foods to your child's diet depends on his or her rate of development, so check with your pediatrician before making any changes. Generally, when your baby is between 4 to 6 months old, you can introduce supplemental (non-breast-milk or formula) foods such as creamy cereals, fruits, and veggies into his or her diet. Creamy rice cereals, fortified with iron, are often among the first soft foods given. Later, you can add other cooked and blended grains, like oats, quinoa, or barley to the repertoire, followed by mashed or puréed fruit and veggies and good sources of protein such as beans and creamy tofu.

Some organic vegan baby foods can help fill the gap when you aren't able to cook something yourself. Just take a look around and read some labels!

Raising Vegan Children

As a vegan parent, you may come under fire for choosing to raise your child vegan. Those who are under the impression that vegans are sickly and malnourished will be doubly concerned about the safety of your child, and they may say rude things or act inappropriately toward you. Many misconceptions about vegans abound, as you might well already know, so it's best to try to patiently and honestly address their concerns.

As you raise your child, teach her about eating properly and nutritionally as a vegan, in addition to explaining why you don't "eat like everyone else." Be honest with your child, and try to explain things in ways she can understand at her particular age. Your conversations and explanations will evolve and develop as your child grows older and understands more about life.

Also, keep in mind that your talks will also provide your child with the means to handle questions from her friends, her friends' well-intentioned parents, and other adults such as teachers and family members. If you explain to your child why a certain food is beneficial when you're serving it, she'll absorb the information and often pass along the information to others. A child's mind is amazingly quick and absorbs information from outside sources with little effort. Without even knowing it, you may be raising a young vegan advocate who is armed with tons of great knowledge!

Healthy and Nutritious Vegan Diets

From the time you start to include supplemental foods or wean your child off breast milk or formula, you have to be concerned about what goes into her mouth and not just what goes into yours anymore. Just feed her like you do yourself, only in much smaller quantities.

Health experts agree that a varied, well-rounded diet that's free of meat, dairy, and eggs is the healthiest way for children—as well as adults—to eat. A vegan diet is more than adequate for children, and actually, it's far superior in terms of vitamin, mineral, and antioxidant content to the standard American diet (SAD), especially to those containing lots of animal products.

HOT POTATO

Most children who follow the SAD get excessive amounts of saturated fats, salt, and sugar. Compound that with the fact that they get inadequate amounts of whole grains and fresh fruits and vegetables, and it's not surprising that juvenile diabetes and obesity are on the rise.

On average, vegan children eat more healthily than most of their nonvegan friends. After age 2, the standard American child's diet consists mainly of highly processed foods like hot dogs, pepperoni pizza, grilled cheese sandwiches, fried chicken and nuggets, hamburgers, and french fries. Some children actually consume these foods at several meals throughout the day.

In contrast, a vegan child consumes several sources of fruits and vegetables, lean sources of protein, and complex carbohydrates from grains in his daily meals. And if these foods also contain organic ingredients, the child will be exposed to fewer genetically modified foods, pesticide and chemical fertilizer residue, and none of the growth hormones and antibiotics contained in animal-based products.

Dietary Suggestions for Youngsters

As a parent, be very conscious of what your child is eating. Start her off with a good breakfast, and sustain her with a nutritious lunch and filling dinner. Have healthy snacks such as fresh fruits, raw vegetables, nuts, dried fruits, and whole-grain granola bars and cereals around for her to munch on. Feeding her healthful foods teaches her good eating habits, which will serve her well throughout her life.

Children are basically little versions of the grown-ups they'll one day become. Their nutritional needs and nutrient concerns are the same as adults, just on a smaller scale. Throughout the day, they need to consume several servings of complex carbohydrates in the form of whole-grain breads, pasta, rice, or cereals, in addition to good sources of calcium, vitamin-rich fruits and vegetables, and protein-dense foods.

IN A NUTSHELL

When feeding children, remember: their little stomachs get full quickly, so it's best to give them foods that have multiple nutritional benefits such as leafy greens, beans, nut butters, cruciferous vegetables, citrus, and whole grains.

As children grow and start to exercise their independence, their tastes in activities, clothes, and foods will most likely change. Once-healthy eaters often become picky eaters. Foods they once loved and eagerly ate may become unappealing, unappetizing, and plain old icky to them. It's best not to fight them. It will only fuel the problem and may lead to others.

Instead, ask your child what foods *she* would like to eat. This will make her feel that she has more control over her food choices and what she's eating. After you know what her current favorite foods are, you can then bargain with her to fill out the rest of her nutritional needs.

For instance, if your daughter is currently into eating peanut butter, encourage it. Just try to get her to pair it with a healthful jelly or fruit spread on whole-grain bread, and she'll get a serving of fruit, protein, and, depending on the size, one or two servings of whole grains. Or if she smears it on celery sticks, she'll get a serving of vegetables and protein. The servings and sources can add up quickly, and even though it may not be a varied diet for the time being, it can meet many of her nutritional needs with a little coaching and coaxing.

As with vegan adults, it doesn't hurt to give your child a supplement. That supplement doesn't have to be a mega-multivitamin if your child is a healthy eater and eats a variety of foods. Just be sure it's a vegan supplement that contains significant amounts of calcium, iron, zinc, B vitamins (especially B_{12}), and vitamin D. Vegan children's supplements come in chewable pill forms, in liquid formulas, and recently, in candy-like shapes such as gummy bears and lollipops. Look for vegan vitamins made by Freeda, VegLife, Gummi King, Yummi Bears, YummyEarth, Rhino, and Nature's Way in your local pharmacy or natural foods store.

For additional nutritional guideline information and kid-friendly eating tips for vegan children, check out *The Complete Idiot's Guide to Vegan Eating for Kids* by Dana and Andrew Villamagna.

Vaccinations: The Issues

For the vegan parent who wants to raise a child according to vegan ideals in every way possible, vaccines are an issue that needs to be considered. Vaccines are designed to help build a child's immunity to various diseases, but a good deal of controversy surrounds their use, side effects, dangers, and efficiency. And they're not in the least bit vegan.

Vaccines are made using various animal ingredients. Most of the viruses used in vaccines are cultured on animal and human tissues, including embryos, cells, and organ tissues. Vaccines routinely contain things such as pus, urine, and serum from horses and calves—obviously none of which are consistent with a vegan lifestyle.

Vaccines also contain viruses, bacteria, and other substances intended to help bolster a child's immunity to diseases. Some vaccines even contain thimerosol, a mercury-based preservative, as well as aluminum, phenol, and formaldehyde. You're probably already aware of the many dangers of mercury, and phenol and formaldehyde are both known carcinogens. Many people are convinced that the mercury and other harmful substances in vaccines are responsible for many childhood health problems and disorders, including autism, and that the risks outweigh the potential benefits.

Many problems and complications are associated with vaccinations: pain and infection at the point of injection, respiratory problems, asthma, sudden infant death syndrome, convulsions, diabetes, autism, multiple sclerosis, meningitis, and various forms of cancer, not to mention chances of developing a toxic reaction or death as a result of the exposure to the live viruses contained within the vaccines. Often, an outbreak of an inoculated disease is traced back to the live viruses contained in the vaccines themselves. Government and medical sources have reported that up to 65 percent of all occurrences of diseases for which people are routinely vaccinated (such as measles and tetanus) occur in people who have already been vaccinated for them.

HOT POTATO

Many state laws require that a child be immunized before entering public school or that parents sign a waiver acknowledging they have refused vaccination. It's very important to remember that all 50 states have exceptions to mandatory vaccination requirements; however, the sorts of permissible exceptions (medical, philosophical, and religious) vary from state to state.

We recommend that you take some time and do your own research into the safety and efficacy of vaccines and the ingredients they contain before you decide to expose your child to them. Become an educated parent and advocate for your child by researching each and every vaccination your doctor recommends. Always ask to see the package insert that comes with the vaccine, and read the warnings on the insert. Research the issues surrounding vaccines on the internet and at your local library and then decide for yourself how to handle the vaccine issue.

The Least You Need to Know

- A vegan mother-to-be can more than adequately nourish herself and her growing baby during pregnancy; still, a supplement is recommended for peace of mind.

- Breast-feeding is the optimal way to nourish your baby, as breast milk provides everything your child needs to grow strong and healthy.

- Eating a well-rounded vegan diet—rich in whole grains, fruits, and veggies—is the healthiest way for a child to eat and is a big improvement over the standard American diet.

- Vaccines have become a controversial issue, so educate yourself by researching each and every vaccination your doctor recommends, as some contain non-vegan and potentially harmful ingredients.

Vegan Raw Foodists

In This Chapter

- Reexamining cooked foods
- Reaping the benefits of raw foods
- Maintaining beneficial live enzymes
- Juicing and dehydrating raw foods
- Growing your own sprouts

Have you ever seen a pack of lions sitting around a fire roasting their prey? Or a rabbit boiling a carrot before eating it? Humans are the only creatures to harness fire for food preparation. Cooking does make some foods more digestible and more enjoyable, and when it comes to meat, it also helps reduce the possibility of food-borne illnesses.

But is regularly subjecting our food to extremely high temperatures beneficial to our long-term health? Many people feel the answer to that question is a resounding "no," and in this chapter, we take a look at some of the issues surrounding cooked foods and some of the raw vegan alternatives.

The Cooking Crock

Sometimes keeping things simple is the best way to approach life. We humans can really make eating too complicated, compared to our fellow members of the animal kingdom. They know to eat all their foods in a simple and raw manner. That's fortunate for them because they're able to avoid all the drawbacks of cooked foods. The notion that you must cook your food before eating it really is a crock—pun intended.

Many studies have shown that cooking meat in particular causes big problems in terms of health. Cancer-causing chemicals known as *heterocyclic amines* are of major concern. These carcinogens are formed when the natural sugars (which cause carmelization on the outer surface), amino acids, and creatine present in the meat are exposed to high cooking temperatures. Fortunately, this isn't a concern when you're roasting a pepper or other veggies.

HOT POTATO

Digestive leukocytosis, or an increase in the number of white blood cells in the blood, can occur soon after eating cooked foods but does not happen when eating raw foods. In 1930, Dr. Paul Kouchakoff, at the Institute of Clinical Chemistry in Switzerland, was studying the effects of eating on the immune system. He noted this strange phenomenon and attributed it to the body's viewing the cooked food as an invader and sending in white blood cell "reinforcements" to defend against it.

Raw foodists, who only eat foods in their natural, uncooked state, believe eating raw foods is truly the best way to nourish our bodies. When we eat foods just as they come from the ground—raw and uncooked—our bodies can retain and utilize vitamins and nutrients better. Eating raw also leaves all the beneficial fiber intact, which is good for the GI tract and colon.

The Cold, Raw Facts

Fortunately, eating raw and vegan does come quite naturally for us humans. There's no denying the desirability of a freshly picked apple or cluster of fresh grapes. Go with your cravings for fresh produce, and you could reap some great rewards. It's a good idea to try to fit in as many sources of raw fresh fruits and vegetables as possible every day.

Eating an all-raw or mostly raw foods diet is nothing new. Many great thinkers who were ahead of their time ate this way, including Hippocrates, who recommended a raw diet to provide relief from disease and cancer to the people of his day. It makes sense that eating fresh, whole, raw foods can improve your overall health in many ways, giving you increased energy, better skin tone, mental clarity, loss of excess weight, and reduced and reversed symptoms of disease.

So what exactly would you eat if you wanted to consume a raw vegan diet? You would eat the same as most vegans, enjoying all fruits, vegetables, sprouts, nuts, seeds, grains, sea vegetables, and other organic/natural foods that haven't been cooked or overly processed. Raw foodists do soak (germinate), sprout, dehydrate, pulverize, and chop their foods, but they do not expose them to high temperatures or excessive processing.

Heavily processed foods that have been canned, bottled, or packaged are generally out of the question for those on a raw diet. Usually these types of foods have been heated to high temperatures or pasteurized or contain additives, preservatives, artificial colorings and flavorings, and refined sugar. These foods are often not considered raw, and many raw foodists avoid them.

However, many natural foods stores do sell some fresh fruit or vegetable juices and fermented foods, like kimchi and sauerkraut, which have been bottled or jarred without having been pasteurized or exposed to excessively high temperatures. These can still be considered "raw foods."

"Alive" Brings Life

A common philosophy many raw foodists share is that from life comes life, or that eating raw foods, with all their vital enzymes and nutrients intact and alive, has an incredibly healthful effect on the consumer.

Raw foods that have been freshly picked are at the height of their nutritional value, as vitamins and minerals found in plant foods are most absorbable and available to your body in their uncooked state. The live enzymes provide energy to your cells and assist in the digestion and absorption of food sources. When you heat foods, you destroy or diminish many vital vitamins, minerals, and enzymes. Eating raw foods can also be less stressful on your body in terms of digestion.

The more raw foods you eat, the stronger your body becomes. Your immune system also becomes stronger, making you better equipped to fight off allergies, illness, and disease. Raw foods also help cleanse your body of toxins and mucus, which helps your inner workings run better, provides you with more energy, and improves your breathing and overall appearance.

It may seem a little intimidating at first to think of yourself adopting an all-raw diet. That's why most people begin it in small steps. Your body also adjusts better that way, especially as you detoxify yourself of all the years of bad eating habits. Just make whatever changes feel comfortable to you, and try to approach it one meal at a time.

A good goal is to include one or more sources of raw fruits, vegetables, or nuts in each meal. An apple, banana, or fruit smoothie for breakfast; a leafy green salad with lunch or dinner; and a crunchy snack of some raw sunflower seeds or nuts helps you incorporate more raw foods into your diet without much effort. Before you know it, your raw food intake can soon exceed the cooked with a little effort and thought.

Preserving "Live" Enzymes

Those who eat as true raw foodists do not cook their foods. If they do expose food items to high temperatures in some way during the preparation process, they are cautious to not exceed 115°F. Temperatures hotter than 105°F alter vital *enzymes*, and temperatures hotter than 115°F kill them.

> **DEFINITION**
>
> **Enzymes** are proteins that act as catalysts for specific biochemical reactions of other substances, and do so without the enzyme itself being destroyed or altered in the process. Each enzyme is designed to initiate a specific response with a specific result, as in digestion of food. Enzymes are vital to the body for achieving and sustaining optimal health.

When foods are heated, free radicals are created. The free radicals bombard your cells, altering, destroying, and infecting them with disease, especially cancer. How do you fight free radicals? Raw plant-based foods are full of antioxidants, and consuming as many as you can in your daily diet helps you win the battle of good health. Plant foods that are concentrated calorie sources—such as avocados, bananas, mangoes, and other fruits—are high in enzymes that can also help keep illness at bay.

Three basic types of enzymes are needed to sustain life: metabolic enzymes, digestive enzymes, and food enzymes. Metabolic and digestive enzymes are produced within the body, but food enzymes are not, and therefore must be provided in the foods you eat.

Metabolic enzymes are produced within the walls of each cell and help with the functioning of your brain, heart, lungs, kidneys, organs, and all your other muscles and tissues. These enzymes are the sparks that get your motor running. Your body uses digestive enzymes to break down the foods you eat into essential nutrients which can then be immediately metabolized, such as essential fatty acids, amino acids in the form of proteins, and glucose or sugars in the form of complex carbohydrates.

Food enzymes are needed in the body's digestive process, but generally, only help digest the particular type of food that contains them.

Digestive enzymes are found in many fruits, especially those from tropical locales. Pineapple contains bromelain and papaya contains papain, both of which help digest proteins. They also have anti-inflammatory and cancer-combating properties. It's best to consume digestive enzymes in their fresh fruit forms, but some people opt for supplements. You can find these in most pharmacies and natural foods stores.

Cooking destroys or depletes most of food's naturally occurring enzymes. As a result, the body pulls enzymes from other areas within itself to pick up the slack in diges-tion. This endless cycle of take, take, take when eating mostly cooked foods wears down your system and opens the door for disease to invade your body. If you can manage to eat 50 to 75 percent raw foods as part of your daily intake, you can help your body keep up with processing and eliminating the cooked foods you eat.

A Few Things to Chew On

If you're curious as to what your daily diet would consist of if you choose to eat a raw or mostly raw vegan diet, wonder no more.

A Raw Menu

Most raw foodists like to begin each day by eating fruit. Eating fruit in the morning helps cleanse your system. Often undigested foods or waste still remain in your sys-tem from the day before, and eating an apple with all its fiber whisks it all away. This is actually quite a smart way for everyone to start off his or her day.

How about a smoothie or glass of fresh juice, made with several servings of fruit, for breakfast? Maybe add a few dates, nuts, or seeds, especially some hemp, flax, or chia seeds, to your smoothie for a boost in flavor and nutrition. Got you thinking, or making you thirsty?

You could also eat some soaked grains or nuts early in the day. Ever heard of muesli? Europeans have enjoyed it for a long time. Muesli is a mixture of whole grains, dried fruits, and nuts that are soaked overnight in water (or in your favorite nondairy milk if you prefer), and eaten like a porridge or breakfast cereal. If you use water, you can leave the covered container on your countertop, but if you're using nondairy milk, you should place the muesli in the refrigerator to soak overnight. A bowlful of muesli for breakfast provides great sources of complex carbohydrates and protein for a constant supply of slow-burning energy throughout the day.

Figuring out what to eat for the rest of the day isn't too hard either. Munch on raw fruits and veggies, or get creative with your ingredients. You can enjoy some raw soup (like gazpacho), or you might dive into a crisp and crunchy tossed salad, with lots of veggies cut in all different shapes and sizes, nuts or sprouts scattered over the top, and topped with a tantalizing raw dressing.

> **IN A NUTSHELL**
>
> You can make a raw veggie burrito by mixing veggies with a raw dressing or sauce and then rolling them up in a crisp lettuce or cabbage leaf!

Pull out the heavy equipment such as a dehydrator or food processor, and you can create some gourmet appetizers, snacks, loaves, pâtés, desserts, or whatever else your imagination and creativity inspire you to try. Eating raw is tantalizing and revitalizing and certainly not bland and boring!

The Joys of Juicing

No one knows when humans first discovered the joys of juicing. References to the enjoyment of fruit nectars, juices, and fermented beverages exist throughout the literature and artifacts of many ancient cultures, including Babylonian, Egyptian, Greek, Roman, Hindu, and Buddhist. After all, wine—which is nothing more than fermented grape juice—is often referred to as the "drink of the gods."

Dr. Norman Walker was a pioneer in the medical field commonly referred to as juice therapy. You're probably familiar with the saying "physician, heal thyself," and that is precisely what Dr. Walker did. Born in 1867 and plagued with illness early in his life, he cured himself with a diet of raw foods and fresh juices. He went on to live to the ripe old age of 99.

Dr. Walker was the author of many books, including *Fresh Vegetable and Fruit Juices, The Vegetarian Guide to Diet and Salad, The Natural Way to Vibrant Health*, and *Become Younger*. He helped provide treatment to thousands throughout his 70-year career, which lasted until 1984, and used a raw juice diet to help cure many people of cancer.

We also have Dr. Walker to thank for inventing the first modern juicer. In 1934, he developed the Norwalk Hydraulic Press Juicer, which made it possible for people to efficiently turn fresh produce into healthful, vibrant juice. His juicer is still on the market and is considered among the finest because it processes without overoxidizing and preserves all the food's vital nutrients. The Norwalk Hydraulic Press Juicer works by finely cutting and grating fruits and vegetables and then squeezing out the juice via a hydraulic press.

You can find many different brands of juicers available on the market. Most of them fall into four categories:

- Juice presses, such as a manual hand press or the Norwalk Juicer

- Twin-gear presses, which have two gears that shred the food between the gears and then squeeze out the juice

- Masticating juicers, such as the Champion, that work by first grating and then masticating into finer pulp and finally pressing out the juice

- Centrifugal ejection juicers that use centrifugal force, or rotation at high speeds, to force the foods against a cutting screen that separates juice from solids

IN A NUTSHELL

The Champion juicer was introduced in 1954 and was the first masticating (grating) type of juicer. It remains one of the most popular brands.

The Norwalk Hydraulic Press Juicer allows for the least oxidation or destruction of enzymes. The centrifugal-type juicers mix in tremendous amounts of oxygen during the juicing process, so you must drink juices made in these juicers immediately to retain most of the nutrients. Juicers vary in price, so analyze your needs and anticipated usage to help determine which juicer best suits your needs.

Juicing is an easy way to get enough servings of fruits and vegetables each day. Juicing veggies also separates the pulp solids from the liquid nutrients, and not having to process the fiber enables easier and faster digestion. The enzymes that were just alive a minute ago in the fresh fruits and veggies are still active when you ingest them. This means added nutrition, increased energy, and rejuvenation of each of your body's cells, organs, and tissues.

When juicing, pretty much anything goes, so experiment! Feel free to combine fruits or vegetables to create your own blends. A mix of carrots and apples can make a good base, and add in some cucumbers, celery, or parsley to help cleanse your system. A clove of garlic boosts your immune system, fights off infections, or relieves the symptoms of a cold. Adding a little piece of ginger in the juicing process results in a spicy flavored beverage that speeds up your metabolism and helps reduce any inflammation you may be experiencing. Wheat grass is one of the most popular juiced items. This vibrant green nectar is full of live enzymes and rich in chlorophyll. It cleanses your system, boosts your immune system, and improves the condition of your hair and skin.

Sprouting a New You

The tiny seeds of plants germinate and sprout forth as new life and then go on to grow, each in their own individual ways, into plant life. Nearly all grains, legumes, nuts, and seeds naturally contain dormant *enzyme inhibitors*, which help seeds survive until growing conditions are optimal for them. In nature, enzyme inhibitors like oxalates (compounds that prevent oxygen from penetrating) and phytates (natural insecticides) are easily removed when there's enough rain for the seed to germinate and sunshine for it to grow into a plant.

DEFINITION

Enzyme inhibitors are present in plants' seeds or nuts to aid in self-preservation. The enzyme inhibitors protect the seed so it has a better chance to germinate and reach full maturity before being gobbled up.

You can replicate this natural occurrence by soaking and sprouting grains, legumes, nuts, and seeds. Soaking them in water for a length of time starts the germination process, bringing them to life as tiny sprouts. This also helps neutralize enzyme inhibitors, convert starches to simple carbohydrates, and break down proteins into amino acids. Soaking and sprouting increases the nutritional value and digestibility of these foods as well. In fact, tender, young sprouts are one of the most significant sources of dietary live enzymes and often contain 10 to 100 times more than the fully developed foods.

You can soak and sprout many varieties of vegetables, grains, legumes, nuts, and seeds, and each has its very own distinct flavor, from sweet red clover to spicy radish. When it comes to sprouts, most people usually think of alfalfa sprouts, which adorn many healthy sandwiches, or mung bean sprouts, which are a staple in Asian cuisine and found on many salad bars. Recently new strains of sprouts have hit markets, including broccoli, red clover, spicy radish, and mixed sprouts made with a mixture of beans, grains, and seeds.

You can sprout other legumes as well, such as lentils, peas, mung beans, black beans, or chickpeas. Grains such as wheat, rye, oats, buckwheat, quinoa, and rice are made more digestible by sprouting. Don't forget about your nuts and seeds, like almonds, sunflower, and pumpkin; you can soak them for 6 or more hours to make them more easily digestible, let them air-dry or dehydrate them to enjoy as a snack, or sprout them for 1 to 3 days. You can use your soaked and sprouted foods to add a tremendous amount of flavor and texture to salads, sandwiches, sides, and main dishes.

It's really quite easy to start your own sprout garden. Special sprouting bags and jars are available in hardware stores, natural foods stores, and through online sources. You can also use a large jar, such as a Mason jar; use a piece of cheesecloth or mesh, with the ring lid or a rubber band over it, to hold it in place over the mouth of the jar.

You can find sprouting seeds in packages and bulk bins in most natural foods stores and through online sources, and we recommend using organic seeds whenever possible. Be sure to pick through the seeds and discard any debris that may be among them. It doesn't take a lot of seeds to yield a quart of sprouts, and depending on what you sprout, you only need from 1 to 4 tablespoons seeds per batch.

The following table provides you with a breakdown, by variety, of how much sprouting seeds you need, how many days they take to sprout, and their yield.

Seed	How Much You Need	Days to Sprout	Yield
Alfalfa	3 tablespoons	3 to 5 days	approximately 3 or 4 cups
Broccoli	2 tablespoons	3 to 5 days	2 cups
Buckwheat (hulled)	1 cup	1 to 2 days	2 cups
Clover and red clover	3 tablespoons	4 to 6 days	approximately 3 or 4 cups
Chickpeas	1 cup	2 to 4 days	4 cups
Fenugreek	¼ cup	4 to 6 days	3 cups
Mung beans	⅓ cup	4 to 6 days	4 cups
Pumpkin seeds	1 cup	1 to 2 days	2 cups
Radish	3 tablespoons	3 to 5 days	3 or 4 cups
Red lentils	½ cup	3 or 4 days	3 or 4 cups
Sunflower seeds	1 cup	1 or 2 days	2 cups
Wheat	1 cup	2 or 3 days	3 cups

Start by placing your sprouting seeds in a sprouting jar. Cover with 3 inches of water; secure the cheesecloth, mesh screen and/or lid on the jar; and leave to soak for 6 hours or overnight. After the seeds have soaked, drain off and discard the soaking water. To rinse the sprouts, fill the jar with enough fresh water to cover seeds, drain, and repeat the procedure two more times. Invert the jar at an angle in a small bowl, and set aside to drain away from direct sunlight or overhead lighting. Repeat the rinsing and draining procedure two more times throughout the day.

Continue the rinsing and draining procedure for the next few days or until your sprouts begin to have small leaves and several-inch-long stems. Now you're ready to put the jar in direct sunlight to develop the chlorophyll and turn the tender young leaves green. When that happens, you can begin to enjoy your sprouts! Store any unused sprouts in the refrigerator and enjoy for 2 or 3 days.

IN A NUTSHELL

Many ancient cultures understood the nutritional value of soaking and sprouting grains, legumes, nuts, and seeds. Plant foods that have been soaked and sprouted provide us with the most concentrated sources of minerals and vitamins A, B, C, E, and K, as well as amino acids and beneficial enzymes.

Although you can sprout nearly anything, there are some things you shouldn't try to sprout. Never eat tomato or potato sprouts! Both are members of the nightshade family and contain an extremely toxic chemical called solanine. Sorghum sprouts could contain toxic levels of cyanide.

Also, in the last few years, alfalfa sprouts have been recalled after cases of E. coli and salmonella were attributed to their consumption, which undoubtedly could be traced back to poor food handling and sanitation. All the more reason for you to grow your own sprouts!

DIY Dehydrating

Dehydrating is a popular food preparation technique raw foodists and others use and is an inexpensive way to preserve excess produce as well as make some tasty simple or gourmet treats. Also, a large amount of the nutrients and enzymes remain in the food as long as they're dehydrated at temperatures cooler than 105°F. Basically, you just want to remove as much water from the food as you can, which prevents bacteria or mold from developing. Always store your dehydrated foods in an airtight container in a cool, dry, and preferably dark place or in the refrigerator.

Electric dehydrators have become more than just a way of preserving foods; they are now used to make gourmet raw cuisine and healthy snacks. Pulverized sprouted grains, nuts, or seeds, as well as some seasonings can be transformed into dehydrated crackers or flatbreads. Fruit purées become instant dried fruit strips. You can infuse foods and then dehydrate them for a slightly roasted flavor. Shoyu-flavored cashews and ginger-covered mango slices are both quite delicious.

The biggest advantage of using an electric dehydrator is that you can dry many items at one time—depending on the brand, dehydrators usually have 5 to 10 racks. You can place thin slices or small pieces of food on the drying racks, load them into the dehydrator, turn it on, and leave it to do its thing. Check on your food periodically to see how it's drying. Drying times vary from machine to machine and the size and moisture content of the items being dried.

IN A NUTSHELL

To speed up the drying process, cut or slice foods into small pieces and turn them over after a few hours of dehydrating.

Uncooked Cuisine Takes Off

Eating raw foods has gone from simply grazing on a piece of fruit or a carrot stick to one of the hottest—or make that the *coolest*—trends in food cuisine.

You don't need to spend a lot of money to get started, either. Just work with what you already have in your kitchen. Pull out your knives, cutting board, peeler, grater, blender, and food processor. These tools can help you create some amazing raw vegan foods that can mimic many of the cooked foods you're used to.

If you love tinkering around with raw foods, you can expand your collection of culinary tools as you need and desire them. Juicers, spiral slicers, special sprouting jars, and dehydrators may one day find themselves on your list of must-have equipment. Then you can experiment with making your own dried fruits, treats, crackers, or interesting salads and entrées with your new slicing capabilities. These tools can really help spark your creativity!

IN A NUTSHELL

A food processor, spiral slicer, or vegetable peeler can turn fresh zucchini, carrots, or other vegetables into long, noodlelike strands. Make a sun-dried tomato sauce or herb pesto, toss it with the vegetable "noodles," garnish or embellish it as you like, and you have a raw gourmet "pasta" dish!

For further information and inspiration, check the internet for raw foods websites, cookbooks, potlucks, support groups, and restaurants. You can find raw foods restaurants all across the United States and throughout the world. They range from simple juice joints and deli-style places to casual and fine gourmet dining. Some raw restaurants have become hot spots with the media and public, such as Lydia's Lovin' Foods Restaurant, Café Gratitude, Cru, and Planet Raw, all in California; Blossoming Lotus in Portland, Oregon; Karyn's Fresh Corner in Chicago; and Pure Food and Wine in New York. These restaurants have proven that eating raw is not bland and boring but exciting, nutritious, and delicious!

If you're interested in learning more about the benefits of eating raw foods, as well as some tasty and easy raw foods recipes, we also recommend checking out *The Complete Idiot's Guide to Eating Raw* by Mark Reinfeld, Bo Rinaldi, and Jennifer Murray.

The Least You Need to Know

- Increasing the amount of raw foods in your daily dietary intake provides you with numerous health benefits.
- Consuming foods in their raw state preserves their vital nutrients, including vitamins and important enzymes.
- Eating too much cooked food has drawbacks, including digestion difficulties and wasted energy.
- Juicing and sprouting are excellent ways to give your body high concentrations of the nutritional benefits of raw veggies.
- Dehydrating removes the moisture content from foods while retaining most of their vitamins and live enzymes.

Maintaining a Vegan Lifestyle

As you meander through your transition into the wonderful world of veganism, living a meatless and cruelty-free life should become easier and easier for you. To be armed with a little know-how helps, so in Part 4, we give you some tips for things such as handling the veg-curious you may encounter, surviving family gatherings and parties, cooking to impress others, and getting a vegan meal when dining out.

Going vegan often means getting rid of your old animal-based stuff and bringing in new plant-based replacements. You can do this at your own speed, a little at a time, or in one fell swoop in the form of a major spring cleaning. Don't worry, we give you some advice on shopping wisely to restock your cabinets, pantry, and closet. We also give you some travel tips to help make you a wise and well-fed vegan traveler!

Handling Nonvegan Family and Friends

In This Chapter

- Answering questions about veganism
- Being a good example
- Arming yourself with knowledge
- Getting through the rough spots
- Co-existing with nonvegans

Living as a vegan on a day-to-day basis, you'll encounter lots of questions—and lots of confusion—about what it means to be vegan. Being informed about the issues is really important in handling your veg-curious friends, family, or co-workers. Be ready to occasionally have to field some really silly, sometimes insensitive, and often personal questions about your vegan lifestyle. You'll be asked about what you eat and wear and how you live your life, and it will help if you can answer these questions and others with a healthy, happy glow about you.

Questions and Answers

Grasping what vegan life is all about, and why, can be a bit tricky for some, and it will require some patience and understanding on your part as those around you deal with the changes you're going through.

Be ready for questions of all sorts and from all sides. Some questions may be strange or even bizarre, but try to answer them as honestly as you can and to the best of your ability. Try not to laugh, either, which can be hard, particularly when you get a real off-the-wall question like, "Don't plants feel pain, too?" or "Can you eat animal crackers?" or "You can eat fish, because fish isn't meat, right?" Some questions will be more serious in nature and more difficult to answer.

HOT POTATO

Before Vatican II put an end to it in the early 1960s, the Catholic Church had long prohibited the eating of meat on Fridays and certain holidays. Eating fish on those days was permitted, however, and this gave rise to the widespread belief that fish are somehow not meat. Many people you encounter will probably still share this belief, so don't be surprised!

More often than not, how you answer these questions is just as important as what you actually say, in terms of what your inquirers take away from the conversation. The more you learn about the many issues surrounding vegan living and the more experienced you become, the more gracefully you can answer questions about your lifestyle.

Being a Vegan Ambassador

When dealing with questions friends, family, and the veg-curious ask, you'll inevitably find yourself in the position of answering on behalf of the entire vegan community when you try to explain why vegans think the way they do. It's like you become a vegan ambassador to the rest of the nonvegan world. But in reality, you're just one person explaining your particular view of the world.

The best way to deal with questions is with well-reasoned answers, and be sure to put your responses in terms that are easy to understand. For example, when asked about what a vegan is and why you think the way you do, you can say something like this:

> I eat fruits, vegetables, beans, grains, nuts, and seeds, but I don't eat anything that comes from animals, including meat, fish, dairy products, eggs, and honey, because I feel that no animal's life is less important than my own. I try to apply that thought to what I put on and in my body and to all other aspects of my life. I'm just trying to make a difference for animals in whatever way I can. You can say I'm a big animal lover.

When asked to explain your choices about clothing and personal items, you can keep it simple again:

I like to wear man-made fabrics and natural fibers instead of items that come from animals, like leather, suede, wool, and even silk. There are some great nonanimal alternatives out there, and it makes me feel good to not involve animals in what I wear.

Expect that as you say this, they will be checking out your wardrobe choices from head to toe and will most likely comment on your footwear or your belt, particularly if those items look a little too leatherlike.

Of course, the reasons for being vegan are often personal and vary from person to person, so only you can explain what brought you to this way of approaching the world around you.

Avoiding the Shock Treatment

When talking about veganism with the veg-curious, you can have more of a positive impact on their overall view of what you're saying if you take it slow and don't shock them too much right off the bat. It's best to save those shocking and disturbing facts—and there are lots of them—for when you feel someone is ready to hear them.

There may be times when you'll be conflicted between hitting someone with the cold, hard facts they probably aren't in the mood to hear and holding your tongue until a more appropriate time when they may be more receptive. The longer you live as a vegan, you'll probably learn that lots of in-your-face preaching doesn't usually have the intended effect and that getting a little more creative in the way you spread the vegan message can have surprising results.

Alleviating Their Concerns

Many people have problems with or fears about veganism that stem from inaccurate perceptions of what it's really all about. Their misconceptions can come from many different areas, including the media, whose portrayals of vegetarians and vegans in various movies and TV shows has led some to believe that vegans and vegetarians are more than a bit strange, with their "really weird beliefs" and choice to "not eat properly."

It may help to inform people with such concerns about the sound nutrition and added health benefits of an all-plant-based vegan diet, as mentioned in Chapter 3. Personal stories of weight loss and your obvious robust appearance and healthy glow can help further illustrate your points.

It can also help to present them with examples of veg-heads, past and present, and their contributions to society. If you think it will help, name-drop vegan celebrities like Woody Harrelson, Alicia Silverstone, Brandy, Prince, Joaquin Phoenix, Alec Baldwin, Ellen DeGeneres, Portia de Rossi, and Moby, as well as some of the illustrious vegans and vegetarians throughout history we mentioned in Chapter 2. Knowing that someone they admire and respect is also a vegan may lessen their concern for your new vegan lifestyle and hasten their acceptance of it. For a great list of famous vegans and vegetarians, and lots of other interesting stuff, go to famousveggie.com.

Certainly, not all people will be opposed to your new lifestyle and ways of thinking. Many will be curious and want to know more. You'll undoubtedly have some great conversations with those who are really interested in what you're saying and want to learn more about it. These conversations can be very rewarding to everyone involved—and downright empowering. They can also go on for hours, as we can say from experience!

Knowledge Is Power

After going vegan, many feel so completely inspired and empowered by what they've learned, they're a little like a butterfly emerging from a cocoon. They feel like spreading their wings and flying all around to spread the good word about being vegan. For some, it's like being clued in to one of the big secrets of the universe, and they feel compelled to share their knowledge and acquired wisdom with others.

That's fine, but remember, the key is knowing the right time, place, and method of doing so, and that will come with experience. (We talk more about that later in this chapter.)

HOT POTATO

Putting people on the defensive is an easy way to get them to close their hearts and minds to what you're saying. If you can phrase what you're saying in a nonjudgmental way and not make the other person feel as if they're being challenged, you'll have a more receptive audience.

Be both prepared and eager to engage in conversations about being a vegan. Being an informed vegan really helps you handle some of the opposition and comments that may come your way. If you're going to quote something, be sure you have your facts straight to avoid someone calling you out and exposing your mistake during an exchange or to prevent a conflict or altercation from arising in the first place. Being prepared for inquiries, as well as insults, keeps feelings on both sides from being hurt and prevents you from being labeled as a vegan troublemaker.

Checkin' Out the Library

Doing your own research and reading from as many different sources as possible helps shape your views as well as expand your knowledge base. Your local library is one of the easiest and most economical ways to educate yourself and open your mind to new concepts and to the world around you. Armed with nothing but a library card, you can gain access to stacks and stacks of books on all sorts of topics from animal rights to nutrition to how to make your own vegan soap. It's also a great way to check out books for content before purchasing to determine which ones are just what you need to fill out your own home library.

If there's a book you really want to read and your local library doesn't own a copy, they might be able to special order it for you from a neighboring library for free. For that and any other issues or questions you may have about resources and how to obtain them, ask the friendly people at your local library.

Surfin' the Web

The internet can really mean the difference between vegan isolation and vegan support. With a few clicks of your mouse or smart phone, you can have a wealth of information at your fingertips on any subject imaginable. And there's definitely no shortage of information about veganism on the web! Use it to find out the latest health information for vegans, get nutritional advice, pick up a few vegan recipes, connect with other vegans, or even shop for cruelty-free items and vegan baked goods. The web can be an incredibly useful tool for vegans, so be sure to make the most of it.

The internet can also make you feel less alone as you start your new life as a vegan. You can log on to find message boards and chat rooms where you can share your views and concerns with other like-minded people. Or use it to track down veg-friendly businesses, restaurants, organizations, or groups that may be of interest to you. In Appendix B, we share information on various online resources to locate vegan products, support, and information about global and local vegan and vegetarian communities and groups.

If you don't have internet access, have no fear. Your local library probably has some internet-connected computers you can use free of charge, although there will most likely be some time restrictions on your use. You might also be able to find internet cafés in your area or friends willing to let you log on from their computers.

Exemplify Sound Nutrition, Not Malnutrition

You may encounter some people who think your going vegan is some sort of new trendy diet. After all, by going vegan, you naturally lose weight and begin to look healthier and more robust after cleaning your system of animal-based products. Those around you who may want to lose a few pounds or get their health together a little more may look to you and your new way of eating with renewed curiosity. So be sure you are living and eating as a positive example, and try to be a good vegan role model.

Of course, you want to show others that living and eating as a vegan is based on sound knowledge and nutrition, not on a whim or because you have an eating disorder or are plunging head-first into malnutrition. Be a positively glowing example of good vegan health—it's one of the best things you can do to influence those around you at home, at work, or at school to want to adopt a vegan approach to eating.

Eat Your Fruits and Veggies

It's best to show people a healthy and happy vegan, so be sure you're taking good care of yourself by eating right and getting enough exercise and sleep. Through your food choices, you can deliciously show others the wide variety of nutritious foods available to vegans. On a daily basis, it's ideal to eat a well-balanced vegan diet, one composed of several delicious and nutritious meals throughout the day full of fruits, vegetables, beans, and whole grains. Simply by making good food choices and eating right, soon your body will start looking and feeling better and better.

If you eat well on a regular basis and have no serious medical issues, you can take a more "moderation rather than deprivation" approach to your vegan diet by allowing yourself to give into a craving for something "not so healthy" once in a while or indulge your sweet tooth. So on an occasional basis, it's fine to have junk-food types of snacks around to indulge in a little and show other people that vegan versions do exist of many of their comfort foods and favorite foods from youth. Your friends and family may even prefer these veganized versions to their regular brands, and this can be an easy way to show them that eating vegan is not at all bland or boring and that it's actually quite an exciting and delicious way to eat!

HOT POTATO

Having only a plate of french fries and a soda when you're at lunch with friends may be vegan, but it certainly isn't healthful. Why not set a better example and have a veggie-packed salad with a bowl of soup or a slice of whole-grain bread? You might just encourage others to eat right, too.

The Protein Issue: Resolved

Expect to get a lot of questions from nonvegans about protein: where you get it, how you can do without meat and dairy sources of it, and more. By familiarizing yourself with the facts, you can easily and intelligently answer their questions.

In your reply, mention that plant-based foods are better sources of lean protein for your body—and are lower in fat and calories and higher in fiber and calcium—than meat and dairy sources. Then throw in that plant-based sources provide no cholesterol whatsoever to your diet. Be ready to mention plant-based protein-rich foods such as broccoli, leafy greens, beans, nuts, seeds, and grains, which are all affordable, delicious, and nutritional powerhouses.

You also could point out that fruits and veggies supply all the vitamins, minerals, and key nutrients you need, while animal-based foods provide very few in comparison. You could mention that animal foods often only pass on to us what the animals took in through their own plant-based diets.

If your questioners challenge the accuracy of any of your statements, be prepared to back them up with some of your newly acquired facts and offer to direct them to where they can learn more for themselves.

Fit by Example

Besides living as a positive example of sound vegan nutrition through what you eat and what you say, it's important for your overall inner well-being to look healthy on the outside as well. It's best for anyone to avoid being overweight or obese if he or she wants to fend off chronic disease and live a healthy and happy life. But making dietary changes isn't always enough for some people to maintain an optimal weight.

Remember, if you don't move it, you will lose it, and in this case "it" is good health and a lean and trim figure. Getting off your butt and getting some regular cardio-vascular exercise is good for getting your heart pumping, blood flowing, and taking excess inches off your hips or belly. Exercise is essential for staying in shape and truly being healthy, not just looking healthy.

Exercise can be as simple as taking a walk, preferably outdoors where you can also breathe fresh air into your lungs and be a part of nature instead of just watching a nature show on a screen. Riding a bike is also one of the best forms of exercise as it provides many different health benefits while being gentle and low impact.

Relationships Put to the Test

Upon becoming vegan, your personal relationships may become challenged, especially if those nearest and dearest to you don't seem to support your decision to go vegan. How you decide to handle this greatly determines whether it will be an "us versus them" situation or an amicable one.

Some people feel threatened by the concept of veganism and vegetarianism and think that somehow your vegan lifestyle choices affect or challenge them directly. They may feel their own lifestyle choices are being called into question. These perceptions can have a tremendous impact on your relationships and interactions.

Most vegans do not usually find themselves surrounded by only vegans or lucky enough to have been raised in a vegan family. So naturally, your circle of friends and family and those you encounter in your everyday life will be made up of those who may completely understand and support your being vegan, those who will be slightly confused by your lifestyle but still accepting, and those who think you're nuts or going through some kind of "thing" and hope you'll eventually and quickly give up on being vegan.

Expect Some Opposition

Family members (especially well-intentioned parents) who are unfamiliar with veganism and uninformed about all the health benefits of a plant-based diet might put up some resistance to your new lifestyle. They may view you as being "difficult" or rebellious, or they may simply fear that you're embarking on a dangerous diet that will leave you lacking nutritionally. Some just won't understand why you can't just stop all this silliness and be "normal" like them. Many have also been influenced by a lifetime of negative, unflattering, and inaccurate portrayals of vegetarians and more recently vegans on TV and in the movies.

You should always feel confident and secure in your decision to become a vegan (or whatever your life choices), and don't let other people have an effect on you. Let your compassion for your fellow living creatures extend to those you deal with on a daily or personal basis. Try to have patience, compassion, and understanding, even for those who don't show it to you. Answer their questions as best and as tactfully as you can, and most importantly, live by positive example.

Needing a Little Extra Support

Joining a support group—such as a vegetarian, vegan, or animal rights organization—may also help with answers and support, especially if you face opposition to your new vegan lifestyle from your friends and loved ones. Many such groups exist, and with a little searching, hopefully you can find one in your area.

Nowadays, because vegans don't usually live in the same geographic proximity as lots of other vegans, a bulk of the communication we have with one another is electronic in nature. The internet really helps bring lots of vegans together!

IN A NUTSHELL

To begin your search for a veg-related group, check your local newspaper, bulletin boards, and even your local natural foods stores. Your best bet, though, is probably online. You can search the net for groups in your area and even join a virtual pro-vegan group online. One such helpful website is vegan.meetup.com.

Finding Common Ground

If you encounter antagonism or a lack of support from those closest to you, don't let it get you down or discourage you. Try seeking out common ground. Having an open and honest conversation can often prove that opposing sides really aren't that far apart when it comes to many aspects of life. This can be as simple as stating that you both want the same things—to be happy and healthy—and that living this way does that for you.

Because veganism is a lot like a moral code upon which we base our decisions and actions stemming from compassion, some vegans choose to compare their vegan views to the kind of belief systems that exist for religions. Putting it in that light can help others better understand the level of commitment you have toward being vegan. They probably wouldn't put down someone for his choice of religious denomination and most likely wouldn't want someone to do that to them either. When they understand how deeply your vegan beliefs are rooted and they're not going to change your mind about it, hopefully they'll back off.

Ideally, respect should flow from both sides, and when it does, it can help open lines of communication. Show respect, and ask for the same in return. Live by positive example, and show patience and understanding when faced with diversity and opposition. Command respect in your demeanor and words, and you most likely will receive it. Having a sense of pride can be contagious. Those around you will pick up on your self-confidence and self-esteem, and hopefully you will have a positive effect on them as well.

The Least You Need to Know

- Being well informed about the issues surrounding being vegan is essential, so take advantage of educational resources available to you.
- The internet can be an invaluable resource for vegans for everything from connecting with others with similar views, swapping vegan recipes, to finding vegan goods and services and locating veg-friendly businesses, restaurants, and organizations in your area.
- Looking healthy and happy is one of the easiest ways to convince people that going vegan was the right decision for you, so be sure to take good care of yourself in every way.
- It's important to have understanding and patience when dealing with questions friends and family members have about the whys and hows of being vegan.

Dining, Vegan Style

In This Chapter

- Avoiding problems at mealtime
- Co-existing in the kitchen
- Holiday survival tips for vegans
- Eating out and ordering vegan meals
- Traveling, vegan style

Mealtime should help nourish the soul as well as the body, and when you go vegan, it can take on quite a few new aspects. For one, you'll now have to give quite a bit more thought to where and what you'll eat. Add other people to the mix, and it can take on another dimension completely. Most of us aren't lucky enough to be surrounded by friends, family members, and colleagues who share our vegan perspectives on eating, so it takes a little extra thought and effort to keep everything, including our relationships, working smoothly. And what about going out to eat now that you're vegan?

This chapter gives you some tips that hopefully will make the world of vegan dining, both in and out, a little easier.

Communal Time, Not Battle Time

Dinnertime should never be battle time; for one thing, it's bad for your digestion. Being aggravated can cause your stomach to get upset, which can lead to indigestion, loss of appetite, or worse, gobbling down your food without chewing properly just to quickly remove yourself from an unpleasant situation.

Informing your dinner companions about the negative aspects of factory farming right as they're about to dig in to the meal before them only leads to conflict. There's no doubt they'll feel threatened by you and your dietary choices, which can lead to a lot of unpleasantness during mealtime. Save the arguing for later, if necessary, and hopefully others will approach it that way as well.

> **HOT POTATO**
>
> Talking about hot-button topics often avoided in most social situations—politics, religion, and moral beliefs—can be extremely touchy at mealtimes and family gatherings.

"Can't You Just Pick It Off?"

As a vegan and dining with others, you'll likely hear one question over and over when nonvegan food is served: "Can't you just pick it off?" Or its companion, "There's barely any on there. Can't you just eat around it?" Some take it a step further with "Can't you just eat it anyway? It's just a little." Well-intentioned relatives often make these comments, but they probably don't realize that it makes most of us a bit nauseous just being in close proximity to the meat or dairy on *other* peoples' plates, let alone on our own. Just sigh to yourself, consider they just really haven't thought about the issue, and try to find something suitably vegan to eat.

Many people forget, or aren't aware to begin with, that being vegan goes beyond dietary choices. If they had thought about it for a minute, they might not have suggested it in the first place. They would probably never tell someone who is Jewish or Hindu to "pick off" an offending item or "eat it anyway," especially if it conflicted with their religious or moral code. Using this example at the opportune time could be advantageous and illustrate your point in a simple manner they can understand and accept.

You can also file away the incident for when you prepare some vegan delicacy you're eager for them to try. After all, what goes around, comes around. Trying to force that pepperoni on me may result in tofu for you later!

Sharing the Space

We feel for vegans in meat-eating households. It can really be tough at times and often makes the transitioning process even harder if you don't have any support for your newly adopted lifestyle—or worse, face open opposition to it. It's best if you take your meals and the preparation of them into your own hands. If you live at home with your parents, leaving it up to them to try to prepare something to your vegan standards may result in you eating a lot of salads and packaged foods.

As you get more into veganism, you'll have to substitute many of your basic necessities for vegan-friendly versions. Ask for a special space for your items, if need be. In the kitchen, it can be a big help to have your own cabinet, or part of the refrigerator or freezer, to stock all your vegan foodstuffs. You may also want to invest in your own utensils and cookware or designate already-existing items as exclusively your own. You'll probably find it unappetizing (to say the least) to think that a piece of meat had previously been cooked in a pan you now need to use to stir-fry your veggies.

Making Your Own Meals

Being sure you're eating a well-balanced diet and getting all the servings and nutrients necessary for fueling your body is important for everyone, not just vegans and vegetarians. Taking control of your meal preparation is the best way to ensure good health and proper nutrition as a vegan. And as mentioned in previous chapters, making a conscious effort to prepare well-balanced meals for yourself helps alleviate any health concerns your friends and family may have about your eating as a vegan.

Preparing your own meals also means there's less chance of cross-contamination or intentional or unintentional sabotage (adding animal products) of your vegan meals, which can happen. When you're first starting out eating as a vegan, you may have to watch out for Aunt Sally or Grandma trying to add a few bits of meat into your dish or a little chicken broth to "enhance" the rice. So stay on your toes! Leaving your meals up to others, when they don't thoroughly understand veganism and its confines, could lead to problems on multiple levels.

Some might think preparing your own separate meals is a hassle, but it's certainly warranted and well worth it. After not consuming meat and dairy for some time, your body will start to adjust, and you may no longer be able to properly digest those types of foods when they're slipped by you unexpectedly. Some vegans experience symptoms of lactose intolerance and nausea when they unintentionally consume animal products. The symptoms can hit suddenly and without much warning.

Strutting Your Vegan Stuff

One of the best ways to sway your family toward accepting your new vegan lifestyle is to create some phenomenally delicious vegan food and entice them to try it. If you have limited kitchen skills, start by making a salad or side or main dish first, and when you've gained some kitchen confidence, move on to making a whole vegan meal for everyone to enjoy!

To prepare for your meal, go shopping and pick up a wide variety of produce and your favorite vegan ingredients. Try making a salad vibrant with mixed leafy greens and colorful and crunchy vegetables, and tossed with a tantalizing dressing. It will blow away the typical boring iceberg lettuce salad.

For something more substantial, make a pasta, grain, or main dish that's flavorful, eye-catching, and hearty enough to satisfy even the largest of appetites. Then pull out all the stops by making a fabulous vegan dessert, whether it's as simple as some cherry-chocolate-chip nondairy ice cream and some vegan cookies or a homemade decadent vegan cake or pie.

IN A NUTSHELL

Check out Part 6 for vegan recipe ideas. We give you 5 chapters full of more than 110 delicious vegan recipes. The internet and your local library are also good sources for recipes and cookbooks to help give you some inspiration. See Appendix B for some useful websites, and also check out the plethora of free vegan recipes on Beverly's website at veganchef.com.

You'll find that most people are very curious about what vegans eat, and a good way to open some eyes to vegan food is by filling their stomachs with something tasty and satisfying. Some may be skeptical about your offerings at first, but don't let that put you off. You know it's good, and so what if they don't? They're the ones missing out—plus that leaves more for you! Maybe they'll be more receptive to trying something new next time, so don't give up.

Taking time to learn how to cook a wide variety of healthy and delicious vegan food is really helpful when it comes to eating right and being well nourished. It also gives you an advantage when dealing with meat-eaters at mealtime. After all, when you make it yourself, you have total control over what goes into it and what doesn't, whether it's the amount of oil or salt used, or the rogue piece of mystery meat your mom might be tempted to add in if she was making it.

With a little practice and patience, you'll soon go from having one vegan dish in your repertoire to several and then on to preparing entire vegan meals for the whole family to enjoy. As your culinary repertoire expands and your talents progress, you'll be able to serve some amazingly vegan dishes that will be hard for anyone to resist. Soon you'll need very little coaxing to get people to try your food!

Generally it's not a good idea to push your beliefs on others, but turning them on to a little delicious vegan food can, at times, be welcomed with much enthusiasm. Who knows—it might even help change some attitudes toward being vegan!

Friends, Family, and Food

You have an active social life, and with it come invitations. Being vegan, some of those invitations will be for restaurants or events where you may no longer feel comfortable being because what they serve either doesn't appeal to you, conflicts with your vegan beliefs, or can no longer accommodate your new dietary requirements. For example, the smells in restaurants and other gathering places where meat is served now might make your stomach churn instead of making your mouth water.

This may prove to be difficult when going out to eat with friends and family members. It will be easy to avoid these places on your own, but problems may arise with invitations from friends and family. Let your instincts and personal choices guide you, and hope that those around you will understand when something conflicts with your vegan values.

HOT POTATO

Some vegans refuse to go to any restaurant that serves meat, refusing to give their money to support the meat industry. Others find that being in close proximity to meat, especially the smell of it cooking, is disturbing and unappetizing. Instead, these vegans support the restaurants that more closely embody their own vegan values.

Handling Invitations

Dining out can be a treat. It can be a nice change of pace, especially after having put in a long day at work or being overwhelmed by the chaos of everyday life. Anticipation of a wonderful meal, out with friends and family, can really get your juices flowing. But that anticipation can turn to dread quickly when your friend invites you to come along and you no longer feel comfortable with the establishment they chose.

What to do? If the circumstances conflict with your vegan values, explain fully and clearly why you no longer feel comfortable going along. Honesty is the best policy. Use tact, and remember that you're explaining your position, not making excuses for it. You have a right to your opinions and beliefs, just like anyone else, and so bravely stand by your vegan convictions. People who truly care about you will understand and support you no matter what you do or eat.

Handling invitations to dine out can be a bit tricky. Your acceptance may be influenced by *who* is going but will definitely be influenced by *where* you're going. In ideal situations, those inviting you along will consider your veganism and allow you to have input on picking a place to dine. Chances are they won't feel adventurous enough to try your favorite veggie place, but you never know.

Being informed about your local eateries and their menus can be vital, if not crucial, in determining whether you will be dining on an entrée, à la carte, or only a salad. Nowadays, most restaurants post their menus online, which can give you a sneak peak of what your menu options might be. You might also get an idea of whether or not they might be willing to prepare something special for you that's not on the menu.

To check the vegan friendliness of a restaurant, you can always call ahead or ask fellow vegans or vegetarians for recommendations of veg-friendly places. Calling ahead can be particularly helpful if your dining companions insist on going to a certain meat-oriented place and you have decided to go along anyway. If the kitchen staff is worth their salt, they'll be able to feed you something vegan, whether that's something already on the menu or something they have to create specially for you. Calling a day or even several hours in advance should be sufficient for most places to do this.

IN A NUTSHELL

For help locating veg-friendly places, check out happycow.net. This website contains tons of helpful pro-veg and healthy-eating information, and also includes great detailed listings of vegan and vegetarian restaurants and natural foods stores, broken down by region, country, state, and city.

Parties and Potlucks

Handling invitations to someone's house for dinner, a potluck, or other type of gathering is also cause for some contemplation. It's best to be honest with your host right away and address any concerns you may have. They may or may not know you're a vegan, much less what you do or do not eat. Try to stick to the basics: fully spell it out, but try to be tactful when inquiring about what they'll be serving and what may be suitable or available for you.

Again, prior notice is best, as your host probably won't appreciate having to scramble at the last minute to see if she has something more than a salad or handful of raw veggies to feed you. If you wait until the last minute, your host may have already tossed the salad with a nonvegan dressing or adorned it with cheese or bacon bits.

Offering to bring something of your own, with plenty to share, often works well and is usually appreciated. Bringing your own dish can also be a great way to show off how delicious eating vegan food can be. Many vegans enjoy "wowing" people with their vegan culinary creations, especially delicious desserts.

Hosting Your Own Gathering

After attending one too many get-togethers where you are the odd vegan out, you may be inspired to host your own all-vegan shindig. This is the best way to showcase the benefits of being vegan and all the wonderful culinary possibilities the lifestyle has to offer. Depending on your culinary talents, start with something simple like having a few friends or family over for dinner. Then if that goes well, try hosting a dinner party or a holiday meal made of several vegan courses.

Go for your tried-and-true recipes first, but if you get stuck for ideas, enlist the help of the recipes in Part 6, some vegan cookbooks, or the internet. Try the recipes for yourself first as sort of a practice run. This way, you'll know how they taste and look before trying something beyond your current level of culinary expertise. Remember, you want to impress your guests, not distress them.

This is also a great way to assure Mom and Grandma they can stop worrying that you'll waste away and starve to death eating a plant-based diet. You'll feel so empowered as a vegan while strutting your stuff, healthfully filling their bellies, and positively showcasing your new lifestyle. You may even open the lines of communication between yourself and those most opposed to or threatened by your being vegan. Many a mind has been swayed by a full stomach!

Advice for Holiday Get-Togethers

Holiday gatherings can cause headaches and squabbles on their own, but throw veganism into the mix, and you're looking at a whole new dimension. How you handle it could mean the difference between chaos and quality time.

Many holiday gatherings are associated with either family or cultural traditions, and most have eating involved somewhere in the festivities. In America, that often means meat and dairy foods are served.

> **IN A NUTSHELL**
>
> Whenever we're invited to a holiday gathering, we offer to bring something and often bring several little things. This ensures we'll eat as well as everyone else, and we also like to tantalize the other diners with some vegan treats. It also makes it easier for our "special diet" to not be a problem for our host, and it's a great way to open the eyes of others to the possibilities of meatless alternatives and substitutions.

The Meat in Front of You

Even though you may feel baited into it or you may just *want* to, resist the urge to condemn or negatively comment on the animal-based food that sits on the table. Remember, even though you don't want or need to eat it, someone did work very hard to prepare what they considered a good meal for their guests, and it would undoubtedly hurt their feelings to have you criticize their food during the meal. After all, you could have chosen not to take part in the meal to begin with, and you can always politely excuse yourself from the table if need be.

You can also try to situate yourself away from meat dishes and other such items, as well as from any arguments that may ensue during mealtime. Conflict is bad for relationships and everyone's digestion, and no matter how things go down, likely you will be blamed. After all, you are the vegan, and they may already view you as different. Don't give them any more ammunition to use against you by ruining the meal with your comments. If you want to talk about why you choose not to eat meat, wait until the right time—preferably away from the dinner table.

A Few Holiday Dining Tips

Many holiday meal traditions revolve around a roast of some sort, but that doesn't mean you can't start some new traditions of your own. You can make hearty casseroles and entrées from all-plant-based ingredients to replace meat-based offerings. A vegan lasagna, pot pie, or stuffed squash makes a wonderful centerpiece for a winter holiday meal, instead of Tom the Turkey or Babe the Pig.

As vegans, we're often asked what we eat for Thanksgiving instead of turkey. We eat most of the normal things, such as mashed potatoes, gravy, stuffing, and so on, in addition to whatever we choose to have as our main entrée. When you really think about it, the best part of the typical Thanksgiving dinner is all the trimmings and side dishes! Yams, with their vitamins A, C, and beta-carotene; mashed potatoes and stuffing full of complex carbohydrates; and cranberries bursting with all kinds of antioxidants are all foods that give you energy. Sure, turkey has protein, but it also contains tryptophan, which tends to knock you out after the big meal instead of revving you up.

IN A NUTSHELL

If you want to really impress your guests, make Harvest Stuffed Pumpkin. Combine bread stuffing, cooked grains, sautéed onions, celery, and apples, and season as you would your favorite stuffing recipe. Pack the mixture into a hollowed-out pumpkin (the kind for eating, not carving) and bake at 350°F for 1 hour or more or until the pumpkin is tender. Place it on a large platter and serve the stuffing, as well as the pumpkin flesh, to your hungry guests. It looks impressive, tastes delicious, and will win you some rave reviews!

"May I Take Your Order?"

When it comes to dining out as a vegan, the first bit of advice we can offer you is don't be intimidated. If you're lucky, you'll have a vegan, vegetarian, or veg-friendly establishment to frequent. Check your local paper and phone book for possible options, as well as online sources. If you have any vegan or vegetarian friends, ask them for some good restaurant recommendations, too.

Eugene, Oregon, where we live, has several all-vegan or vegetarian restaurants, and vegans who live here feel so fortunate. Most establishments and people in the community are familiar with the terms *vegan* and *vegetarian*, which means we don't have to give a long explanation every time we mention we're vegans.

But living in such a progressive community is not the norm for most newbie vegans. If you live in a community without *veg-friendly* places to eat, you'll have to make full use of your vegan survival skills.

> **DEFINITION**
>
> If an establishment is **veg-friendly,** the owners or employees understand the basics of vegan and vegetarian dietary guidelines and philosophies and provide appropriate options.

Begin by assuming that when you go to a restaurant, you'll have to spend some time looking over the menu if you haven't already checked it out online ahead of time. First, look to see if the menu has a vegetarian section or selections. If it does, you're in luck, as it's usually very easy to leave off cheeses and other dairy products used as garnishes to accommodate vegan tastes. If not, check for salad and side-dish options you can combine to create your own vegan meal.

Server Suggestions

After looking over the menu, your server is a helpful ally. Be very friendly and polite as you ask your server for help. First let him know you're a vegan and don't eat any meat or dairy products as well as eggs, gelatin, and honey. He may or may not be familiar with veganism, so it will only benefit you in the long run to spell out your exact dietary no-no's.

Don't be afraid to ask your server for any menu suggestions. You can ask how things are prepared and what ingredients are in a specific dish, especially some that may be hidden or not obvious from the menu description. If he doesn't know, ask if he would be so kind as to check with the chef for further clarification. A little checking ahead of time can save having to send something back that you aren't able to eat, and more importantly, prevent you from ingesting hidden animal products.

> **IN A NUTSHELL**
>
> If you tend to dine out a lot, you may want to write out a card listing the foods you avoid as a vegan and pass it to the chef or cook via your server when ordering. Nothing ruins a good evening faster than an unexpected bout with lactose intolerance!

On the Lookout for Hidden Ingredients

Being a vegan means staying on your toes, especially when you have to rely on others to eat. When cooking for yourself, you know exactly what ingredients you used and how you prepared the food. But when dining out, you don't exactly have access to a precise ingredients list or know the path your food followed on its way to your plate. As a vegan dining out at a nonvegan restaurant, you must be aware of the possibility of hidden animal ingredients in your food.

Some servers easily overlook the chicken broth used to cook the rice, the sprinkle of cheese, or the added dollop of sour cream when attesting that the offering is suitable for a vegan. So use a little common sense. If the name of the recipe includes *fromage*, *au gratin*, *Alfredo*, or *cream* of this or that, it probably contains dairy or cheese.

When in doubt, ask what exact ingredients are in the dish. Be polite and friendly because you don't want your server to think you're difficult, or he may just start telling you what he thinks you want to hear just to appease you. If you discover there really isn't anything suitable for a vegan on the menu, you can find out if the kitchen would be able to prepare something special for you. Often, you can make an impromptu entrée by combining vegetable side dishes with grains or pasta.

"Service" Is Their Middle Name

Don't forget, it's called the food *service* industry, and service is and should be their middle name and a big part of what they do. Restaurants are there to serve you, the customer, and any decent establishment should have a chef or cook who is able to whip up something special with a little advance notice and instruction. And for many, this allows the chef to be creative and deviate from the standard menu items. Prior notice gives them a better chance of serving you something spectacular instead of just plain boiled or steamed veggies and white rice.

Hopefully, these tips will help make your dining experiences pleasant ones, as they should be. Be sure to let your waiter know if you were satisfied, ask him to give your compliments to the chef, and be sure to reward his efforts with a generous tip or a kudos to the manager on his behalf. Working in food service is extremely hard work and often goes underappreciated. Waiters remember who gave them a generous tip, who gave them an adequate tip, and who was a cheapskate. If you frequent a place often, you'll become recognized. If you're known as being generous, their level and quality of service will likely know no bounds.

Dining Expectations

Of course, eating at an all-vegan restaurant is the ideal dining experience for a vegan. The first time you eat at one, you'll feel incredibly spoiled, being able to peruse the menu knowing you can order anything and not worry about what may or may not be lurking in the dish. It's pure bliss. But you can't always be so lucky as to have even one completely vegan restaurant in your area.

The type of establishment you dine at can greatly influence your chances of having a satisfactory vegan meal. The level of service and experience of the kitchen staff varies greatly from restaurant to restaurant, and you can expect this to be reflected in your choice of selections, means of preparations, possibilities of substitutions, and encounters with hidden ingredients.

> **IN A NUTSHELL**
>
> Some restaurants gladly share ingredient lists, especially when special diets are an issue. It's helpful to call ahead of your arrival, at a nonbusy time, to fully address all your specific questions and concerns.

Fine Dining

Most people who are not independently wealthy can only afford to eat at fine-dining restaurants—you know, those places that have several stars to their credit—on special occasions or when the boss is treating. Such restaurants usually have tons of animal-based dishes on their menus, but some are becoming more progressive and offering vegetarian, vegan, and even raw meals or "tastings," as they're currently being called.

If a fine-dining restaurant is on top of its game, it will try to stay up on the latest food trends, and plant-based dishes are becoming the in thing lately. If the menu doesn't offer something suitable, someone in the kitchen might be able to whip up something vegan and delicious for you. Expect that your creation may take a little longer to arrive at your table, so be patient and appreciative, remembering it's being specially prepared for you.

Speaking of food trends, another growing trend in the restaurant biz is including Meatless Monday specials on the menu. Meatless Monday is a grassroots campaign based on the voluntary meatless days encouraged by Presidents Wilson, Truman, and Roosevelt during both world wars. The purpose of this campaign is to encourage people to avoid eating meat on Mondays because just cutting out meat once a week can have far-reaching effects, both for your health and for the planet. Many restaurateurs have publicly embraced the Meatless Monday message, including Mario Batali, who insists that every one of his 14 restaurants serve at least two vegetarian options each Monday.

> **HOT POTATO**
>
> You'd think wine, made from grapes, would be vegan, but that's not always the case. Clarifying agents, used to remove cloudiness as well as yeast and other substances from the wine, are often of animal origin. One example is isinglass, a gelatin made from the swimming bladder of fish. Fortunately, many manufacturers produce vegan wine. One all-vegan, added-sulfite-free brand of wine is Frey Vineyards (freywine.com).

The Average American Sit-Down Place

Eating at the average American sit-down restaurant can prove to be a bit tricky for vegans. First, check to see if it serves any vegetarian offerings that could easily have the dairy or eggs omitted. If not, check the salads and side dishes for possibilities.

Use your common sense, though, when deciding what a safe vegan option is. For instance, if they have fried fish or chicken on the menu, there's a good chance that the french fries you ordered will be fried in the same oil, in the same fryer. Or the hash browns could possibly be cooked on the grill next to some meat item. The same goes for a veggie burger, or anything fried or grilled. Some vegans request that their veggie burger or veggies be cooked in a skillet or the microwave just to eliminate the possibility of coming into contact with meat.

Salads without dressing and plain baked potatoes are usually safe choices. A drizzle or two of olive oil or a squeeze of lemon makes a tasty vegan addition not only to your salad but to your potato as well. Some margarines, especially those small, individual serving packaged varieties, often contain casein, whey, or some other dairy-derived ingredient, so don't automatically consider them a dairy-free option. And of course, be sure to read their ingredients label.

White and brown rice are usually fine, but check for the addition of butter. Most restaurants usually don't have a problem steaming, sautéing, or oven-roasting some veggies for you, so don't be afraid to ask even if it isn't listed on the menu. When in doubt about how something is prepared, ask the waiter to ask the kitchen staff. Better safe than sorry!

The Global Diner

Certain types of cuisine are more veg-friendly than others. We find that many Italian, Mexican, Chinese, Japanese, Mediterranean, and Middle Eastern restaurants seem to be more accommodating of vegan diets and offer many traditional vegan or vegetarian dishes to begin with. You still might have to ask for the cheese or dairy to be left off as a garnish or sauce, and remember to inquire about whether or not an item has any other animal ingredients that aren't obvious.

Vegans do need to be careful when dining on Thai or Indian food because they like to use ghee, which is clarified butter, or fish sauce to add flavor to their dishes.

You should also keep in mind that the means of preparation attributed to a certain cuisine or style of cooking may determine if you will actually be served a vegan meal or one with a few meat remnants from the meal cooked before or beside yours.

Feasting on Fast Foods

Eating on the go seems to be becoming more and more the norm for an increasing number of us, and it's often the result of trying to fit too much into our everyday lives. That's why many Americans are turning to fast food on a weekly, and for some, a daily basis. And no wonder; fast-food joints are everywhere you turn, and their advertising on TV, radio, and online is relentless. Many of the more popular and heavily advertised franchises have locations across the globe, in remote places, with much the same menu as the one just down the street.

Unfortunately, these major fast-food chains have very little to offer vegans or the health conscious. Their menu selections are made of mostly meat and dairy-oriented foods and contain lots of simple carbohydrates; fried and heavily processed foods; and excessive amounts of fat, salt, and sugar. To say that the fruit and veggie options are limited is a massive understatement. Eating too many fast-food meals could easily lead you down the path to poor health and obesity.

There's really no reason why nutritious, whole vegan foods can't be served quickly and healthily to fit in with people's busy lives. Look for fast-food places that offer build-your-own options; this allows you more control over what goes in your meal, and you can load up on the items you like best.

Another fast meal option is to hit the grab-and-go section of your local natural foods store. Many sell prepared salads, sandwiches, soups, and main and side dishes.

Fortunately, the food service industry is responding to customer's requests for more veg-friendly options, and as a result, several vegan and vegetarian fast-food-type restaurants have already opened throughout the United States and elsewhere. Hopefully more will follow.

Eating on the Road

It can be challenging to be vegan in familiar surroundings like your home, your town, and your workplace, but being on the road can take that challenge to a whole new level! Suddenly, you are without your safety nets—your trusty natural foods store, your refrigerator packed full of nutritious and delicious vegan foods, and your local restaurants where you know exactly what's suitable to order and what isn't.

As a vegan, finding yourself in a strange town where you don't know the veg-friendly establishments can be a bit intimidating … unless you plan ahead and take some precautions.

Planning Ahead

One of the best things you can do as a traveling vegan is to research your destination town or city before your trip. You can go online and find a list of vegan, vegetarian, or veg-friendly restaurants, natural foods stores, and even bed and breakfasts in the vicinity.

If you happen to be flying to your destination, call the airline and ask about vegan meal options available for your flight. Several of the major airlines do offer vegan, vegetarian, kosher, and other special meals on request. Just be sure to request your meal ahead of time because if you wait until you're already on the plane to think of it, it will be too late.

Packing Your Own Food

Bringing your own food with you can be a real lifesaver in the event that you aren't able to find something vegan-suitable on the road, in the air, or at your destination. You could easily find yourself stuck with only a few pieces of iceberg lettuce or a carrot stick at a restaurant or at the mercy of the fast-food restaurants prevalent at most rest areas, terminals, depots, and stations.

Consider packing food items that are portable, easy to eat, and will provide you with something nutritious to hold you over until your next meal. If you have an insulated lunch bag, you could make some veggie wraps or sandwiches, a big salad, or even a hearty noodle or rice dish with lots of veggies. Just throw in a cold pack or some ice to keep things cool. Another great-tasting and filling option that doesn't require refrigeration is the classic PB&J (or other nut butter–and–fruit spread sandwich). Make it on some whole-grain bread to boost its nutritional content.

Be sure to pack a few pieces of fresh vegetables such as carrots or celery sticks, or a piece of fruit like an apple, pear, or banana. These will give you energy and help boost your immune system as you travel. It's also a good idea to pack some easy-munching snacks, such as nuts, seeds, raisins, trail mix, crackers, pretzels, or rice cakes. You can make up your own small containers or buy them in small packages through natural foods stores. If you include some items such as protein and nutrition bars, granola bars, fruit leather snacks, and a few juice boxes or bottles of water, you'll be ready for just about anything!

The Least You Need to Know

- Preparing your own meals—and creating a space in the kitchen for your vegan ingredients, foods, and cookware—can make it easier for a vegan to live in a meat-eating household.

- Bringing a tasty vegan dish or two of your own to a gathering can be a great way to ensure you'll have something vegan and nutritious to eat—and might entice nonvegans to open their mouths (and minds!).

- Mealtime isn't a good time to argue about vegan issues, even if you're baited by others; try to save any debating for a more appropriate time.

- Explaining your vegan dietary restrictions to a server or cook can make your dining experience in a nonvegan restaurant more successful and enjoyable.

- When traveling, it's wise to research vegan options in your destination city ahead of time, and be sure to bring along some convenient and nutritious food just in case.

Buying Your Vegan Eats

Chapter

15

In This Chapter

* Buying your vegan bounty
* Making a difference with organics
* Super shopping tips
* Snacking and satisfying your sweet tooth

Being vegan means putting your beliefs and compassion into action through the things you do, wear, say, and eat. It's a way of approaching the world around you and can certainly have a great influence on what you buy and who you buy it from.

Supporting those businesses, individuals, and products that most closely embody and support your values as a vegan can be a way to make your presence known and your economic influence felt. When it comes to the way you spend your money on goods and services, your actions could end up making a world of difference to everyone involved.

Where and How to Shop

Your money, and how you choose to use it, is quite important. Informed vegan consumers who spend their dollars wisely can have a huge effect on the kinds of products manufactured, as well as the kinds of companies that become, and remain, successful. Consumers don't just greatly affect the market; they *are* the market. And if enough of them want to, they can help effect positive change for animals through the way they approach shopping.

Think of each dollar you spend as a vote for the product you're buying and for the merchant you're buying it from. Choose to support shops and businesses that more closely reflect and support your vegan ideals first and foremost, especially the small independent companies that need you as a loyal customer to stay competitive against the big corporations.

You can also make statements with your purchases by not supporting certain businesses or large retailers that support animal cruelty and the use of resulting products, in addition to employing unfair and child labor practices. For vegans, showing compassion and opposing the abuse and suffering of others is extended to fellow human beings as well, and not just members of the animal kingdom.

Take a look around your local grocery, and you'll be amazed at the number of foods on your supermarket shelves that are vegan and you didn't even know it. Your local market may even stock organic produce next to the conventional produce, although they may have a limited number of organic and vegan product selections in other areas. That's where a natural foods store can be your best bet.

Check your phone book or online. Most large towns and cities have at least one natural foods store somewhere in the vicinity. As you'll soon learn, natural foods stores have a larger selection of products that fall within your new dietary guidelines. You'll undoubtedly discover vegan products you didn't even know existed—as well as those you couldn't have imagined in your wildest vegan fantasies! Shredded meltable cheeses, vegan marshmallows, organic peanut butter cups, whipped toppings, coconut-based ice creams, chickenless nuggets, and even soy jerky are just a few of the vegan products available from coast to coast.

You may be lucky enough to have a natural foods cooperative, or co-op, in your area. A co-op is a not-for-profit organization of members, usually families, who join together to combine their purchasing power and share the labor of purchasing, displaying, and storing items. The main idea is to buy in bulk and share in the costs and savings. Becoming a member of a co-op gives you access to foods and products you normally wouldn't be able to find in your area, and at a reduced rate. If you have the opportunity to join a co-op, by all means do so!

If no natural foods stores are nearby, have no fear—the internet can help. You can find many different sources for purchasing items to stock your vegan pantry or fulfill your personal or household needs online, as well as learn where you can find a particular product or service in your area. Just use your favorite search engine to get started, and see Appendix B for some great website suggestions.

IN A NUTSHELL

Three of the most popular online vegan merchants are veganessentials.com, veganstore.com, and differentdaisy.com. Each has a wide assortment of vegan products, from snacks to clothing to supplements—even vegan marshmallows and marshmallow fluff, doughnuts, or the ever-elusive vegan gelatin!

When shopping, whether you're in the grocery store or a natural foods store, start in the produce section. Here you'll find the best sources of good, wholesome, plant-based foods and a large selection of fresh and dried fruits and vegetables in all shapes, colors, and textures. Many stores also feature specials or discounted produce sections, so use these to your advantage.

Another good tip is to buy fruits and veggies when they're in season and abundant. Not only will they taste better, they'll also be more affordable. And of course, opt for organic over conventionally grown produce whenever possible.

After checking out the produce section, move on to filling your dry goods and pantry needs.

Always make your freezer and refrigerated selections last. You don't want these items exposed to room temperature for any longer than they need to be, and you don't want to risk spoilage or other problems that arise from refreezing. Keep in mind your transit time, especially in warm summer months, and consider keeping a cooler in your trunk to carry frozen or refrigerated foods home in. Fewer dangers are associated with improperly refrigerated veggie-based items than with meat-based ones, but you still need to be conscious of these things, especially when it may result in the unthinkable: a half-melted carton of your favorite nondairy ice cream.

Organics: The Natural Way

One of the best things you can do for yourself, your family, and the environment is to support organic farming practices and purchase organic and non–genetically modified products whenever possible. Better sustainability of crops and gentler use of the land is better for farmers and for you. No pesticides or chemical fertilizers used on crops means none are passed on to you or the environment. Choose organics, and you're choosing wise, Earth-friendly agricultural practices over widespread pesticide usage and environmental harm.

By purchasing organic products whenever possible, you can use your purchasing power to vote in favor of the organic approach to farming and sustaining ourselves, while voting against polluting the earth, and your body, with dangerous chemicals and pesticides.

Purchasing organic over conventionally grown produce is optimal, but not always viable or practical, especially for those on a tight budget. To aid you in your picking and choosing, the Environmental Working Group has compiled lists of produce with the most and least pesticide residues. The "Dirty Dozen" list includes apples, celery, strawberries, peaches, spinach, nectarines, grapes, bell peppers, potatoes, blueberries, lettuce, and kale/collards. We recommend buying organic of these items because their conventional counterparts often have high levels of pesticide residues. The "Clean Fifteen" tend to have fewer traces of pesticides, and this list includes onions, corn, pineapples, avocado, asparagus, peas, mangoes, eggplant, cantaloupe, kiwi, cabbage, watermelon, sweet potatoes, grapefruit, and mushrooms.

> **IN A NUTSHELL**
>
> Don't be put off by slightly higher prices for organic goods. The extra money you spend on organic food now saves you many more times that money in the future, in the form of prevented medical bills arising from conditions caused by exposure to pesticides and chemical fertilizers. Look at it as a wise investment in your future health!

Shopping at Natural Foods Stores

Natural foods stores or health-food stores are places of wonderment and havens for vegans, vegetarians, and those who have to follow special diets. Natural foods stores have really come a long way in the last 30 years in terms of selection, pricing, and availability of goods and services, and as a result, they now make up a multibillion-dollar-a-year industry. Many stores started out as supplement stores and juice joints and then branched out to include produce as well as personal- and home-care products.

One of the best ways to judge the caliber of a natural foods store is by what it more prominently features: food items or supplements. Those stores that emphasize food first for good health and supplementation second as a backup are the true gems of the industry and should be your first choice for where to shop.

A good natural foods store provides customers with all the ingredients necessary for sustaining themselves as healthfully as possible, and in return, has loyal, healthy, repeat customers, not those who just come back for a refill of pills every so often.

Shopping at natural foods stores has several advantages over shopping at your local supermarket:

- A larger selection of organic products

- Fresher all-organic or mostly organic produce sections

- More support of local produce and products

- A wider selection of vegan and vegetarian alternative products

- A more expansive and inclusive bulk section

Natural foods stores stock many meat and dairy alternative products that can assist you in preparing your vegan meals. Check the package labels for ingredients, and analyze the nutritional information when comparing brands if you have an option. Of course, seek out organic products and ingredients whenever possible.

Natural foods stores also stock packaged foods such as veggie pizzas; vegan meals; meat alternative products; nondairy frozen desserts and novelties; and frozen fruits, vegetables, and juices, just to name a few. All these products can make transitioning easier and come in handy when you come home hungry and too tired to cook.

Some stores may also give you a discount, usually 5 or 10 percent, if you purchase a product by the case. Call in advance to ask about whether or not a store offers case discounts and check availability. The store might even be able to order you a case of a product you don't see on the shelves if it has more products available via distributors than it has shelf space for.

Savvy Vegan Shopping Tips

Now that you have some ideas on where and how to shop as a vegan, it's time to learn how to be a wise vegan food shopper. Some people dread shopping for groceries, but it can actually be quite fun, with so many different vegan products available on the shelves as well as a never-ending supply of products you may have never even known existed. Be an informed consumer when you go shopping. Know what you came for and what you like and dislike, buy from companies and stores you like and trust, take advantage of sales or use coupons, and don't let fancy packaging mislead you.

Be sure to read all packaging to know what you're actually getting and paying for. When purchasing packaged foods, start by reading the label. Some companies that market to the natural foods community clearly note on the label if their foods are vegan, low in fat or sugar, wheat or gluten free, nut free, or dairy free. It really makes your shopping process easier and quicker when products are already labeled vegan or in a similar manner. Let's get ready to go shopping, vegans!

Veggie Wonderland

Most conventional grocery stores have fairly large produce sections but generally only have a small area containing organic produce. You'll find just the opposite at natural foods stores. Most carry all-organic or mostly organic produce, and many stock seasonal and specialty items you may not find anywhere else in your area. It really is like a veggie wonderland for a vegan!

Many natural foods stores stock locally grown produce when it's available. If you have a farmers' market in your area, shop there first for your produce needs and then move on to your local natural foods or grocery store. Buying produce from local sources means getting the freshest and best quality, as well as contributing to the livelihood of the small farmers in your community. Foods taste their best when eaten in season and picked at their peak of ripeness and not long before. Prices are usually more affordable at those times as well.

As you learned in Chapter 9, it's best to eat a wide variety of fruits and veggies in a rainbow of colors to ensure you're getting enough sources of the mighty antioxidants and phytochemicals in your diet. Strolling through a well-stocked farmers' market or produce department makes this all very easy because you should find a wide assortment of colors and textures to choose from there. Taking it all in, visually, can fill you with wonder and excitement. It can also give you some ideas about what you might want to eat for your next meal. Go with what looks good and is affordable, and build the rest of your meal around that.

Wholesome Whole Grains

Vegan or otherwise, consuming and purchasing wholesome products whenever possible is a good rule to follow. Choose cereals, grain dishes, snacks, baked goods, and dessert items made with whole grains and not heavily refined ingredients. Whole-grain items contain the entire seed or kernel of the grain, with all the important nutrients and fiber still intact.

Eat grains either in whole, cracked, split, or ground forms. Look for the words *whole grain* on the label, and seek out products, especially breads, that contain 100 percent whole-grain ingredients to ensure you're getting all the nutritional benefits. Manufacturers often also use molasses or other natural sweeteners, which are better choices for your health and your body than high-fructose corn syrup and bleached sugars.

You'll find multigrain products—those made from a mixture of grains—on the shelves of most stores. They're a great way to increase your consumption of grains such as amaranth, buckwheat, barley, or rye, which most of us consume rarely if ever at all. However, keep in mind that many whole-grain baked goods and breads contain no preservatives or artificial additives and are more susceptible to attracting mold. Such items last longer if stored in your refrigerator.

Sprouted-grain products like breads, crackers, and other baked goods are also becoming more popular and readily available. Grains are soaked, rinsed, and sprouted; grinded together; and processed and baked accordingly. Sprouting increases and retains the availability of vital nutrients such as vitamins, minerals, amino acids, and digestive enzymes, which help keep your body functioning as smoothly and efficiently as it should. Sprouted-grain products tend to have more protein, fiber, and complex carbohydrates than other grain products.

Ezekiel 4:9 bread by Food for Life is a commercially available organic sprouted-grain bread made from a mixture of sprouted whole grains and beans such as barley, millet, wheat, spelt, soybeans, lentils, and others. The bread, based on a Bible verse, is full of complex carbohydrates and protein to sustain you. If you're feeling a little adventurous and want to try making your own sprouted-grain bread, look for recipes online.

> **VEGAN VOICES**
>
> Take thou also unto thee wheat, and barley, and beans, and [lentils], and millet, and fitches, and put them in one vessel, and make thee bread thereof, according to the number of the days that thou shalt lie upon thy side, three hundred and ninety days shalt thou eat thereof.
>
> —Ezekiel 4:9 (King James Version)

Buying in Bulk

Being able to purchase items in bulk quantities from bins is one of the best things about shopping at natural foods stores. Buying in bulk is good for you and the environment. It's good for you because you often pay a third to half of the price for the same product out of a bulk bin as you would in packaged form. Check the quality of bulk items, as with any ingredient you use, to ensure freshness and turnover rate.

Many stores offer paper or plastic bags for dry goods or encourage you to bring your own. They might also sell containers to use for bulk liquid and solid ingredients such as oils, nut butters, and syrups. Buy in useable-size quantities to prevent spoilage and to keep from overstocking your pantry. However, if it's something you use often, and you have room for it, then by all means stock up on those 10-pound bags of organic brown rice and quinoa!

Buying in bulk saves you money because it helps manufacturers reduce packaging and advertising costs, in addition to cutting down on the store's cost expended and shelf space needed for restocking. The conservation of packaging materials has a ripple effect on our environment: buying items with little or no packaging means less waste added to our landfills and less petrochemicals used in the creation of environmentally unfriendly packaging. Many organic product manufacturers prefer to use Earth-friendly packaging materials, including recycled paper and soy-based (instead of petroleum-based) inks for their labels.

Deciphering Food Labels

When buying any packaged product, whether it's a box of veggie burgers or a bag of chips, be sure to read the ingredient list. Items are listed by their volume as contained within the product, from largest to smallest. If you see whole-wheat flour listed first, you know there's more whole-wheat flour in the item than any other ingredient. If salt is listed last, salt is the least used ingredient by volume.

Use these tips to know what to look for—and what to avoid—on a label. Look for the word *organic* before as many ingredients as possible. Favor foods that contain whole grains, unrefined sweeteners, and other wholesome ingredients. Avoid partially hydrogenated or hydrogenated oils whenever possible, and instead look for cold-pressed or expeller-pressed oils. (We discuss proper oil choices and the reasons behind them in Chapter 17.)

Watch out for animal ingredients in the most unlikely foods. Manufacturers use gelatin; eggs; dairy products such as cheese, butter, and casein; and animal-based broths and oils in many packaged foods. Whey, the liquid that results from cheese-making, is also a commonly used flavor enhancer. It is a cheap way for food manufacturers to give foods a creamy or cheesy flavor.

Natural flavorings is actually a catch-all term used in ingredient lists to hide secret blends of herbs and spices or other ingredients. These "natural flavorings" can be from animal- or plant-based sources, and this phrase on a label can be very tricky for vegans. When you see it among the ingredients, don't buy the product unless you know the natural flavorings are vegan in origin. When in doubt, call or email the manufacturer to ask whether or not its natural flavorings are suitable for vegans.

In fact, when you wonder about any ingredient or aspect of a product, contact the manufacturer and ask about it. Most are usually happy to clear up any confusion about their products and answer your questions, particularly if they can put your mind at ease about animal products being involved, and gain or keep a customer in the process.

Enriched foods can also contain animal-based sources of nutrients. As mentioned in Chapter 10, the supplement form of vitamin D_3 used to fortify foods is only derived from animal-based sources. So if you see vitamin D_3 or cholecalciferol listed on your box of fortified breakfast cereal, it definitely isn't vegan (look for D_2 or ergocalciferol instead).

Avoid ingredients you don't recognize or can't understand because they're usually synthetic chemical additives, artificial preservatives, or other ingredients that are far from wholesome and natural. Avoid artificial colorings and flavorings, too. Many are not only derived from animal sources, but may be actually harmful to your health and have been linked to various health problems.

It can also be easier to avoid bad ingredients if you buy all organic or mostly organic packaged foods because they tend to be free of these unwanted and controversial additives.

HOT POTATO

Beware of foods that have been dyed red, as they may contain ground-up bugs! Carmine, also known as carminic acid and cochineal extract, is a red dye made from ground cochineal beetles. These beetles eat prickly pears and other cacti and absorb and concentrate their bright red juices in their bodies. The red dye is used to color lipsticks and other makeup, candy and confections, baked goods, maraschino cherries, spreads, juices, and other products. This takes finding a bug in your food to a whole new level!

Finally, check the sugar, fat, and sodium contents for an individual serving. Some manufacturers try to fool you into thinking their product is better for you than it actually is by considering a serving size an unrealistically small amount no one would actually limit him- or herself to in one sitting. Be sure to multiply the fat content and other nutritional aspects by the amount of servings in the item to get the full picture of what you'd consume.

Helping Hands: Convenience Items

Once you go vegan, you're really going to be inspired by the foods you eat. And if you don't already cook for yourself, be prepared for that to change very soon, out of sheer necessity if nothing else. Unless you live in L.A., New York, or some other large veg-friendly city and can afford to dine out at veggie restaurants for all your meals, you're going to have to learn to cook. Cooking for yourself is essential to vegan survival. Don't be intimidated. Just get some cookbooks or go online for some recipes, and dive right in!

If entering your kitchen seems foreign to you or feels a little like entering a lab with all its gadgets, metal, hard surfaces, and sharp utensils, then start small with simple dishes such as soups, salads, sandwiches, one-pot meals, or pasta. Don't be afraid of trial and error because experimenting can often be very rewarding. Even if your finished product seems to border on the inedible, remind yourself that it's vegan and you made it yourself!

Not everyone can work quickly in the kitchen or has time for making every meal from scratch on a daily basis. With our hectic lifestyles, it's understandable and even practical to have some packaged foods in your pantry, refrigerator, or freezer. There's nothing wrong with using a few helping-hand convenience items now and again. They can help you eat a nutritious and healthy vegan snack or meal—not a fast-food meal—during a busy workweek or weekday schedule. Remember then, when you have more time, to prepare for yourself some homemade vegan foods and goodies from scratch.

In this chapter and in Part 5, we share recommendations to help stock your pantry, refrigerator, and freezer with delicious and nutritious vegan food items. To start you out slowly, we begin with quick-fix ideas to help you through your transition into eating as a vegan on a daily basis. Applying all your newfound vegan nutritional advice immediately to your daily diet may seem intimidating at first, but it shouldn't be. Just take it meal by meal, and day by day.

IN A NUTSHELL

Veg-friendly companies with a conscience do exist! Here are some of our favorite companies: Eden Foods, Road's End Organics, Amy's, Purity Foods, Small Planet, Lumen Foods, Westbrae Naturals, Annie's Naturals, Green & Black's, Wildwood, Turtle Mountain, Endangered Species Chocolate Company, and Plamil. Look for them in your natural foods store. In Part 5, you learn more about how to specifically use some vegan food items that may be new to you, like dairy and meat replacements, in addition to picking up some easy vegan baking tips.

Boxes and Mixes

So what kinds of quick-fix vegan foods can you expect to find on your store's shelves to make your life easier? Starting with breakfast, you can find boxed and bulk dry cold and hot cereals that are full of hearty whole grains, nuts, seeds, and dried fruits. You can also discover, in mix and boxed forms, vegan baked goods such as quick breads, muffins, cornbread, cookies, and cakes. Some stores even offer these types of mixes in gluten- and sugar-free varieties as well.

For lunch and dinner, try boxed and bulk grain, rice, and pasta selections. Natural meals-in-a-cup or -bowl are also available, made with grains or pasta, veggies, beans or tofu, and a sauce, which are great starts for lunches and light meals. You can find seitan mixes, veggie burgers, and soy-based loaves and sandwich fixings in boxes and bulk, too. These enable you to quickly whip up your own semi-homemade creations.

Shortcut Ingredients

You can also buy precooked ingredients to help speed up your meal production time. Organic canned goods run the gamut from plain cooked beans, seasoned beans, and veggies, to soups, veg-based chilies, and mock meat products. These can really come in handy when you're short on time but still want to eat something healthful.

> **HOT POTATO**
>
> When using precooked or packaged foods, be sure to read the ingredient and nutrition facts labels, and be conscious of sodium levels. Many prepared canned goods contain rather large amounts of sodium per serving. Drain and rinse canned beans to remove any brining liquid and its excess sodium before cooking.

Look for bottled sauces and condiments that can turn simple vegetables and grains into exotic coconut curries, tempting teriyaki stir-fries, or new twists on comfort food. Using canned tomato products and sauces, many of which come preseasoned and in a wide variety of flavors, paired with your additions of veggies, beans, or mock meats, requires very short simmering times but can give you the same rich flavors of slow-cooked meals.

Also check your produce department for precut and prewashed fruits and veggies. If cutting and chopping aren't your favorite tasks and often keep you from eating better, then by all means, pay a little extra to have someone else do it for you.

In the produce department, you'll also find bags of prewashed organic greens, lettuces, and salad mixes, all of which come in a variety of blends and make salad munching so amazingly easy. They not only make meal preparations easier; they also help ensure you incorporate more fresh produce into your daily diet. Use them quickly because fruits and veggies become more perishable as more surfaces are cut and exposed to air and light.

If the store has a salad bar, you can often find precut vegetables, marinated or cooked vegetables, olives, and small amounts of greens, sprouts, and other assorted ingredients you can use in your recipes. When you buy off the salad bar, you can often get the exact amount of a veggie you need and with no labor involved on your part. With a quick stroll down the aisle, you can have the makings of a great stir-fry or veggie burrito in no time.

> **IN A NUTSHELL**
>
> If you don't like to use canned goods, why not cook large amounts of foods, divide them into useable portions, and freeze them? You can do this with beans, grains and pasta, veggies, fruits, sauces, spreads, soups, stews, and casseroles. Putting a little extra aside for another time takes very little effort, and you'll thank yourself when you're in need of a quick, healthful meal and don't have the time to prepare it from scratch.

Prepared Deli and Grab-and-Go Items

As an ever-increasing and expanding part of the retail market, more and more grocery and natural foods stores are including in-store bakeries and delis. If your local store has these, check to see what whole-grain breads and vegan baked goods may be available. Most natural foods stores have a larger selection and more options for you and your wallet. A hearty bread can make for some great morning toast with jam, as the base of an awesome sandwich with a yummy spread and tons of veggies, or a juicy portobello mushroom sandwich or veggie burger.

For those who have little confidence in their baking skills or who may have food allergies, the bakery in your natural foods store could be an eye-opening experience. Following the current food trends, many stores are developing new products to suit vegans, special diets, and food allergies. You should be able to find cookies, cakes, pies, and other baked goods, and some even accept special orders to alter recipes to fit your specific needs. Just ask at the counter if you don't see something vegan that suits your taste.

Some stores have even developed their own lines of prepared grab-and-go items, which you can usually find in either the store's deli section or with the other refrigerated items. These can be anything from prepared sandwiches, salads, spreads, side dishes, and main dishes, to entire meals. It's kind of like a healthier version of fast food! Many of these items are made with all-natural and organic ingredients—you can't find that in the average burger joint.

Packaged Refrigerated and Frozen Items

After checking for fresh options in the deli area of your local grocery or natural foods store, be sure to check for vegan foods in the refrigerated and frozen-foods sections. In addition to premade meal items, you can find vegan dairy substitutes; beverages; mock meats of all kinds; vegan mayonnaise substitutes; vegan puddings; and other condiments, oils, and refrigerated products.

Look in the freezer section for frozen harvested delights such as organic juices, berries and cut fruits, vegetables, and mixed blends. Organic food companies are now even marketing such foods as french fries, onion rings, and tater tots, and many stores stock them. Freezing captures a food's freshness, halts its decay, and, barring any mishaps in the freezing process, helps it retain more of its nutrients. These frozen items can help you whip up a delicious smoothie, toss together a stir-fry, or round out your plate with a veggie option.

Vegan products are often stocked in specialty areas or right next to their animal-based counterparts in many conventional supermarkets. Check for frozen waffles, veggie burgers, soy sausages, veggie burritos, appetizers, and specialty dessert items near their nonvegan counterparts. You can also find many vegan meal-type foods such as noodle or grain bowls with veggies, heat-and-serve entrées, frozen vegan pizzas, and even frozen holiday alternatives like mock turkey with all the vegan fixings.

Last, but certainly not least, you can find vegan versions of ice cream in the freezer cases of your natural foods store and even some regular grocers. Just because you go vegan doesn't mean you have to give up your sundaes and ice-cream cones! Many stores carry several types of nondairy frozen desserts to choose from, including sorbets; soy, rice, coconut, hemp, and even a few nut-based nondairy ice creams; and other frozen treats.

In the freezer cases, you should be able to find at least one type of vegan sorbet, produced by manufacturers such as Howler, Natural Choice, Double Rainbow, Turtle Mountain, and Cascadian Farms. You'll also find one or more of the following brands of nondairy ice cream: Soy Cream, So Delicious, Purely Decadent, Rice Dream, Soy Dream, Almond Dream, Whole Soy Cultured Soy Yogurt, Coconut Bliss, Tempt, Wheeler's Black Label, and Tofutti. You can also find all sorts of frozen vegan novelty treats as well, like frozen chocolate-covered bananas, ice-cream bars of all varieties, fudgey frozen bar treats, fruit bars, ice-cream sandwiches, and even ice-cream cookie sandwiches.

When purchasing packaged refrigerated and frozen foods, be sure to read the labels before you buy. Look for wholesome and organic ingredients in the list, and check sodium, sugar, and fat contents. This greatly helps you make smarter choices for fueling your engine. It really does pay to put the best-quality foods into your body if you want to get positive results out of it in the form of good health and vitality.

Smart Snacking

Most people love to munch on a little something here and there throughout the day. It's only natural. In fact, nutritionists say it's fine to snack on the right foods at the right times. Some take it a step further to say we should have five to seven small meals or snacks throughout the course of the day instead of three large meals. They feel that it makes better nutritional sense for your body to receive a more steady supply of nutrients throughout the day, and it's easier for your body to digest smaller meals. Snacking could have a positive effect on any stomach or regularity issues you might be having, in addition to helping even out spikes and dips in your blood sugar levels.

Be sure to snack wisely, though. Small meals or leftovers, a piece of raw fruit or veggies, a handful of nuts, or a few whole-grain crackers are all examples of good snacks or between-meal munchies. Chomping down on an entire bag of chips or cookies at one sitting isn't good for your waistline, skin, or physical or mental health. And you'll probably regret the indulgence later on.

You can find more healthful versions of chips and snack foods on many store shelves. As always, check the labels to discover the ingredient and nutritional information and to help you choose between brands, if necessary, to get the best deal for your money. Baked snacks tend to have less fat and calories, so buy baked varieties over fried whenever you have the choice. Avoid snacks that contain hydrogenated and partially hydrogenated oils; they contain tremendous amounts of saturated fats, especially harmful trans-fatty acids, and consumption of these types of fats contributes to developing heart disease and obesity.

Good Snacking Ideas

Start with a nutritious breakfast or early morning meal to get started in the right direction, because how you start your morning affects your nutritional and physical snacking needs later in the day. If you eat well, you might only need a handful of nuts or dried fruit to keep you going until lunch. If you eat light or hardly anything at all, then maybe reach for a granola bar, energy or protein bar, or some raw veggies and a savory dip to help satisfy your food cravings. You can repeat this pattern of eating a larger meal followed by a smaller meal or snack throughout the day to keep eating right and satisfy your caloric and nutritional needs as well as your appetite.

Of course, at times you will want to eat a little junk food–type snack instead of a piece of fruit or other healthful treat. You may be having a party or inviting friends over to watch a movie, or maybe you are just in need of a little crunchy munching. If you take a careful look at the store shelves, you can find some great-tasting snacks that are better for you than others.

Many food companies use organic ingredients in their snack foods. A few of the companies that produce healthy savory snacks include Alpsnack, Bearitos, Garden of Eatin', Guiltless Gourmet, Newman's Own, Robert's American Gourmet, Late July, Mary's Gone Crackers, Kettle, Terra, Boulder, Hain, Stacy's, and many others. You can find these products in conventional or natural foods stores from coast to coast.

Snacks to Avoid

When buying packaged snacks, always read the label carefully. Steer clear of animal-based flavorings and ingredients—this is more obvious with some snack foods than with others.

Many product flavors such as sour cream, honey Dijon, nacho cheese, cheddar cheese, chili and cheese, and buttered, just to name a few, are obviously not vegan. Avoid products that contain the animal ingredients we've already mentioned, too, including "natural flavors," carmine, whey, and casein. Some bean dips, fried foods, and baked snack cakes could even contain lard or beef fat. Many other products have animal ingredients buried within a long list of ingredients, so put on your reading glasses and check out the whole ingredient list. Where and when these ingredients and others pop up keeps you on your toes when shopping for food items.

If you stick with wholesome organic products, you can better avoid artificial colorings and flavorings as well as animal-based ingredients. Try to also look for low-fat and baked, not fried, snacks. Choose naturally sweetened or unrefined sugar–based snacks instead of those full of high-fructose corn syrup and bleached sugar. And don't forget fiber-rich, whole-grain, or multigrain snack foods to help kick your metabolism into high gear!

Satisfying Your Vegan Sweet Tooth

A few fortunate souls out there don't really favor sweets, but most of us do have a sweet tooth and feel obliged to satisfy it from time to time. Too many of us actually let our sweet tooth *control* us in making most of our food choices, though. Sugary sodas, chewing gums, candies, cookies, cakes, pastries, doughnuts, and other sweet treats are part of almost everyone's daily diet in one form or another. Many of these foods are loaded with empty calories, excessive amounts of sugar and fat, and, all too often, preservatives and artificial ingredients.

You can find many wholesome vegan baked goods in natural foods stores. Some may be made in-store while others come packaged. A few of our favorite brands are Alternative Baking Company, Uncle Eddie's, Goodbaker, Nana's, Health Valley, Liz Lovely, Fabe's Natural Gourmet, Sun Flour Baking Company, and Newman's Own.

Sometimes you can also find vegan baking mixes for cakes, cookies, and other baked goods. Dr. Oetker's Simple Organics and Bob's Red Mill make many such products; look for them and others in the baking aisle of your local natural foods store. In Chapter 23, we give you recipes for making a few homemade vegan baked goods and desserts that hopefully will inspire you to become your own vegan baker!

If you suffer from food allergies, natural foods stores often feature baked goods to help you satisfy your sweet tooth as well. Read labels and ingredient lists carefully to avoid unwanted ingredients, and also be aware of the nutritional information for each serving.

Vegan Chocolate

It's a common misconception that you have to give up chocolate when you go vegan. This couldn't be further from the truth because, traditionally, chocolate is made without the use of milk or other dairy products. Most fine-quality dark chocolate is still dairy free. (Just take a look at the ingredient list to be sure.)

Many chocolates are now made with milk, although many connoisseurs would argue such products really shouldn't be considered chocolate if milk is added to the equation. U.S. manufacturers rely on heavy amounts of cream, milk, and even butter to make their chocolaty confections. However, many European and fine chocolatiers use dairy-free dark chocolate more often in their products.

Chocolate is made from chocolate liquor, which is made up of a 50-50 blend of cocoa solids and cocoa butter. The higher the percentage of cocoa solids, the finer and darker tasting the chocolate. Dark chocolate contains up to 75 percent cocoa solids and sometimes a sweetener such as sugar is added. (Really good dark chocolate has a slightly bitter taste as it melts on your tongue.) Additional flavorings can be added if desired, along with a stabilizer such as lecithin to help the chocolate form into a bar or mold.

If you look, you can find some really excellent vegan chocolates and chocolate products. For use in baking, you can find vegan chocolate chips in most stores. Many semisweet brands are already dairy free, and in natural foods stores, you can find brands such as Sunspire, Dagoba, Tropical Source, and Enjoy Life. You may even be able to find some of these brands in bulk as well.

For stocking stuffers, Valentine's Day, Easter, special occasions, or whenever you need a chocolate fix, check out any of several yummy vegan chocolate bars available. They come in all sorts of flavors, such as almond, hazelnut, peanut butter, raspberry, truffle, espresso, orange, mint, and chile from brands like Endangered Species, Theo Chocolate, Green and Black's, Newman's Own, Tropical Source, Conscious Creations, Ecco Bella, Chocolate Decadence, Cloud Nine, Terra Nostra, and Rapunzel. You can chop these bars and use them to garnish desserts, top nondairy ice creams, or use in place of chocolate chips in your vegan baked goods.

Vegan Candy

Most candies are nothing more than sugar, flavoring, and coloring, yet they can trigger childhood memories and bring instant delight. And you might be surprised to learn plenty of your childhood favorites are vegan. They're not necessarily good for you or made with wholesome ingredients, but they are free of animal products.

Here's a partial list of "old-school" vegan candy options for the sugar fiend, according to PETA's petakids.com website: Airheads Taffy, Charms Blow Pops and Lollipops, Chick-o-Sticks, Cracker Jack, Dots, Dum-Dums, Fireballs, Goldenberg's Peanut Chews (original), Hot Tamales, Jolly Ranchers, Jujubees and Jujyfruits, Lemonheads, Mambas, Mary Janes, Mike and Ike, Now and Later, Pez, Ring Pop Lollipops, Smarties (U.S. brand), Sour Patch Kids, Starburst, Super Bubble, Swedish Fish, Sweet Tarts, Twizzlers, and Zotz.

Many natural foods stores now sell a new wave of candies flavored with fruit juices and other unrefined sweeteners instead of sugar. Let's Do Organic makes vegan Gummi Bears in several flavors. Sharkies Organic Fruit Chews are a similar gummy-style chew. St. Claire's makes mints and tarts to flavor and freshen your breath, and Yummy Earth makes hard candies of many flavors.

For those who like chewy candy treats, check out fruit strips and rolls, Wha Guru Chews, Panda or Tubi's licorices, and ginger candies made by several companies, including Ginger People and Reed's. You can even find sprinkles for your sundaes and desserts by Let's Do Organic in chocolate and multicolored confetti varieties.

As you can see, sweet vegan options abound!

IN A NUTSHELL

Allison's Gourmet is a wonderful online source of completely vegan baked goods, including scrumptious cookies, brownies, fudge, and more recently, gourmet chocolates. Her goodies are made with organic ingredients and are available in different varieties each month or as samplers. She even uses eco-friendly packaging! Visit Allison's Gourmet at allisonsgourmet.com.

The Least You Need to Know

- Support shops and businesses that most closely reflect and support your vegan ideals.
- A good natural foods store has just about everything you need to sustain your vegan diet and lifestyle.
- Choosing organics is best for your health and for the planet's.
- Many prepared and packaged vegan food options at your local market can make it easier for you to eat right when you don't have much time to cook.
- When reading product ingredient lists, be on the lookout for animal ingredients labeled as "natural flavors," cochineal extract, whey, gelatin, and others. Instead, look for products with organic and wholesome ingredients.
- When you're in the mood for a vegan indulgence, many vegan options are available in most grocery and natural foods stores, like healthy snacks, vegan cookies, cakes, and chocolates, and even nondairy ice creams, sorbets, and other frozen novelties.

Successful Substitutions

If you don't eat meat and dairy, what *will* you eat? Have no fear! Many plant-based substitutes are available, with an endless array of uses.

In Part 5, you learn about the amazing soybean, which you can use to replace meat, dairy products, eggs, and flours and starches while providing protein, carbohydrates, calcium, and many other vital nutrients. You learn how to mimic with mock meats, nondairy milks, and cheese substitutes and discover some of the available packaged brands. We also give you some pointers on revamping baking recipes; hints on replacing eggs, butter, and milk with ease; and tips to make things "gel" as a vegan and sweeten your treats to perfection!

Using Plant-Based Proteins

In This Chapter

- Preparing beans, grains, and greens
- Suggestions for using soy products
- Substituting with seitan
- Using mock meats

It's our hope that by the time you reach this point in the book, you've already begun to feel secure about the issue of getting enough protein and are also familiar with which vegan foods can supply it.

In this chapter, we take a look at using store-bought plant-based protein sources in your cooking, and we clear up any confusion you may still have about the products on your grocery store or natural foods store shelves. Armed with this information, plus the recipes in Chapters 19 through 23, you'll be able to make some of your own homemade vegan protein powerhouses.

Cooking with Beans, Grains, and Greens

Many cultures, past and present, have sustained themselves on a diet that relies heavily on beans, grains, and greens as sources of protein, among other nutrients. Italians often eat polenta, rice, and pasta with stewed beans such as cannellini, chickpeas, Roman beans, and peas. Greens such as escarole, spinach, or rainbow chard are enjoyed with aromatics, seasonings, fresh herbs, and olive oil. Eastern Europeans and those who live in the British Isles nourish themselves with kasha, oats, and noodles, plus kale, cabbage, and other hardy greens. They also use peas, lentils, white beans, and red beans in many of their standard dishes.

In the Pacific, rice and noodles are eaten at most meals with vegetables and greens such as spinach, bok choy, and cabbage. Cooks there use soybeans in thousands of ways, and black beans and aduki beans are also used whole and to make sauces and desserts. In the Americas, a majority of foods use corn, wild rice, quinoa, and other wild-growing seeds and grains. Many native peoples developed and harvested hundreds of varieties of beans, root vegetables, and grasses. Flavorful items such as carrots, onions, herbs, dandelion, cress, and chicory are used to flavor and supplement the cooking pot.

Beans, grains, and greens are often thought of as simple and hearty "peasant foods." However, you can also use them to make gourmet fare, such as bean and roasted veggie croquettes on a bed of millet, basmati, and wild rice pilaf, with a side of chard and radicchio sautéed in chile-flavored olive oil with shallots, garlic, and sliced almonds. Sounds yummy, doesn't it?

Or you can make a simple lentil and spinach soup flavored with tarragon and thyme. Stir in some small orzo pasta or brown basmati rice toward the end of the cooking time.

And don't forget the traditional New Year's good luck meal of black-eyed peas and greens simmered with the "holy trinity" of Southern cooking: onions, celery, and peppers. Serve this delicious concoction with rice and cornbread—yum!

The Noble Bean

Many people are intimidated by cooking beans, maybe because they experienced gas after eating them or maybe because they didn't season them well or fully cook them the last time. Beans do get a bad rep, but they shouldn't. They're delicious when prepared with care; nutritiously high in protein, complex carbohydrates, and B vitamins; and low in fat and calories. They're also extremely affordable in cost-per-pound comparison with nonvegan protein sources such as meat, eggs, and dairy.

You can find precooked beans in cans at most stores, and they're good to keep on hand for making quick and easy meals. However, buying dry beans in bulk or packaged is really the cheapest way to purchase them. Remember to sort through your dry beans to remove dirt, rocks, and other debris. Some people like to do this in a colander. We like to sort beans on a large plate, in small batches, moving small amounts from one side to the other. This way we can easily and fully see any foreign material. After you've sorted through the beans, place them in a colander and rinse them under running water.

Here's how you can make a basic batch of beans:

1. Start with the largest and heaviest pot you have in your kitchen. Place your beans inside, cover them with at least 4 to 6 inches of filtered water, and bring the water to a boil over high heat.

2. Reduce heat to low, cover, and simmer for 1 to 3 hours or until the beans are tender. Add more water, as needed, while the beans cook so they remain covered with water.

> **IN A NUTSHELL**
>
> Some people like to add a piece of kombu, a sea vegetable, to the pot when cooking beans because it can help reduce gas and make beans more tender. Some people also like to soak their beans first, discard the water, and then start with new water when cooking them. Soaking can reduce cooking time and potentially eliminate excess gas, but it is not a necessary step. Also, using a pressure cooker to cook beans can be a time-saver if you happen to own one.

A big mistake some people make while cooking beans is not cooking them in enough water or for long enough to get them fully tender. Eating undercooked beans can cause gas, abdominal pains, or both. The size and variety of the beans you cook determine the length of cooking time needed to fully cook the beans until tender. The best ways to tell if your beans are tender are to taste them or squish a cooked bean between your fingers. When the beans are fully soft, they're done.

You can fully cool cooked beans, portion them into small containers, and freeze them for use in quick meals later. For convenience, freeze cooked beans in 1½- and 3-cup portions—these are the same amounts you get from using 1 or 2 (15-ounce) cans. This is a great economical alternative to using canned beans, particularly if you're using organic beans.

Deeply Ingrained in Grains

Cooking grains is a lot like cooking beans because it requires a good deal of water or other liquids to soften the grains or kernels. Preparing grains is based on ratios of moisture to dry product; sometimes it's 1:1, others call for 1½:1 or 2:1 or a variation thereof when you're cooking large quantities of grains.

Don't be afraid to try new grain varieties you may never have eaten. Instead of buying long-grain rice every time, why not try a different variety, such as basmati, jasmine, arborio, wild, Bhutanese red, or the black forbidden rice, or a completely different type of grain altogether? When you're feeling a little adventurous, explore your store's bulk or packaged grains sections, and see what appeals to you.

Most grains packages list cooking directions; when buying in bulk, check for directions near the bin. Also use cookbooks and the internet for inspiration and ideas. Some people like to toast their grains, in a dry pan or with some oil, to bring out a nutty flavor. They then add the liquid and proceed with the cooking procedure.

You can cook your grains in filtered water, fruit or vegetable juices or purées, vegetable stock, or plant-based milks like soy or coconut. Feel free to add seasonings and herbs, either prior to or after cooking. Tossing in some vegetables, greens, beans, or other ingredients can turn a simple pot of grains into a one-pot meal.

> **IN A NUTSHELL**
>
> Lundberg Family Farms was one of the early pioneers of organic rice growing in the United States. Since the 1960s, Lundberg has produced their rice using organic and sustainable growing practices they call "nutra-farming." Today, they sell a wide variety of healthy rice varieties, including brown, wehani, basmati, black japonica, jasmine, and many others. They also offer a wide assortment of other rice products like brown rice syrup, rice-based pasta, rice cakes, and yummy rice tortilla-style chips, many of which are suitable for vegans.

Greenery Gastronomy

Greens and all their wonderful fiber are a vegan's and dieter's dream. No matter what the variety, greens are low in fat and loaded with flavor and vitamins. Greens such as spinach and broccoli, for example, are surprisingly high in protein. Eating greens raw preserves most of their nutrients, so nibble on raw greens whenever possible. Chop raw greens to make salads and slaws or add crunch to other dishes. You can even make a raw burrito by using large leaves to encase a wide assortment of your favorite raw fillings.

You could also sauté or stir-fry them in a little oil, alone or with other vegetables, until crisp tender or just tender. Their colors should remain bright and not turn drab and dull. Most greens are delicious when sautéed in a little olive oil with garlic and seasoned with salt, pepper, and red pepper flakes for a little kick!

Some people like to stew or simmer greens in broth or water for a long time to make them so tender they fall apart. If you do this, don't discard the cooking liquid (a.k.a. pot liquor). It contains many vitamins the cooking greens released. Drink it, sop it up with bread, or use it to add flavor to soups and stews.

Demystifying Soy Products

Soy is extremely versatile, easily grown throughout the world, capable of filling many of our nutritional needs, and very affordable as a food source. There's no wonder, in an effort to fight world hunger and malnourishment, more and more people across the globe are adding soy products to their daily diets and food supplies.

Soy products confuse many people because they come in so many different forms. You can purchase soy milk, soy sauce, miso or fermented soybean paste, soy flour, soy grits or flakes, edamame, tofu, and tempeh. Soy products appear as meat analogues and mock meats, soy-based cheeses and other dairy replacements, sauces and soups, and flavorful and frozen novelties and ice creams.

Gettin' Saucy: Soy Sauce

Soy sauce is a commonly used condiment and flavoring agent made from a fermented soybean mash. It comes in several varieties:

- Tamari, a rich-tasting soy sauce made from fermented miso, or from soybeans, salt, water, and koji (a beneficial mold), and usually aged for 2 years

- Shoyu, made the same way as tamari, but with the addition of wheat

- Nama shoyu, a raw version of shoyu with many live enzymes still intact

- Bragg Liquid Aminos, used as a substitute for traditional soy sauces, it contains all essential and many nonessential amino acids

In general, you can freely substitute any of these soy sauces for another in recipes.

The Incredible Tofu

Tofu is one of the most amazing soy foods. A coagulant is added to creamy soy milk and then the curds and whey are separated, as in traditional cheese-making. The result is silky, protein-rich tofu. This soft-textured tofu—often packaged as soft or silken-style tofu—is used to make purées and desserts (which we discuss in Chapter 18).

Other blocks of tofu are pressed to varying degrees to remove excess water to form firm, extra-firm, and super-firm varieties. These denser styles of tofu are more suitable for making cubes, strips, cutlets, and substantial fillings, sandwiches, and entrées.

If you've never tried tofu or cooked with it before, don't be intimidated. Tofu is easier to work with than you might think. First squeeze out as much of the water it was packaged with as you can. Cut the tofu into cubes, strips, big cutlet-size pieces, or whatever you desire. You can then bake it, broil it, fry it, grill it, or use a combination of these methods.

IN A NUTSHELL

Tofu is often referred to as being spongelike, for several reasons. It does have a spongelike texture; tiny holes are often visible within the soybean curd. Also, like a sponge, you can squeeze out excess moisture from tofu and soak up other liquids with it.

You might have heard people say tofu is bland, scary looking, and tasteless. These folks must have just had a badly prepared tofu dish or tried to eat it straight from the package. Well-prepared and flavored tofu can be heavenly, amazingly pungent and chewy, and a wonder to behold when prepared by a tofu master or talented chef!

When it comes to flavoring ideas, remember tofu's spongelike qualities. It absorbs whatever you throw at it or marinate it in, and the tofu takes on and further develops those flavors during the cooking process. You can't go wrong with using a little tamari or other form of soy sauce. Then choose an oil such as olive, toasted sesame, or a hot chile or other flavored oil to prevent sticking during cooking and to add flavor.

Sea salt, black pepper, turmeric, chile powder, and dried and fresh herbs such as basil, parsley, dill, and thyme all impart great flavor to tofu. But don't stop there! Shake on a little of this, a dash of that, and you can come up with some new combinations of your own. Use barbecue sauce, tomato sauce, gravy, and other creamy toppings to make some savory flavor combinations and hearty meals when paired with some grains and veggies.

Nutritional yeast gives your tofu—or tempeh, for that matter—a nutty, cheezy, or savory flavor. You can add it to marinades, sprinkle it on top of a dish, add it to dry breading ingredients, or use it as part of a seasoning mixture. (See Chapter 6 for more on nutritional yeast.)

Tempting with Tempeh

As you first gaze at tempeh through its plastic packaging, you may think it has gone bad, with its colorful marbling and odd texture. But don't be scared. It may look like a child's science project gone awry, but it tastes absolutely wonderful! Think of it as the blue cheese of the soy world; after all, it is injected with mold spores and fermented in much the same way. The result is a highly digestible, fermented soybean cake that has an earthy flavor often described as being meaty, beefy, or mushroomy.

Tempeh is fabulous when crumbled or cubed and used in recipes commonly calling for beef. Try it in tomato sauces, chili, stroganoff, and hearty stews. Flavor and season it very much like tofu, with tamari and olive or toasted sesame oil. It can also easily handle more assertive herbs and spices such as rosemary, tarragon, cayenne, and curry powder. Large cutlets of tempeh make for delicious sandwiches, either baked or fried, and they can become great burgers, hoagies, and patty melts. In Chapter 19, you'll even learn how to turn tempeh and a few other ingredients into some spicy meatless sausages.

> **IN A NUTSHELL**
>
> Want to make a tempeh Reuben? Start by mixing soy mayonnaise, a little ketchup and relish, and some seasonings to make the creamy dressing. Then cook some tempeh cutlets that you've marinated in tamari and oil, toast some rye bread, and begin assembling your sandwich. Add your choice of toppings such as sauerkraut, tomato slices, lettuce, spinach, onions, avocado, soy cheese slices, or soy mock bacon or Canadian bacon. You can eat it after assembling or place it under a broiler for a few minutes. Then roll up your sleeves, tuck in your napkin, and dive in to one fantastic vegan sandwich!

Playing Tricks with TVP

Textured vegetable protein, or TVP, is one of the easiest meat substitutes to use and keep on hand. You can purchase dry TVP in the bulk section of many stores in small flakes or granules or big, chunklike pellets. Store this type of TVP in airtight containers for long periods of time and rehydrate in liquid—perfect for traveling or camping. As soon as you rehydrate TVP, refrigerate it and treat it as you would any perishable cooked food.

Also, in the mock meat section of your local store you can find products marketed as "ground" or "crumbles" by several brands such as Boca, MorningStar, and Yves Veggie Cuisine. These come ready to use, flavored, in several varieties, and can be found refrigerated or frozen in many stores. You can use them as ground meat replacements; in making burgers or loaves; or stir them into sauces, stews, chilies, and entrées. The texture and flavor of these products in dishes will fool most people who will swear they're eating meat, not a soy substitute.

Seitan in Your Supper

Seitan, also known as wheat meat, is a delicious meat substitute made from the protein portion, or gluten, of wheat flour. It's nutritious, has zero cholesterol, and has little or no fat. Seitan has a firm, chewy texture that works well in recipes that call for meat.

You can find several varieties of prepared seitan, either plain, seasoned, or in sauces, made by companies such as White Wave and Lightlife Foods, in the refrigerated and freezer sections of many stores. Use them to make sandwiches, spreads, and salads. Toss in some seitan strips or chunks in your stir-fries, soups, stews, pasta or grain dishes, and entrées for a chewy and nutritious addition.

You can even make homemade seitan with vital wheat gluten, available in most baking aisles or bulk bin sections. In Chapter 21, we give you a recipe to make your own Baked Seitan Roast. The roast also makes a fabulous sandwich: thinly slice and layer the roast onto a large roll, and serve it with the seitan cooking liquid, *au jus* style. Or forego the bread and serve slices with some creamy gravy like the Groovy Onion Gravy (Chapter 22), along with a side of Mouthwatering Mashed Potatoes (Chapter 21) for a fantastic family-style meal. Or cut the roast into cubes, strips, cutlets, make it into breaded treats, and on and on. Seitan has endless uses!

IN A NUTSHELL

You can easily make a mock chicken salad by mixing cooked seitan chunks, diced celery, onion, and herbs with a little vegan mayonnaise. Add some sliced almonds or shredded carrot for color and texture, and serve on whole-grain toast!

Mimicking with Mock Meats

If you miss the meaty-tasting items in your diet, you don't have to do without. In your grocer's freezer or refrigerator cases, you can find vegan replacements for many of your childhood favorites.

Craving a hot dog or hamburger? No problem! Simply choose from several brands of soy-based hot dogs or burgers made with ingredients such as vegetables, mushrooms, grains, nuts, and soy products. You can also find sliced deli "meats" in bologna, ham, or turkey flavors. How about a few slices of mock Canadian bacon, pepperoni, meatballs, or sausages in spicy Italian, breakfast, or brat styles? Or maybe you're hankering for some jaw-stiffening vegan jerky? You can find that as well.

Want to have a supersize vegan hoagie, or throw a tailgate party or other casual get-together? Vegan sliced deli meats are the answer. Start with some hearty bread or rolls and layer different varieties of slices, alternating with vegan sliced cheeses and crunchy vegetables. Sprinkle on some seasonings, and pour a great dressing over the top. You can't find anything like that in your neighborhood sub shop!

You can also turn the same ingredients into a mock-meat-and-cheese platter or an antipasto tray. Or use them to create some snazzy appetizers such as the classic pepperoni-cheese-cracker combo or a fancy version of "pigs in a blanket" using vegan ingredients. For a show-stopper, take a spear of asparagus, wrap it in Canadian bacon or a ham-style slice with a little soy cheese and a smear of Dijon mustard, encase the entire little package in phyllo dough, and bake until crispy. This is guaranteed to wow the eyes and taste buds!

You can even host your own vegan barbecue bash by grilling veggies, ears of corn, veggie burgers, and vegan hot dogs. Make a big pasta, potato, or green salad with a wide assortment of colorful raw veggies and fresh dressing. You can even have s'mores for dessert by using vegan graham crackers (try Health Valley Amaranth Graham Crackers), vegan marshmallows (purchase in natural foods stores or online), and your choice of vegan chocolate. Prepare them like you did when you were a kid, and enjoy!

When Thanksgiving and other such holidays roll around, mock meats can help round out your menu. Tofurky is a widely distributed brand of tofu and seitan-based turkey alternative that manages to look and taste a lot like turkey. The manufacturer even sells a complete vegan holiday meal, including gravy, stuffing, "wishstix," and dumplings. It's quite popular among vegetarians and vegans who are looking for a good turkey substitute at holiday time. Tofurky also markets an assortment of vegan deli slices, sausages, and jerky.

The Field Roast Grain Meat Company makes "grain meats" such as vegan sausages, deli slices, loaves, cutlets, and a stuffed celebration loaf suitable for the holiday season as well. Similar to seitan, it's made with a mixture of vital wheat gluten and other grains, vegetables, legumes, and seasonings.

The Least You Need to Know

- Cooking with beans, grains, and greens is an easy and delicious way to add whole, natural sources of protein and other nutrients to your vegan meals.
- Using an assortment of available soy products such as tofu, tempeh, and TVP can make it easy for you to prepare convenient and protein-rich meals.
- Using seitan in your meals, either purchased frozen or made at home, is a great way to add a "meaty" texture to your meatless dishes.
- Prepared mock meats can provide vegan replacements for many of your meaty childhood favorites; look in your grocer's freezer or refrigerator cases to see what's available.

Doing Without Dairy and Cheese

In This Chapter

- Comparing butter, margarine, and oils
- Demystifying hydrogenated fats
- Replacing and substituting dairy products
- Sampling various vegan cheeses
- DIY cheezy creations

Often, while talking with someone about what you do and don't eat as a vegan, they'll say something such as, "Oh, I could probably give up meat, but not cheese and ice cream. I would miss them too much!" By now, you know how to enlighten such people about the vegan alternatives that exist for all these products, including what's available and their health advantages over the traditional versions.

In this chapter, you learn more about how to substitute for dairy ingredients in your day-to-day eating, cooking, and baking. Some ingredients such as butter and milk are easy to replace, but others may be a bit trickier or take some getting used to. Don't expect to have the exact same end results with vegan substitutes you may have had with dairy products (like the browning or stringy characteristics of melted cheese, for instance). Some vegan items are very close, though!

Butter, Margarine, and Oils

It takes more than 2 gallons milk to make 1 pound butter. Everything that's bad about whole milk is multiplied many times over in butter. It's got a high concentration of saturated fats, and indulging in it can raise your cholesterol levels, increase your risk of cardiovascular disease (among other diseases), and lead to obesity. It's no wonder, then, that there's such a huge market for healthier alternatives to butter.

Unfortunately, most commercially available margarines made with hydrogenated oils aren't any better than butter and can contain just as much saturated fat—and worse! Read labels to be sure of what you're actually getting. Some margarine brands even contain whey or other dairy derivatives, so don't assume a product is vegan just because you see the word *margarine* on the label.

Instead, look for vegan brands such as Earth Balance that contain little or no trans-fatty acids and are nonhydrogenated. Such products are available both in sticks and plastic tubs of whipped spread in several varieties, including soy-free and even a coconut oil–based spread. Another tub-style product is palm oil–based vegan shortening, which some vegans like to use in baking, especially for flaky pie crusts and fluffy frostings that hold their shape when piped.

HOT POTATO

A growing number of people are avoiding products that contain palm oil due to some controversy surrounding its production of palm oil: human rights violations and devastating and often irreversible damage to the natural environment, such as deforestation, loss of habitat for endangered species like the orangutan and Sumatran tiger, and significant increase in greenhouse gas emissions.

An alternative choice over margarine and butter is the use of plant-based oils such as olive, safflower, flax, sesame, sunflower, or pumpkin seed. You can use these in many forms of baking and cooking, often with better results than with hardened fats such as margarine or vegetable shortening. If you were going to melt them down anyway in the preparation of your recipe, using a liquid form actually saves you time and effort. You can use margarine in cookies, piecrusts, and frostings, if you want, but oils (especially if chilled) also work well in most cases.

Choose your oil by the recipe, the other ingredients you're using, and the preparation technique. Olive oil works well in and on practically everything, so you can't go wrong keeping it well stocked in your pantry. Buy extra virgin and organic for the best flavor and the most health benefits. Store it away from light, keep the bottle tightly sealed, and don't keep it for more than a year because it can turn rancid.

What's *Hydrogenated* Mean?

Food labels contain some very confusing ingredients, particularly when it comes to fats. *Cold-pressed, expeller-pressed, unrefined, partially hydrogenated, hydrogenated, nonhydrogenated*—all these terms can appear before oils and other fats on the nutritional labels of your favorite foods.

Cold-pressed, expeller-pressed, and *unrefined* are all desirable terms describing how the oil was processed, so seek out products with these words on the label whenever possible.

But when you get to *hydrogenated*, read carefully because what comes before it can be very important. If the word appears at all, you want it to read *non*hydrogenated. Hydrogenated fats, or trans fats, are the man-made "bad fats" that clog your arteries and lead to heart disease. Back when scientists were playing around with the development of margarine, they learned to use hydrogen to suspend fat molecules to make them become more saturated and hardened. Hardening was important to the nature of the product, and suspending molecules to hold or bind food together seemed all right in theory.

IN A NUTSHELL

Many natural foods companies are aware of the negative effects of hydrogenated fats and don't use them in their production. They often proudly draw attention to the presence of minimally processed expeller-pressed, cold-pressed, nonhydrogenated, and organic oils in their products on the front labels, which makes healthy and wise vegan shopping that much easier.

Unfortunately, because hydrogenated fats were something completely new, the end result was quite harmful. Our bodies were and continue to be confused by hydrogenated fats. They don't recognize them as normal fats, so they don't process them accordingly for energy and fuel. Instead, these fats go directly into fat storage supplies and end up clogging arteries and adding inches to hips and waistlines. They also raise bad cholesterol levels and decrease good cholesterol levels. They're basically the worst kind of fat you could possibly put into your body!

The Functions of Fats

The slick characteristic of fats makes them useful in dressings, marinades, and sauces, where they provide flavor and mobility to ingredients or emulsify if vigorously blended. In baking, fats add layers between the starch or grain molecules that provide flavor and flakiness to cookies, pastries, and piecrusts.

Fats also provide a certain richness, or mouthfeel, to foods. But you don't need a lot of fat in your foods to achieve this sensation, which is where many cooks go wrong. Fats should flavor and not overpower or overwhelm the food. Excessively oily or greasy foods are unappealing, unappetizing, and usually bad tasting. Start with small amounts of fat, and add more only as needed.

You could cut part of the fat called for by replacing it with other liquid ingredients such as water, juices, plant-based milks, or fruit purées (like applesauce or mashed bananas) that would complement the recipe. Cutting out additional fats in foods wherever possible is good for your waistline and your heart. It can also allow for a more guilt-free consumption of dessert if you pass up the greasy french fries or chips with your meal.

Using Nondairy Substitutes

As we mentioned in Chapter 6, and as you may know from your own purchases, some truly amazing alternatives to milk, cream, yogurt, sour cream, cream cheese, and other dairy products fill grocery store shelves. You can find products made from soy, rice, coconut, hemp, nuts, grains, or combinations thereof in most dairy cases, right next to their animal-based cousins. Availability varies from store to store and from state to state, so those living in more veg-friendly areas will have more of a selection.

Read labels and compare brands to see which ones best suit your personal tastes and needs. Some are thicker than others, and some come sweetened or unsweetened, plain or flavored, so you're bound to have fun in the sampling process. These vegan versions work as fine substitutes and can help provide a thick, creamy texture to beverages, smoothies, light sauces, soups, stews, curries, and desserts.

Measure for Measure

You won't have to do a lot of tinkering with or altering measurements when using vegan ingredients, especially when you use soy milks, rice milks, and other nondairy beverages. They usually work measure for measure as a milk substitute, and they impart the same thick and creamy texture to your dishes. Likewise, vegan sour creams and cream cheeses usually cause few problems when used measure for measure for their dairy counterparts. The same can be said for the creamy almond, coconut, rice, and soy-based vegan yogurts. They can be used in both sweet and savory recipes or eaten on their own as a tasty treat.

If you don't think you'd be able to use an entire container of soy milk, for example, you're in luck. If you check your store shelves, you're bound to find a wide assortment of soy, rice, hemp, and even pea-based protein powders you can use as needed when making sauces, beverages, dressings, soups, savory dishes, and desserts.

HOT POTATO

Using powdered soy beverages in recipes may yield slightly different results than when using the liquid versions. Powdered beverages tend to be a bit watery, so you may need to increase the amount of powder to create a thicker version.

Using What, Where?

So how do you know what type of nondairy substitute to use and in what recipe to use it, particularly if you're new to cooking in general? Start with the liquid beverages because they're easy to use. They add creaminess to your soups, sauces, and libations just as milk or cream would. You can thicken them with a roux or starch, or thin them to suit your needs.

Use soy yogurt just like regular yogurt in recipes such as curries, raitas, desserts, and smoothies, or enjoy it with your morning granola and fruit. Look for vegan yogurts manufactured by So Delicious, Amande, Ricera, Whole Soy, White Wave, and Nancy's. Tofutti, Galaxy Foods, Follow Your Heart, WayFare, and several other private label companies make vegan versions of sour cream and cream cheese. You can also use soy yogurt, sour cream, and cream cheese to add creaminess to sauces and dressings or in dessert recipes in place of their dairy counterparts.

Whether you buy sweetened or unsweetened nondairy milks is a personal choice, but consider these thoughts: for use in soups, stews, and baked goods, it's best to stick with a plain variety or perhaps even vanilla in some cases. The other flavors, such as chocolate, carob, or nut varieties, all work well in beverages, smoothies, and desserts. But feel free to experiment. Cooking and baking is all based on personal preferences and tastes, so have fun and enjoy!

Packaged Vegan Cheeses

Americans are obsessed with cheese. They melt it on everything; nibble it in chunks, slices, and wedges; and use it as everything from a sprinkled garnish to a heaping stand-alone side dish. Fortunately for vegans, a vast array of nondairy cheeses are on the market, although availability varies from region to region. Nondairy cheeses really come in handy when you're missing the taste and feel of cheese or when you're craving a creamy addition to your meal.

Soymage Vegan, Tofutti, Follow Your Heart, and WayFare also make a vegan cream cheese and soft and cheezy-flavored spreads and dips. Soymage and Parma both make several varieties of Parmesan-style cheese suitable for sprinkling on pasta or pizza. Some nondairy cheeses come sliced (Tofutti, Vegan Rella, and Soymage Vegan) and ready to be placed between slices of whole-grain bread for an incredible vegan grilled cheese sandwich or with other vegan goodies for a patty melt sandwich.

The best unsliced vegan cheese we've found so far is a brand called Vegan Gourmet Cheese Alternative, made by Follow Your Heart. Most vegans want a cheese that melts and tastes delicious, and this one does both. It comes in mozzarella, cheddar, nacho, and Monterey Jack flavors. You can cut it into slices, strips, or cubes, or shred fine strands onto your next pizza and bake it until browned, bubbling, and gooey!

Speaking of shredded vegan cheese, one of the best-melting, shredded-style nondairy cheeses widely available today is Daiya, which comes in mozzarella, cheddar, and pepper Jack. It tastes, melts, and looks a lot like its dairy counterpart when used on pizza, on nachos, or as vegan fondue. You can also find it on top of some brands of frozen vegan pizza.

IN A NUTSHELL

The average American cheese lover consumes more than 30 pounds of cheese per year. The average vegan probably doesn't even come close to eating that quantity of vegan cheese in a year's time, but even if you tried, you'd only get a fraction of the saturated fat and none of the cholesterol. Some natural foods stores make their own brand of vegan cheeses or carry their own private label products, so take a look around and see what may be available!

Making Your Own Cheese Alternatives

If you don't have access to vegan cheeses in your area or you don't like the varieties available locally, you can always try making your own. It's actually pretty easy, and you can control what ingredients go into your vegan cheese.

You can usually find recipes in vegan cookbooks available in your local library and bookstores. These can help you get started making vegan cheese. Joanne Stepaniak has written several great books with recipes for homemade vegan cheeses, sauces, dips, and spreads. Our favorites are *The Nutritional Yeast Cookbook* and *The Uncheese Cookbook*.

You can also find many helpful vegan recipes online, including at vegsource.com and veganchef.com. For additional homemade vegan cheese recipes, check out Beverly's other books in *The Complete Idiot's Guide* series (see Appendix B).

Getting Saucy

The simplest cheese substitute to make is a mock cheese sauce. In Chapter 22, we give you a basic Vegan Cheezy Sauce recipe to get you started. It's rich and creamy and flavored with oh-so-cheezy nutritional yeast.

You can jazz it up with a little hot sauce, chile powder, wine, or additional shredded vegan cheese. Adding more paprika or chile powder deepens the color of the sauce; leaving them out makes it lighter. Stirring in a little Dijon or whole-grain mustard or black or white pepper gives it zip. The sauce takes on a more savory flavor with the addition of fresh herbs such as parsley, thyme, dill, and basil.

Vegan Cheezy Sauce is excellent as a dip for bread, like a fondue, or as a sauce over veggies, pasta, grains, mashed potatoes, or tofu. Or drizzle it over sandwiches or pizza for a melted gooey treat!

Firming Things Up

Do you want your vegan cheese spreadable or sliceable? You can vary the consistency and firmness of your vegan cheese by using different coagulants. Nut butters and seed pastes, such as cashew butter and raw tahini, lend creaminess and texture to crock-style vegan cheese spreads. Starches such as *arrowroot*, tapioca, and cornstarch help bind your cheese into a block, suitable for cutting into soft chunks or slices.

DEFINITION

Arrowroot is a starch made from the tubers of the tropical herb *Maranta arundinacea.* Used primarily as a thickener, arrowroot tubers are sometimes also eaten whole as a vegetable. The word *arrowroot* is derived from the Arawak word *aru-aru,* meaning "meal of meals."

Agar-agar, which comes from the sea and is used as a vegan gelatin, is your best choice for firming your cheezy creations. It really solidifies and holds your vegan cheese together to produce nice, even slices when cutting. (We discuss the wonders of agar-agar further in Chapter 18.)

For more recipes to make crock or spreadable types of cheese, blocks, and sliceable cheeses, check out Beverly's other books, Joanne Stepaniak's books, other vegan cookbooks, and online sources. You're bound to find a few cheezy creations you and your family will love!

The Least You Need to Know

- When it comes to using fats, opt for nonhydrogenated margarines or cold or expeller-pressed oils over those high in saturated or hydrogenated fats.
- You can generally substitute vegan versions of dairy products measure for measure.
- Quite a few tasty sliceable, shakeable, and meltable vegan nondairy cheese products are available in stores that can help when you're missing the taste of cheese or craving a creamy addition to your meal.
- It's easy to make your own vegan cheezy creations, from creamy sauces to solid slices, with a little know-how and the right ingredients.

Vegan Baking Substitutions

In This Chapter

- Taking the dairy out of baking
- Firming up without gelatin
- Getting sweet with vegan sweeteners
- Substituting for eggs in recipes
- Using tofu in your baking

Many people believe you have to use butter, milk, and eggs to make delicious baked goods and you simply can't do without those traditional staples. Actually, vegan baking produces a variety of rich and delicious baked goods that could easily rival the best any traditional baker has to offer!

Of course, how well an item turns out has a lot to do with the quality of the ingredients and the skill of the baker. Vegan baking usually begins with high-quality ingredients, so you're already off to a good start. Now all you need to learn is a little about cooking and baking terms and some vegan baking substitutions—that's where this chapter comes in!

Vegan baking relies on a lot of seemingly magical chemical reactions with leaveners, binders, flours, fats, and fat replacements. Don't let that intimidate you; that's how all baking is, vegan or not. With a little practice and patience, you can become the wizard of your vegan kitchen. Then you can enjoy the fruits of your labor and even proudly share your creations with others to show them how delicious vegan eating can be!

Baking Without Butter

It's helpful to understand the role the fat, seasoning, starch, or acid is playing in a recipe, and whether it's an essential part or just a supporting component in the dish. Always start with small changes first when trying out a newly veganized recipe.

> **IN A NUTSHELL**
>
> Don't give away all your nonvegan cookbooks. Instead, why not try to veganize some of your favorite recipes from them?

Fats are the easiest to replace. Olive oil is a great baking substitute, in most instances, for melted butter, ghee, lard, and heavily processed vegetable oils and shortening. You can also use other light oils such as sunflower, safflower, or soybean in baking. Oils work best in cakes, brownies, some drop cookies, breads, and quick breads.

Solid fats work best in pastry recipes because the chilled fat remains separated in layers from the dry ingredients and melts when baking to provide a rich flavor and flaky texture. No wonder butter is so prized by pie bakers for its rich taste, and frugal bakers rely on lard and vegetable shortening to add flake and fat to their piecrusts and biscuits at a fraction of the cost.

But these aren't suitable vegan ingredients, so what should a vegan baker use? Well, for one, don't use just any old margarine. Instead, use nonhydrogenated whipped or sticks or some vegan shortening or coconut oil if you prefer (see Chapter 17).

The best-tasting and most consistent measure-for-measure butter replacement is made by Earth Balance. It comes in several varieties, including Original, Organic Whipped, Soy Garden, Soy-Free, Coconut Spread, Buttery Sticks, and Shortening. Some stores also sell Spectrum Naturals Spread, which is also vegan and nonhydrogenated. Each of these products gives your vegan baked goods a buttery flavor with much less fat than butter and no cholesterol. Use them in place of butter in piecrusts, cookies, chilled pastry doughs, crisps, cobblers, and crumb toppings. They also whip up nicely and make vegan frostings light and creamy!

Leaving Out the Milk and Cream

In most of your baking, you can easily do without cow's milk. All soy milks, rice milks, and grain- and nut-based milks can be suitable replacements in puddings, pastries, cakes, desserts, and even to prepare or thin frostings and glazes. If milk is only providing moisture in a recipe, you can also substitute other liquids such as water or juices.

Cream has a thicker consistency than milk, and the higher fat content also adds richness to recipes. You can usually easily substitute a soy or coconut nondairy liquid creamer in a recipe where cream is providing moisture and creaminess.

You can also use tofu to make a whipped topping replacement for whipped cream. In Chapter 23, we give you a recipe for Tofu Mousse or Crème Topping, which can be used on top of fruit and your favorite desserts.

IN A NUTSHELL

Make a homemade Vegan Cream Alternative by blending ½ cup soy milk and ½ cup silken tofu, or ½ cup soy milk and 2 or 3 tablespoons dry soy milk powder until smooth and creamy. It substitutes measure for measure for the cream called for in most recipes.

Some big-name nondairy whipped toppings are available at your local supermarket, but most of them still contain animal ingredients such as sodium caseinate, along with hydrogenated oils, high-fructose corn syrup, preservatives, and artificial ingredients.

But luckily, several brands of vegan whipped topping are now available. The makers of Soyatoo offer both Soy Whip and soy-free Rice Whip in convenient-to-use pressurized cans, as well as Soy Whip in small cartons, which you beat with an electric mixer until fluffy. Another whip-it-yourself option is Healthy Top made by MimicCreme. Look for these items in the refrigerated case of your local grocery or natural foods stores. Use these whipped toppings to decorate your desserts, pies, and parfaits or provide a light and creamy sweetness to your vegan creations.

Excellent Egg Substitutes

It's quite unfortunate that eggs have become a staple of many people's diets. Not only do the hens pay a heavy price for laying them, but so do those who eat them. According to the American Heart Association, the average large egg contains 213 milligrams cholesterol, which is more than 70 percent of the daily recommendation for dietary cholesterol intake. These numbers make eggs unsuitable for heart patients who have to keep their dietary cholesterol intake below 200 milligrams per day.

Fortunately, you can substitute for eggs in many ways. How you do it depends on the role the eggs played in the original recipe. Basically, the purpose of eggs in a recipe is either to act as a binder, thickener, moistener, or leavening agent. For instance, in veggie burgers, sauces, or casseroles, you want a binding or thickening effect. Starches do the trick here, so try adding some arrowroot, potato starch, cornstarch, flour, oats, or breadcrumbs to reach the desired consistency. Adding a tablespoon or two of nut butter, like peanut butter, cashew butter, or raw tahini, also helps bind or hold ingredients together.

Substituting for eggs in baking can be a bit trickier. If the eggs are part of the recipe simply to provide moisture, you can replace them with the same amount of water, soy milk, or juice. When you need the binding properties of eggs when making cookies, breads, and baked goods, you can use applesauce, puréed bananas, puréed dates, or Ener-G Egg Replacer, which is made with potato and tapioca starch and is widely available in natural foods stores. To achieve the thickening qualities of eggs in pie fillings or custards, you can use agar-agar, kudzu, arrowroot, cornstarch, or flour.

Use these basic suggestions for substituting 1 egg:

- ¼ cup soft, firm, or extra-firm silken tofu, puréed until smooth
- ¼ cup puréed bananas or applesauce, plus ½ teaspoon aluminum-free baking powder
- 2 tablespoons nut butter, such as peanut butter or tahini
- 1 tablespoon finely ground flaxseeds or 1 teaspoon chia seeds, plus 3 tablespoons water, stirred together, and allowed to rest for 10 to 15 minutes
- 1 tablespoon Ener-G Egg Replacer whisked with 2 tablespoons water
- 1 tablespoon cornstarch or flour whisked with 1 tablespoon water

Try experimenting with some of these to see which ones work best in your recipes.

IN A NUTSHELL

Here's a little tip for using Ener-G Egg Replacer: the directions on the box suggest you use 1½ teaspoons Ener-G Egg Replacer plus 2 tablespoons water to replace 1 egg. We've had better results by increasing the amount of Ener-G Egg Replacer to 1 tablespoon, especially when using it as a binder or thickener.

Gellin' Without Gelatin

Gelatin is a very strange food product. It turns liquids into solid or semisolid masses, thickening a little or a lot, depending on the amount used. Some fruits and veggies, including tomatoes, beans, and peas, contain natural gelling properties. (Just look at a leftover pot of split-pea soup for the layer of gel across the top.)

This type of gelatin is based on plant cellulose structure, not the collagen released from animal bones and tissues. That's right—animal-based gelatin is made of leftovers from the slaughtering process. Bones, hooves, skin, tendons, and other miscellaneous parts are boiled in water to release their natural collagen. The extracted gelatin is formed into translucent sheets or strings, or ground into a powder.

The powder is used to thicken sauces, jellies, desserts, candies, ice creams, marshmallows, baked goods, and many other products. Surprisingly, it also is used to clarify soups and stocks, some vinegars, juices, wines, beers, and spirits. You'll also find it in cosmetics, capsules for supplements, personal-care products, and as an industrial stabilizer used in many everyday products. (See Chapter 26 to learn a little more about the uses of gelatin in household items.)

There's some culinary benefit to being able to bind things together or gel them, but you don't have to rely on animal by-products to do it. Vegans and vegetarians have several alternatives to use. A few companies, such as KoJel and Hain, even make boxed plain and flavored vegan gelatin; look for it in grocery and natural foods stores.

You can also experiment with other gelling agents such as flaxseeds, chia seeds, agar-agar, starches, and other all-natural plant ingredients. You'll be amazed by the solidifying results!

Fabulous Flaxseeds

A mixture of flaxseeds and water was once a popular hair-setting solution. After making the standard flaxseed gel recipe of 1 tablespoon ground flaxseeds and 3 tablespoons water, either boiled or blended together, and letting it sit for a while, you'll see why. It turns into a very gummy, gel-like substance.

The most beneficial part of the flaxseed is inside its hard hull, which can be difficult to digest. You can easily access the seeds' healthy goodness simply by grinding them a bit before using them on your food or in recipes. You can grind flaxseeds in a coffee grinder, blender, or food processor to a fine powder for ease of use. You can do this in batches, ahead of time, and keep the ground flax meal in an airtight container in the refrigerator for use as needed.

Flaxseeds have a slightly nutty flavor, and they're especially good paired with recipes that contain nuts and seeds. The gelling properties of the flaxseeds and water can work as a binder or egg replacement in your baking recipes such as quick breads, pie fillings, and cookies.

Flaxseeds are very nutritious because they are high in beneficial omega-3 fatty acids, vitamins, minerals, and protein. They're also a high-fiber and protein-rich food source good for your skin, brain, immunity, and weight control. These tiny seeds are also rich in lignans, which provide so many health benefits and safety nets. They have anticancer, antitumor, antiviral, antibacterial, and antifungal properties as well.

You can purchase flaxseeds in brown and golden varieties, either whole or as ground flaxseed meal, or in liquid form as flaxseed oil, which can be used in sauces, salad dressings, and smoothies. Visit your neighborhood natural foods store to see what's available.

HOT POTATO

Always store your flaxseeds in the refrigerator or freezer, and use them within 6 months or less. Like most seeds, their high fat content can easily lead to rancidity, so keep them cool. Flaxseed oil is sold in dark glass bottles to protect it from light and should be stored in the fridge as well.

Energizing Chia Seeds

Chia is the tiny edible seed that comes from the desert plant *Salvia Hispanica*, a member of the mint family, and has a speckled white, gray, and black appearance. You can even purchase a golden chia seed variety as well.

Chia seeds were first enjoyed by the Aztecs and Mayans, who believed that even a small serving was capable of providing their messengers and warriors with tremendous endurance and energy. Even today, they're appreciated as a superfood worldwide for both their nutritional and medicinal benefits.

Chia seeds are high in fiber, especially beneficial soluble fiber. When they're mixed with liquids or ingested, they begin to swell up and are capable of absorbing more than 10 times their weight in water, which helps make you feel full faster, which can help with weight loss. They're also an excellent source of complete protein, calcium, phosphorus, magnesium, manganese, copper, iron, niacin, and zinc.

Besides being an appetite suppressant, chia seeds provide other health benefits as well, including improving digestion and elimination, building lean muscle mass, supporting cardiovascular health, fighting cancer, and stabilizing blood glucose levels.

> **IN A NUTSHELL**
>
> A 1-ounce serving of chia seeds supplies 4 grams protein, 12 grams carbohydrates, 9 grams fat (only 1 gram saturated), 11 grams dietary fiber, and 137 calories.

So how do chia seeds compare to flaxseeds? Chia seeds contain three times the amount of beneficial omega-3 fatty acids, and unlike flax, they contain naturally occurring antioxidants that help prevent them from going rancid when stored for an extended period of time. They also don't need to be ground to make their nutrients available to the body or to transform into a gelatinous substance.

Chia seeds are very mild tasting and are often undetectable in a recipe. You can simply mix chia seeds with water or juices to create a soft gel for use in thickening or to replace part of the fat or oil in a recipe. Or sprinkle some over your cereal, oatmeal, or salad, or try adding some to your smoothie or salad dressing to not only thicken it but also boost its nutritional content.

You can also make a quick-and-easy sweet treat by mixing together 3 tablespoons chia seeds with 1 cup chocolate almond milk. Let the mixture sit for 15 minutes or more until it thickens, and voilà! A delicious no-cook chocolate pudding!

Amazing Agar-Agar

Agar-agar is a widely used seaweed derivative that's odorless, tasteless, nearly colorless, and has amazing gelling properties. It's available in sticks, flakes, or as a powder, and the amount you use varies with each variety and depends on the amount of gelling required.

Use it to thicken your own fruit juices to make jiggly treats, like kanten! (Kanten is a dish that suspends fruits, beans, nuts, and seeds in a gelled agar-agar mixture and is very much like the gelatin desserts most of us grew up with at family functions and as part of our school lunches.)

Also add agar-agar to thicken sauces, frostings, puddings, fillings, and other custard-like desserts, as well as give your homemade vegan cheese a firmer consistency. You can find agar-agar in many Asian specialty markets, grocery stores, and natural foods stores.

Stiffening with Starch

Many starches are available to help your sauce or pie filling gel. Try a little Ener-G Egg Replacer, arrowroot, cornstarch, potato starch, *kudzu*, tapioca starch, or some flour diluted in some water or other liquid to give substance to your creation. You often need to cook the starch-liquid mixture to begin the thickening process and remove any starchy taste.

> **DEFINITION**
>
> **Kudzu**, or *kuzu*, is a starch-based thickening product made from the tuber of the kudzu plant. In Japan and throughout much of Asia, the leafy foliage is cooked and eaten like other greens, and the large tubers are used as a thickening agent. This quick-growing vine was brought from Japan to the southern United States, where it is referred to as "the vine that ate the South" because it now covers nearly 7 million acres of land!

Arrowroot and tapioca starches give your finished sauce or filling a glossy shine, while cornstarch and flour often leave things dull, cloudy, or creamy looking. Arrowroot also works better with acidic ingredients, which sometimes inhibit cornstarch.

In general, it takes 1 tablespoon starch diluted in 2 tablespoons liquid to thicken 1 cup of a liquid mixture such as a gravy, sauce, stock, or juice.

Perfecting Pectin

Many fruits and vegetables contain a natural dietary fiber known as pectin. Pectin can help keep your digestive system running properly and regulate your blood cholesterol and sugar levels, helping you fight off chronic degenerative diseases, heart disease, and diabetes. In addition to its health benefits, you can also use pectin as a thickening agent.

The following are pectin-rich foods:

- Apples
- Avocados
- Bananas
- Blueberries
- Carob
- Cherries
- Currants
- Grapes

- Oranges and other citrus fruits
- Peaches
- Pineapples
- Raisins
- Raspberries
- Sunflower seeds
- Tomatoes

and baking powder combination. Make them for your friends and family, and they'll find it hard to believe the treats are dairy and egg free!

Sweeteners to Use and to Avoid

Many of us love to eat sweet-tasting foods more than salty, sour, or even spicy foods. Sugars do provide energy, but consuming too much sugar, especially in heavily refined foods, can be detrimental to your health.

White sugar, in particular, is the enemy of the health conscious and the vegan alike. Most of the major sugar companies in the United States bleach their sugar to make it white. Not only do manufacturers strip away beneficial nutrients in the process, but the bleaching process itself is usually not even vegan.

Sugar, Sugar

In particular, sugar produced from sugar cane, also known as cane sugar, is bleached using a special filtration process that cleanses away its nutty brown color and leaves a polished ivory-colored mass. It is often filtered through activated charcoal that can come from animal as well as plant sources. Often, the process uses bone char or boneblack, a charcoal made from animal bones. Using bone char in the bleaching process is only done with cane sugar, not beet sugar. In Europe, the production of almost all bleached cane sugar is done without the use of bone char, and therefore is suitable for vegans. The opposite is true for most of the big U.S. producers, though.

> **HOT POTATO**
>
> Three of the largest U.S. sugar manufacturers—Domino, California & Hawaiian Sugar Company (C&H), and Savannah Foods—use bone char in their cane sugar–bleaching processes. Their sugar is sold as various supermarket and generic brands as well. Wholesome Sweeteners and Florida Crystals are two widely available brands of sugar that do not involve the use of bone char and are suitable for vegans.

Powdered and brown cane sugar are often processed using bone char as well, particularly those produced by manufacturers that normally use bone char in their bleaching process. For them, brown sugar is simply bleached cane sugar with some molasses added in, and powdered or confectioners' sugar is bleached cane sugar that's been finely processed with cornstarch to prevent caking.

Brown or powdered sugar based on beet sugar rather than cane sugar is suitable for vegans, as are those sugars produced by companies that do not use bone char. Wholesome Sweeteners, Hain, and Florida Crystals all make a great vegan powdered sugar as well as several other varieties of sugar, like turbinado, demerara, light and dark brown, and muscovado sugar, a vegan moist brown sugar available at natural foods stores.

To know for sure you're getting a truly vegan sugar, you can contact the company directly and ask them for information. You can also avoid problems by looking for products labeled *evaporated cane juice*, *organic unbleached sugar*, *raw sugar*, *Sucanat*, or *beet sugar*, which are all vegan. You can also substitute maple sugar (made from dehydrated maple syrup), date sugar (made from pulverized dried dates), or coconut palm sugar (made from the nectar of coconut palm flower blossoms) in place of cane or beet sugar. Maple, coconut, and date sugars are especially delicious in cookies that contain nuts or seeds.

Syrupy Sweetness

Some vegans prefer to stay away from granular sugar altogether and stick with using liquid sweeteners such as molasses, maple syrup, barley malt syrup, brown rice syrup, concentrated fruit juice syrups, agave nectar, and sorghum. These sweeteners tend to keep your blood sugar at more even levels, with fewer spikes and dips than those caused by refined cane sugar.

To ensure that your maple syrup is pure, try to buy only certified organic. Also, avoid "maple-flavored syrup," which is usually made from sugar or corn syrup mixed with artificial colorings and flavorings and maybe a tiny percentage of actual maple syrup. There's really no comparison between the two products, and they're only interchangeable on pancakes and waffles, not in cooking or baking.

HOT POTATO

You might have heard that maple syrup isn't vegan because it's clarified using lard. Fortunately, most modern maple syrup producers use a small amount of vegetable-based oil rather than lard. When in doubt about a specific brand, either contact the manufacturer or look to see if it is kosher certified, which would ensure it was not produced with lard.

Stevia is known as the "sweet herb" to the people of Paraguay and Brazil, where it originates. People of these regions have used the leaves of the plant for centuries to impart sweetness to all sorts of foods and beverages, like yerba maté or other herbal tea concoctions. Stevia has been growing in popularity in the United States since the 1990s, and you can find it as liquid and powdered extracts, and even natural cut leaves, in grocery and natural foods stores. Its sweetening capabilities are highly concentrated, so only a very little is needed to replace a cup of sugar or other sweetener. Unlike some of its artificial counterparts, there are no known side effects to its usage.

Honey, You're Not So Sweet

Honey is another sweetener vegans avoid. What's wrong with honey? Simply put, honey is the regurgitation of the food bees eat, and as a result, is not vegan by any stretch of the imagination. Putting other animals, including insects, to work for our own benefit is contrary to what it means to be vegan. Honey was also listed as one of the foods vegans abstain from in the original aims of the Vegan Society.

Vegans consider it cruel to take the honey away from the bees because the bees created it for themselves. Honey is food bees make from the nectar of flowers and flowering trees to feed the hive and sustain the young. The honey production of a single bee, over the course of a lifetime, is only around $1/12$ teaspoon. That's a lot of work to produce very little honey! Each tablespoon of honey represents the life's work of 36 bees.

Also, to obtain honey on a commercial level, the bees have to be smoked out of their hives, which isn't pleasant. Who likes to get smoke in their eyes and respiratory system? Often, bees are also killed in the process of obtaining honey, the comb, and beeswax.

IN A NUTSHELL

Surprising as it may be, honey also sometimes contains botulism, which is why it's widely recommended that honey never be fed to children under age 1. Between 70 and 90 cases of infant botulism are reported in the United States annually, and sudden infant death syndrome has been linked, in part, to infant botulism.

Flour Power

The importance of purchasing whole-grain flours is really apparent in vegan baked goods because they bind, thicken, coat, and encapsulate so many foods and food items.

The nutty, almost sweet flavors of whole-grain flours give more depth to the flavors of your baked goods, in addition to a deep golden brown color after baking. Also, all the vital bran, germ, and other nutritional benefits of the whole grains are all still contained within your baked goods instead of having been stripped away. Because whole grains contain fiber, which is good for your digestion and colon, they can make for some pretty tasty good-for-you desserts.

Try experimenting with using new flours such as whole-wheat flour, white whole-wheat flour, whole-wheat pastry flour, barley flour, and oat flour—alone or in combinations—to replace bleached white all-purpose flour in recipes.

Going Gluten Free

More and more people are discovering that their bodies are sensitive to gluten. Gluten is the protein found in several grains, most notably in all forms of wheat, including durum, semolina, spelt, kamut, einkorn, and faro, and related grains like rye, barley, and triticale. Oats are also included in this list because they're processed on shared equipment, although you can now buy certified gluten-free oats.

Depending on whether you have a gluten intolerance, a gluten allergy, or celiac disease (an autoimmune condition), symptoms of gluten sensitivity can range from fatigue, eczema, weight issues, or gastrointestinal discomfort to vitamin deficiencies, asthma, or severe damage to your GI tract. If you're experiencing any of these symptoms and think gluten may be the cause, consider refraining from eating foods that contain gluten, and check with your doctor about being tested for food allergies, intolerances, and sensitivities.

Fortunately, there are still plenty of gluten-free whole grains to be had, like amaranth, buckwheat, corn, millet, quinoa, and numerous types of rice. To try your hand at gluten-free baking, stock up on some gluten-free flours such as brown rice, millet, quinoa, coconut, sorghum, chickpea/garbanzo bean, and almond meal or other nut-based flours or meals, as well as arrowroot, cornstarch, and potato and tapioca starches, to replace wheat and other gluten-based flours. Use a ratio of 2 parts brown rice flour to 1 part either quinoa, sorghum, or millet flours or potato or tapioca starches, or a combination of two or more of them, along with a small amount of xanthan or guar gum. This works well in most pastries, cookies, cakes, and other baked goods.

> **HOT POTATO**
>
> Flours can go stale and rancid, as well as attract bugs. Always store flour (and starches, too) in airtight containers or zipper-lock bags, either in a cool dark place like your pantry or in the refrigerator or freezer.

Several companies, including Arrowhead Mills and Bob's Red Mill, produce a vast array of gluten-free flours, mixed blends, and packaged products made from assorted grains, nuts, and legumes, and even certified gluten-free oats. These gluten-free flours and baking mixes can often be used measure for measure for wheat flours in your gluten-free baking and cooking. In many of the gluten-free recipe variations in this book, we recommend using Bob's Red Mill Gluten-Free All-Purpose Baking Flour for best results.

You can find all these gluten-free flours in most grocery and natural foods stores, both packaged and in bulk bins. Buy flours and starches in bulk for the best price, and rotate your stock often to ensure the freshest quality.

For more information about gluten-free vegan cooking and baking, as well as tons of recipe ideas, check out Beverly's book *The Complete Idiot's Guide to Gluten-Free Vegan Cooking*, co-authored with plant-based dietitian Julieanna Hever.

Experimenting and Accepting

It may take you a while to get used to using some of these vegan ingredients, but be patient and keep trying, especially if baking and cooking are new to you. Accept the fact that you won't be able to duplicate *everything* with vegan ingredients.

For instance, foods made entirely of eggs, such as meringues and soufflés—forget about it. They can't be done vegan because there are too many eggs holding the mix together. You can make other vegan goodies instead of meringues, or use tofu whipped toppings or Soyatoo whipped topping to sort of replace the meringue on a pie. You can also have some tofu scramble instead of a soufflé for brunch or breakfast or a tofu cheesecake to replace a dairy version.

There will be times when you want to duplicate or imitate a once-favorite food item and others when you'll be inspired to strike out in a different direction with the same ingredients to create a new vegan gastronomical nirvana. Different can be better! Tinker and experiment in your kitchen to accommodate your own tastes or lack or abundance of ingredients. If you stumble upon something really great tasting, be sure to write it down so you'll be able to duplicate the recipe another time. Also, don't forget to share your vegan goodies with others; they can be a great way to spread the joys of veganism and turn others on to this great way of eating and living!

The Least You Need to Know

- Nonhydrogenated vegan margarine, buttery sticks, vegan shortening, and vegetable and coconut oil work extremely well as a replacement for butter in your baked goods, and plant-based nondairy milks can substitute for cow's milk with ease.

- Agar-agar is a vegan alternative to gelatin you can use to thicken sauces, frostings, puddings, fillings, and other custardlike desserts. Several brands of vegan gelatin are also available commercially.

- Tofu is a versatile ingredient you can use in a variety of ways to replace fat, eggs, and cream in your vegan baked goods.

- Bananas and other pectin-rich fruits can act as binders and fat replacers in a recipe. They also add height and moisture to the finished product.

- In the United States, most bleached cane sugar is processed using bone char, a special charcoal made from animal bones. Beet sugar, organic evaporated cane juice, Sucanat, turbinado, or other vegan-friendly types of sugar are not.

- Choose whole-grain flours whenever possible, as they yield the best results for your baked vegan creations while supplying nutritional benefits.

Vegan Food for the Soul

Now that you know how to shop wisely, it's time to stock up on your vegan cooking and baking supplies. Pull out the pots, pans, bowls, colanders, and cutting boards; sharpen your knives; gather your utensils; and get ready to create some delicious vegan goodies!

No matter what your level of kitchen experience, we offer you vegan recipes to suit all your wants, needs, and cravings. We give you the quick and easy, as well as the basics needed to create meals at holiday time or as a special treat for someone you love. From breakfast to dessert, we give you lots of options and ideas for fueling yourself with good vegan foods!

Good Morning Breakfasts

In This Chapter

- Cool and healthy fruity beginnings
- Veganizing breakfast favorites
- Hearty and hot vegan breakfast ideas
- Soy-based selections

Going vegan doesn't mean you have to miss out on delicious breakfasts like the ones you might fondly remember from your childhood. You can easily make vegan versions of dishes such as French toast, scrambled eggs, sausages, and other hearty fare with a little bit of know-how and culinary creativity!

In this chapter, we share recipes for some awesome and filling vegan breakfasts, most of which help you start your day energized and ready to roll, with lower cholesterol and more fruit and veggies than the nonvegan versions. Complex carbs, protein, and calcium—what a great way to jump-start your day!

If you have hectic morning schedules or just don't move so quickly in the morning, we have you covered with recipes for quick fruit-based breakfasts such as a cool and creamy smoothie and even a multilayer breakfast parfait. We also offer a few hearty choices like tofu scramble, potato and veggie home fries, tempeh sausages, and veganized versions of pancakes and French toast. You can make many of the heartier recipes in large batches ahead of time and reheat them in smaller batches as needed to satisfy your morning grumblings with a nutritious breakfast even when you're pressed for time.

Power Up Smoothie

A frozen banana and berries add sweetness and help camouflage the color and flavor of the leafy greens in this creamy hemp-and-flaxseed-enhanced breakfast smoothie.

Yield:	Prep time:	Serving size:
5 or 6 cups	5 minutes	1¼ cups

4 cups packed spinach, kale, chard, or a combination

2 cups fresh or frozen mixed blueberries, blackberries, strawberries, or red raspberries

2 cups almond or other nondairy milk

1 cup *coconut water* or water

½ cup ice cubes

1 large banana, peeled and broken into 3 pieces

2 TB. hemp seeds

2 TB. ground flaxseeds or flaxseed meal

1. In a blender, blend spinach, mixed berries, almond milk, coconut water, ice, banana, hemp seeds, and flaxseeds for 1 or 2 minutes or until smooth.

2. Evenly divide mixture among 4 glasses, and serve immediately.

Variation: For a sweeter smoothie, add 2 or 3 pitted dates. For a **Hawaiian Power Up Smoothie,** replace the mixed berries with 1 cup frozen or canned pineapple chunks and 1 cup frozen papaya or mango chunks.

DEFINITION

Coconut water is the clear liquid found inside young green coconuts. It's mild and sweet in flavor and rich in electrolytes, making it the perfect natural sports drink. You can find it in bottles and cans in most grocery and natural foods stores.

Breakfast Fruit Parfaits

These delicious and eye-catching breakfast parfaits are made of layers of fruit, fruit purée, and granola, similar to an ice-cream sundae. Who says you can't have dessert for breakfast?

Yield:	Prep time:	Serving size:
4 parfaits	5 minutes	2 cups or 1 parfait

1 cup fresh blueberries	3 large bananas, peeled and cut into 2-in. pieces
1 cup fresh blackberries, cut in ½ lengthwise	1 tsp. fresh or bottled lemon juice
1 cup fresh strawberries, hulled and sliced	½ cup unsweetened shredded coconut
1 large kiwifruit, peeled and diced	3⅔ cups granola

1. In a medium bowl, combine blueberries, blackberries, strawberries, and kiwi-fruit, and set aside.

2. In a food processor fitted with an S blade, process bananas and lemon juice for 1 minute or until smooth. Scrape down the sides of the container with a spatula.

3. Add shredded coconut, and process for 2 or 3 minutes or until extremely light and creamy. Transfer mixture to a glass bowl.

4. To assemble parfaits: in the bottom of 4 large glasses or dessert dishes, add ⅓ cup mixed fruit mixture, ⅓ cup granola, and follow with ⅓ cup banana–coconut cream mixture. Repeat layers, ending with banana–coconut cream mixture. Serve immediately.

Variation: For **Fruit, Yogurt, and Granola Parfaits,** in each parfait, replace the banana–coconut cream mixture with a 6-ounce container of plain or flavored vegan yogurt.

IN A NUTSHELL

If you're a raw foodist, you can skip the granola and replace it with some chopped nuts or seeds for added crunch.

Banana-Walnut Bread Oatmeal

Enjoy the great taste of banana bread without turning on your oven! A bowlful of this hearty oatmeal studded with banana slices and chopped walnuts gets your day off to a great start.

Yield:	Prep time:	Cook time:	Serving size:
4 cups	5 minutes	5 to 7 minutes	1 cup

1¾ cups water

1½ cups plain or vanilla soy or other nondairy milk

1½ cups old-fashioned or regular rolled oats

2 large bananas, peeled and thinly sliced

Pinch sea salt

¼ cup maple syrup or light brown sugar, packed

1 tsp. ground cinnamon

1 tsp. vanilla extract

6 TB. raw or toasted walnuts, roughly chopped

1. In a medium saucepan over medium heat, combine water, soy milk, old-fashioned rolled oats, 1 sliced banana, and pinch sea salt. Cook, stirring often, for 5 to 7 minutes or until liquid is absorbed and oats are very soft and creamy.

2. Add maple syrup, cinnamon, and vanilla extract, and stir well to combine. Remove the saucepan from heat, and serve hot, garnishing individual servings with ¼ of remaining banana slices and 1½ tablespoons toasted walnuts.

Variation: If you like your oatmeal really thick, only add 1 cup water. For **Nut and Seed Banana Bread Oatmeal,** sprinkle 1 or 2 teaspoons chia seeds, hemp seeds, or ground flaxseeds over the individual servings.

IN A NUTSHELL

Oats contain beneficial soluble fiber, which helps lower your blood cholesterol levels as well as improve your digestion and elimination processes.

Almond Spice French Toast

Rather than eggs and milk, a homemade sweetened and spiced almond milk base is used to make over your favorite whole-grain bread into a fantastic warm breakfast.

Yield:	Prep time:	Cook time:	Serving size:
8 slices	10 minutes	10 minutes	2 slices

1¼ cups water

½ cup raw whole almonds

¼ cup brown rice syrup or maple syrup

1 tsp. almond extract

1 tsp. vanilla extract

1 tsp. ground cinnamon

½ tsp. ground nutmeg

½ tsp. sea salt

8 slices whole-grain or other bread of choice

1. In a blender, process water, almonds, brown rice syrup, almond extract, vanilla extract, cinnamon, nutmeg, and sea salt for 2 or 3 minutes or until very smooth and creamy. (Alternatively, use a food processor fitted with an S blade, but first process almonds until finely chopped and then process with remaining ingredients until smooth.)

2. Transfer almond mixture to a 9×13-inch baking pan. Place 4 whole-grain bread slices in almond mixture, flip them over to coat other side, and allow bread slices to soak in mixture for 2 minutes.

3. Lightly oil a large, nonstick skillet, and place over medium heat. Or use a griddle.

4. Using a fork, carefully remove soaked bread slices from almond mixture, and place them into the hot skillet. Cook for 1 or 2 minutes or until golden brown on the bottom. Flip over bread with a spatula, and cook for 1 or 2 more minutes or until golden brown on the other side.

5. While first batch cooks, repeat soaking procedure for remaining 4 bread slices. Lightly oil the skillet again, and repeat the cooking procedure for remaining bread slices. Keep cooked slices warm in a 250°F oven while preparing second batch.

6. Serve hot with your choice of jams, preserves, syrups, or fresh fruit.

Variation: For **Happy Hemp French Toast,** replace the almonds and water with 1½ cups vanilla hemp milk, and also replace the almond extract with 1 teaspoon rum extract or additional vanilla extract.

Multigrain Pancakes

These wholesome pancakes are rich in protein and beneficial fiber and have a slightly nutty flavor that results from combining flaxseeds with whole-wheat and barley flours and blended rolled oats.

Yield:	Prep time:	Cook time:	Serving size:
8 pancakes	8 to 10 minutes	15 to 20 minutes	1 pancake

3 TB. water

1 TB. ground flaxseeds or flaxseed meal

⅓ cup old-fashioned or regular rolled oats

⅓ cup cornmeal (preferably medium grind)

⅔ cup whole-wheat or white whole-wheat flour

⅔ cup barley flour

2 TB. turbinado sugar or date sugar

1 TB. aluminum-free baking powder

½ tsp. ground cinnamon

¼ tsp. sea salt

2 cups soy or other nondairy milk

1½ TB. sunflower or other oil

1 tsp. vanilla extract

1. In a small bowl, combine water and flaxseeds, and let sit for 5 minutes.

2. In a blender or food processor fitted with an S blade, process old-fashioned rolled oats and cornmeal for 1 or 2 minutes or until oats are ground to a fine powder. Transfer to a large bowl. Add whole-wheat flour, barley flour, turbinado sugar, aluminum-free baking powder, cinnamon, and sea salt, and whisk well.

3. Add flaxseed mixture, soy milk, sunflower oil, and vanilla extract, and whisk well.

4. Lightly oil a large nonstick skillet, and place over medium heat. Or use a griddle. Pour ½ cup batter per pancake into the hot skillet, and cook for 2 or 3 minutes or until edges of pancake are slightly dry and bubbles appear on top. Flip over pancake with a spatula, and cook for 2 or 3 more minutes or until golden brown on the other side.

5. As needed, lightly oil skillet again and repeat with remaining batter.

6. Serve hot with maple syrup or other toppings of choice.

Variation: Feel free to add fresh or frozen berries, sliced fruits, chopped nuts, or seeds to the pancake batter. For **Gluten-Free Multigrain Pancakes,** replace the whole-wheat flour with buckwheat flour and the barley flour with brown rice flour.

> **IN A NUTSHELL**
>
> Brown flaxseeds are the most readily available, but you can also purchase golden flaxseeds, which are a pale strawlike color. You can use either variety of flaxseeds for preparing these pancakes.

Hearty Home Fries

This skillet-cooked side dish is a savory and colorful combination of potatoes, onions, bell peppers, leafy kale, and seasonings, and pairs well with toast, pancakes, or tofu scrambles.

Yield:	Prep time:	Cook time:	Serving size:
7 or 8 cups	10 minutes	15–20 minutes	1 cup

6 cups (7 or 8 medium) red-skinned potatoes, cut into quarters lengthwise, and thinly sliced

2 TB. olive oil

1½ cups (1 large) yellow onion, diced

1½ cups (1 large) green bell pepper, ribs and seeds removed, and diced

1½ cups (1 large) red bell pepper, ribs and seeds removed, and diced

3 cups kale, stems removed, roughly chopped, and packed, or 3 cups baby spinach, packed

½ cup green onions, white and green parts, thinly sliced

½ TB. minced garlic

1 tsp. dried basil

1 tsp. dried thyme

½ tsp. smoked paprika or chile powder

½ tsp. seasoning salt or sea salt

½ tsp. freshly ground black pepper

⅓ cup chopped fresh parsley

1½ TB. nutritional yeast flakes

1. In a large nonstick skillet over medium-high heat, combine red-skinned pota-toes and olive oil, and cook, partially covered and stirring occasionally, for 7 minutes.

2. Add yellow onion, green bell pepper, and red bell pepper, and cook, uncovered and stirring often, for 5 minutes.

3. Add kale, green onions, garlic, basil, thyme, smoked paprika, seasoning salt, and black pepper, and cook, stirring often, for 3 to 5 minutes or until potatoes are tender and lightly browned.

4. Stir in parsley and nutritional yeast flakes. Remove the skillet from heat, and serve hot.

Variation: Feel free to replace the red-skinned potatoes with Yukon Gold, Russian Blue, Peruvian Purple, or fingerling potatoes. For more traditional **Home-Style Home Fries,** use 2 cups yellow onion, and omit the bell peppers and kale.

IN A NUTSHELL

Even though potatoes are often lumped together with root vegetables like beets, carrots, and turnips, they're actually a tuber. Other types of tubers include sweet potatoes, yams, Jerusalem artichokes (sunchokes), jicama, water chestnuts, and yucca (cassava).

Sammy's Spicy Tempeh Sausages

Forget about those frozen sausage patties! The flavor of these spicy tempeh sausage patties beats them hands down, and you can easily change their seasonings to suit your own tastes.

Yield:	Prep time:	Cook time:	Serving size:
10 sausage patties	5 minutes, plus 1 hour chill time	10 to 15 minutes	2 sausage patties

2 (8-oz.) pkg. tempeh

1½ TB. tamari, shoyu, or Bragg Liquid Aminos

1½ TB. balsamic vinegar

2 TB. olive oil

½ cup whole-wheat flour

1 tsp. dried basil

1 tsp. dried oregano

1 tsp. dried thyme

1 tsp. garlic powder

1 tsp. onion powder

1 tsp. ground fennel

1 tsp. crushed red pepper flakes

½ tsp. freshly ground black pepper

1. Line a cookie sheet with parchment paper.

2. In a food processor fitted with an S blade, process tempeh, tamari, balsamic vinegar, and 1 tablespoon olive oil for 1 minute. Scrape down the sides of the container with a spatula, and process for 30 to 60 more seconds or until tempeh is finely ground. Transfer tempeh mixture to a medium bowl.

3. Add whole-wheat flour, basil, oregano, thyme, garlic powder, onion powder, fennel, crushed red pepper flakes, and black pepper, and stir well to combine.

4. Gently pack tempeh mixture into a ¼-cup measuring cup using the back of a spoon, flip over the cup onto the prepared cookie sheet, and give the cup a tap to release patty. Using a burger press or your hands, slightly flatten patties. Repeat with remaining tempeh mixture, and refrigerate for 1 hour or more.

5. In a large nonstick skillet over medium heat, heat ½ tablespoon olive oil. In batches, add tempeh sausage patties to the skillet and cook for 5 to 7 minutes or until well browned. Flip over sausage patties with a spatula, and cook for 5 more minutes or until golden brown and crisp around the edges. Repeat with remaining ½ tablespoon olive oil and sausage patties.

6. Serve sausage patties hot, warm, or at room temperature as a side dish, sandwich filling, or pizza topping (crumbled); or use to add to sauces, pasta or grain-based salads, or main dishes. Store in an airtight container or zipper-lock bag in the refrigerator for up to 5 days, or freeze for up to 3 months.

Variation: To make **Tempeh Maple Sausages,** replace the tamari and balsamic vinegar with ¼ cup pure maple syrup and 2 tablespoons apple juice; omit all the dried herbs and crushed red pepper flakes, and replace them with 2 teaspoons herbes de Provence, and add ½ cup (1 medium) apple of choice, peeled and grated.

IN A NUTSHELL

You can prepare these tempeh sausage patties in larger batches, cook them, and freeze them in an airtight container. Then, simply reheat in the oven or in a nonstick skillet until heated through.

Tempeh Sausage and Gravy on Biscuits

Transform your leftovers into a fantastic and filling breakfast. To create this classic down-home breakfast, split biscuits are topped with Creamy Onion Gravy that contains crumbled pieces of tempeh sausage.

Yield:	Prep time:	Cook time:	Serving size:
6 biscuits and 2 cups gravy	5 minutes	10 to 15 minutes	1 biscuit wedge and ⅓ cup gravy

4 Sammy's Spicy Tempeh Sausages (recipe earlier in this chapter)

2 cups Creamy Onion Gravy (recipe in Chapter 22)

1 TB. nutritional yeast flakes

¼ tsp. freshly ground black pepper

Hot pepper sauce

6 Soy Buttermilk Biscuits (recipe in Chapter 23)

1. Using your fingers, crumble Sammy's Spicy Tempeh Sausages into a medium saucepan. Add Creamy Onion Gravy, nutritional yeast flakes, and black pepper, and cook over medium heat, stirring often, for 3 to 5 minutes or until gravy is hot and bubbling.

2. Taste and season with hot pepper sauce as desired. Remove the saucepan from heat.

3. Split Soy Buttermilk Biscuits in ½, top with tempeh sausage and gravy mixture, and serve hot.

Variation: You can also serve the tempeh sausage and gravy mixture over Mouth-watering Mashed Potatoes (recipe in Chapter 21), rice, or other cooked grains. For **Seitan and Gravy on Biscuits,** replace the Sammy's Spicy Tempeh Sausages with 1½ cups Baked Seitan Roast (recipe in Chapter 21), roughly chopped.

> **HOT POTATO**
>
> Be sure to keep stirring the tempeh sausage and gravy mixture as it heats. The prepared gravy has already been thickened and could easily scorch on the bottom of the saucepan during heating.

Tofu and Veggie Scramble

One of the most popular vegan breakfast options is the tofu scramble, a tofu-based vegan version of scrambled eggs. This tofu scramble recipe is flavored with bits of red and green onion and green bell pepper.

Yield:	Prep time:	Cook time:	Serving size:
4 cups	5 minutes	2½ to 3½ minutes	1 cup

1 lb. firm or extra-firm tofu	½ cup green bell pepper, ribs and seeds removed, and diced
2 TB. nutritional yeast flakes	
1 TB. tamari, shoyu, or Bragg Liquid Aminos	1 TB. olive oil
	⅓ cup green onions, white and green parts, thinly sliced
1 tsp. onion powder	
1 tsp. garlic powder or garlic granules	3 TB. chopped fresh parsley
½ tsp. *turmeric*	Sea salt
½ cup red onion, diced	Freshly ground black pepper

1. Using your fingers, crumble firm tofu into a medium bowl. Add nutritional yeast flakes, tamari, onion powder, garlic powder, and turmeric, and stir well to coat.

2. In a large nonstick skillet over medium-high heat, combine red onion, green bell pepper, and olive oil. Cook, stirring occasionally, for 3 minutes.

3. Add tofu mixture and green onions, and cook, stirring often, for 5 minutes or until tofu is dry and lightly browned.

4. Stir in parsley. Taste and season with sea salt and black pepper. Remove the skillet from heat, and serve hot.

Variation: You can also add other chopped veggies, such as carrots, broccoli, or zucchini, and fresh herbs to your tofu scramble. For a **Western-Style Tofu Scramble,** replace the red onion with ½ cup yellow onion, diced, and add ½ cup red bell pepper, ribs and seeds removed, and diced.

> **DEFINITION**
>
> **Turmeric** is a spicy, pungent yellow root that's dried and finely ground to a powder for use in many dishes, especially Indian cuisine, for color and flavor. Turmeric is the source of the yellow color in many prepared mustards and curry powder.

Vegan Eggs Benedict

Our Tofu and Veggie Scramble and Vegan Cheezy Sauce recipes work well as delicious, cholesterol-free substitutes for the typical poached eggs and hollandaise sauce in this vegan version of the classic brunch offering.

Yield:	Prep time:	Cook time:	Serving size:
6 cups or 4 assembled servings	10 minutes	10 to 15 minutes	1½ cups or 1 assembled serving

2 plain, whole-wheat, or sprouted-grain English muffins

4 slices Yves Canadian Veggie Bacon

½ batch Tofu and Veggie Scramble (recipe earlier in this chapter)

4 thick tomato slices

½ batch Vegan Cheezy Sauce (recipe in Chapter 22)

Chopped fresh dill

Chopped fresh parsley

1. Split English muffins, toast until golden brown, and set aside.

2. Prepare Yves Canadian Veggie Bacon according to the package instructions.

3. In the center of each serving plate, place ½ toasted English muffin. Top with 1 slice Yves Canadian Veggie Bacon, ¼ of prepared Tofu and Veggie Scramble, and 1 slice tomato. Drizzle with ¼ of Vegan Cheezy Sauce, garnish with dill and parsley, and serve.

Variation: For a handheld **Vegan Scramble and Bacon Muffin Sandwich,** omit the Vegan Cheezy Sauce and tomato, and instead layer the Yves Canadian Veggie Bacon and Tofu and Veggie Scramble between a split Soy Buttermilk Biscuit (recipe in Chapter 23) or English muffin.

IN A NUTSHELL

Yves Veggie Cuisine makes several vegan meatless products suitable for serving for breakfast or for use in recipes. Try their Canadian Bacon, Bacon Strips, Breakfast Patties, and Breakfast Links. You can find them in the refrigerated section of most natural foods stores.

Midday Meals

In This Chapter

- Filling hot soups and chili
- Colorful and nutritious salads
- Layered wraps and cold sandwiches
- Hearty hot sandwiches and burgers

It isn't smart to start your day off on an empty stomach, but due to time constraints and daily routines, many people go without a morning meal. If you skip breakfast, lunch is the first meal of your day, so it really needs to count and provide enough fuel to power you through the rest of your day.

Your breakfast choices influence your lunch choices. If you had a hearty breakfast, you may still feel quite full and want to eat a lighter lunch of a bowl of soup or a salad or a combination of the two. If you had your usual morning bowl of oatmeal and fruit, you should have something more substantial, such as a big bowl of soup or salad, a hearty sandwich or burger, or both if your appetite is up for it.

Making your own vegan meals and taking them to work or school is much more economical, environmentally friendly, and nutritious than buying lunch. And by making your own meals, you know exactly what's in each dish and that it's up to your vegan standards. Leftovers from the night before often make for some of the best and easiest lunchtime options. Chopped leftover veggies, grains, and pasta dishes become impromptu salads with little effort.

To round out your lunch, be sure to pack a healthy snack, too—maybe a few raw veggies or a piece of fruit, or whole-grain crackers or some pretzels, depending on what's already in your lunch basket. You can also pack nuts, fruit strips, or dried fruits such as raisins or figs for an afternoon snack.

IN A NUTSHELL

If you want to make your co-workers or friends jealous, pack one of the hearty burgers or sandwiches with a side of this chapter's Deli-Style Potato Salad. They won't believe they're vegan!

Creamy Vegetable Soup

This creamy soup is studded with pieces of potatoes, carrots, celery, broccoli, and Swiss chard, and blending part of the soup with soy milk and cornstarch quickly and easily thickens the soup.

Yield:	Prep time:	Cook time:	Serving size:
2 quarts	10 to 15 minutes	45 minutes	1½ cups

4 cups low-sodium vegetable broth

2 cups (2 or 3 medium) Yukon Gold potatoes, cut into quarters lengthwise, and thinly sliced

2 cups (1 lb.) fresh or frozen broccoli, cut into small florets

1 cup (1 medium) yellow onion, diced

1 cup (2 large) carrots, diced

1 cup (2 large stalks) celery (including inner leaves), diced

1½ TB. minced garlic

1 bay leaf

1 TB. chopped fresh thyme or 1 tsp. dried

1 TB. chopped fresh dill or 1 tsp. dried dill weed

1 tsp. sea salt

½ tsp. freshly ground black pepper

1½ cups soy or other nondairy milk

3 TB. cornstarch

2 TB. nutritional yeast flakes

4 cups (½ a bunch) rainbow Swiss chard, stems and leaves roughly chopped, and packed

¼ cup chopped fresh parsley

1. In a large pot over high heat, bring vegetable broth, Yukon Gold potatoes, broccoli, yellow onion, carrots, celery, garlic, bay leaf, thyme, dill, sea salt, and black pepper to a boil. Cover, reduce heat to low, and simmer for 20 to 25 minutes or until potatoes are soft. Remove and discard bay leaf.

2. In a blender or food processor fitted with an S blade, process 2 cups soup mixture (not bay leaf), soy milk, cornstarch, and nutritional yeast flakes for 1 or 2 minutes or until smooth.

3. Stir blended mixture back into the pot. Add rainbow Swiss chard and parsley, and simmer for 10 to 15 minutes or until rainbow Swiss chard is wilted.

4. Taste and adjust seasonings as desired, and serve hot.

Variation: For **Cheezy Vegetable Soup,** add 1½ cups Vegan Cheezy Sauce (recipe in Chapter 22) to the finished soup.

VEGAN VOICES

Good soup is one of the prime ingredients of good living. For soup can do more to lift the spirits and stimulate the appetite than any other one dish.

—Louis P. De Gouy, *The Soup Book* (1949)

Seitan Vegetable Noodle Soup

Chewy bits of chopped seitan, aromatic vegetables, and pasta are simmered together in a golden broth to create this vegan version of chicken noodle soup.

Yield:	Prep time:	Cook time:	Serving size:
2 quarts	10 to 15 minutes	30 minutes	1½ cups

6 cups low-sodium vegetable broth

1½ cups (1 large) yellow onion, diced

1½ cups (2 or 3 large) carrots, diced

1½ cups (2 or 3 large stalks) celery (including inner leaves), diced

1½ TB. minced garlic

1 bay leaf

1 TB. chopped fresh thyme or 1 tsp. dried

1 TB. chopped fresh dill or 1 tsp. dried dill weed

1 tsp. sea salt

½ tsp. freshly ground black pepper

2 cups water

¼ cup *nutritional yeast flakes*

¼ tsp. turmeric or *curry powder*

1 cup Baked Seitan Roast (recipe in Chapter 21), roughly chopped

¾ cup whole-wheat spaghetti, broken into 3-in. pieces, or other shaped pasta such as rotini or small shells

⅓ cup chopped fresh parsley

1. In a large pot over high heat, bring vegetable broth, yellow onion, carrots, celery, garlic, bay leaf, thyme, dill, sea salt, and black pepper to a boil. Cover, reduce heat to low, and simmer for 15 minutes. Remove and discard bay leaf.

2. In a blender or food processor fitted with an S blade, process 2 cups soup mixture for 1 minute. Add water, nutritional yeast flakes, and turmeric, and process for 30 to 60 more seconds or until completely smooth.

3. Stir blended mixture back into the pot. Add Baked Seitan Roast, whole-wheat spaghetti, and parsley, and simmer for 10 minutes or until pasta is al dente.

4. Taste and adjust seasonings as desired, and serve hot.

Variation: For added flavor, begin recipe by sautéing yellow onion, carrots, celery, and garlic in ½ tablespoon olive oil over medium heat, stirring often, for 3 minutes. For **Seitan, Vegetable, and Rice Soup,** replace spaghetti with ½ cup basmati, jasmine, or brown rice, and simmer soup for 10 to 20 more minutes or until rice is tender.

DEFINITION

Nutritional yeast flakes are a type of inactive yeast that has a nutty, almost cheeselike flavor, which is why it's commonly used as a cheese flavoring. It's an excellent product for vegans to use to attain their recommended daily dose of vitamin B_{12}. Do not confuse this with active yeast, the type used for making breads and baked goods.

Curry powder is a ground blend of rich and flavorful spices used as a basis for curry and many other Indian-influenced dishes. Common ingredients include hot pepper, nutmeg, cumin, cinnamon, pepper, and turmeric. Some curry can also be found in paste form.

Quick-and-Easy Veggie-and-Bean Chili

This mildly spiced, hearty chili is packed with a colorful assortment of fresh veggies. To save on prep and cook time, it makes use of two kinds of canned beans and tomato products.

Yield:	Prep time:	Cook time:	Serving size:
3 quarts	10 to 15 minutes	30 minutes	1½ cups

2 cups (2 large) sweet potatoes, peeled and cut into ½-in. cubes

½ TB. olive oil

1 cup (1 medium) yellow or red onion, diced

½ cup celery (including inner leaves), diced

1 medium zucchini, diced

1 cup fresh or frozen cut corn

1 cup (1 medium) green bell pepper, ribs and seeds removed, and diced

1 cup (1 medium) red bell pepper, ribs and seeds removed, and diced

1 medium jalapeño pepper, ribs and seeds removed, and finely diced

1 TB. minced garlic

1 (28-oz.) can crushed tomatoes, with juice

1 (15-oz.) can black beans, drained and rinsed

1 (15-oz.) can kidney beans, drained and rinsed

1 (8-oz.) can tomato sauce

1 TB. chili powder

½ TB. ground cumin

½ TB. dried oregano

¾ tsp. sea salt

½ tsp. freshly ground black pepper

¼ cup green onions, white and green parts, thinly sliced

¼ cup chopped fresh cilantro

¼ cup chopped fresh parsley

1. In a large pot over medium heat, combine sweet potatoes and olive oil. Sauté, stirring often, for 5 minutes.

2. Add yellow onion and celery, and sauté, stirring often, for 3 minutes.

3. Add zucchini, corn, green bell pepper, red bell pepper, jalapeño pepper, and garlic, and sauté, stirring often, for 3 minutes or until vegetables are tender.

4. Add crushed tomatoes, black beans, kidney beans, tomato sauce, chili powder, cumin, oregano, sea salt, and black pepper, and stir well to combine. Cover, reduce heat to low, and cook for 15 minutes to allow flavors to blend.

5. Stir in green onions, and cook for 3 more minutes.

6. Remove from heat. Stir in cilantro and parsley, taste and adjust seasonings, and serve hot.

Variation: Feel free to substitute other fresh or frozen vegetables or beans. For **Smoky Veggie and Bean Chili,** use fire-roasted crushed tomatoes. Also, use only 2 teaspoons chili powder, and add 1 teaspoon smoked paprika, and ½ teaspoon chipotle chili powder.

> **IN A NUTSHELL**
>
> This chili is so versatile. Serve it as a side dish, as a filling for sandwiches, mixed with grain dishes for a hearty entrée, or as a chunky dip for tortilla chips or crackers. You can also garnish individual servings with sliced green onions, shredded soy cheese, diced avocado, or tofu sour cream.

Colorful Kale and Chard Salad with Tahini Dressing

Experts agree you should strive to eat foods from all colors of the rainbow, and this colorful salad made with leafy greens, red cabbage, and shredded beets and carrots will help you achieve that goal deliciously.

Yield:	Prep time:	Serving size:
9 to 10 cups	10 to 15 minutes	2 cups

3 large leaves green or purple kale, stems removed, and roughly chopped

3 large leaves rainbow Swiss chard, stems and leaves roughly chopped

1½ cups (½ medium head) red cabbage, shredded

1 cup (1 or 2 medium) beets, shredded

1 cup (1 or 2 large) carrots, shredded

1 cup (2 large stalks) celery (including inner leaves), thinly sliced

3 green onions, white and green parts, thinly sliced

1 cup mung bean or other sprouts

2 TB. raw sesame seeds

2 TB. raw hemp seeds

1 batch Tahini Dressing (recipe in Chapter 22)

1. In a large bowl, combine green kale, rainbow Swiss chard, red cabbage, beets, carrots, celery, and green onions.

2. Scatter mung bean sprouts, sesame seeds, and hemp seeds over top. Drizzle ⅓ to ½ cup Tahini Dressing over salad, and toss gently to coat. Or drizzle dressing over individual servings. Serve immediately.

Variation: Feel free to make this salad with other varieties of leafy greens, such as spinach, collard greens, or arugula, or replace the red cabbage with green cabbage. For **Tahini Slaw Wraps,** toss all the salad ingredients with ⅔ cup Tahini Dressing, and let mixture marinate at room temperature for 30 to 60 minutes or until salad slightly wilts. Place 1 cup marinated salad inside a warmed 8-inch white, whole-wheat, or flavored flour tortilla, fold to enclose filling or roll up like a burrito, and serve immediately.

HOT POTATO

Cruciferous vegetables like kale, cabbage, broccoli, cauliflower, and brussels sprouts contain a lot of insoluble fiber, which can cause digestive problems for many people. This is especially true when they're eaten raw. Be sure to thoroughly chew these veggies before swallowing to help the digestive process.

Vegan Chef's Salad

The popular bistro-style chef's salad often contains many animal-based ingredients like eggs and julienne strips of meat, but this colorful version is 100 percent plant based—and better for you, too!

Yield:	Prep time:	Serving size:
11 to 12 cups	10 to 15 minutes	2 cups

4 cups romaine lettuce or other green lettuce, rinsed, patted dry, and torn into bite-size pieces

4 cups red-tipped loose-leaf lettuce, rinsed, patted dry, and torn into bite-size pieces

1 cup cooked chickpeas

1 cup (½ medium) cucumber, cut in ½ lengthwise and thinly sliced

⅔ cup red onion, cut into ½ moons

1 cup cooked kidney beans

1 cup shredded vegan cheddar cheese

2 medium tomatoes, cut into wedges, or 1 cup cherry tomatoes, cut in ½

⅓ cup sunflower seeds

⅓ cup black olives, pitted, and thinly sliced

Salad dressing of choice

1. In a large bowl, gently toss romaine lettuce and red-tipped lettuce.

2. In rows or in a spoke pattern on top of greens, decoratively arrange, in order, chickpeas, cucumber, red onion, kidney beans, and cheddar cheese.

3. Arrange tomatoes around outer edges of salad. Scatter sunflower seeds and black olives over top.

4. Serve immediately, topping individual servings with salad dressing of choice (such as French, Thousand Island, sweet and sour, or vinaigrette), or chill.

Variation: Feel free to replace the romaine and red-tipped lettuces with a mixed greens blend of choice. For a **Composed Chef's Salad,** assemble the salad ingredients on individual plates: make a bed of the mixed lettuces, place small handfuls of the other ingredients in a spoke pattern on top, and drizzle salad dressing over salads.

IN A NUTSHELL

For an easier preparation, you can simply toss all the ingredients for this salad together in the bowl. Top individual servings with your favorite salad dressing as desired, or if you prefer, drizzle ⅓ to ½ cup of dressing over the salad mixture, and toss well to coat.

Deli-Style Potato Salad

Red-skinned potatoes, red and green onions, celery, and herbs are coated in a vegan mayonnaise-based dressing to create a creamy potato salad you can serve at your next picnic, barbecue, or family get-together.

Yield:	Prep time:	Cook time:	Serving size:
7 or 8 cups	10 to 15 minutes, plus 30 minutes chill time	15 minutes	1 cup

3 lb. (8 or 9 large) red-skinned potatoes, cut into 1-in. cubes

1½ cups Vegan Soy Milk Mayonnaise (recipe in Chapter 22)

1 TB. apple cider vinegar

1 TB. Dijon or spicy brown mustard

¾ tsp. celery seed

¾ tsp. sea salt

½ tsp. freshly ground black pepper

1 cup (2 large stalks) celery (including inner leaves), diced

⅔ cup red onion, diced

½ cup green onions, thinly sliced

¼ cup chopped fresh parsley

2 TB. chopped fresh dill or 2 tsp. dried dill weed

1. In a large pot over high heat, place red-skinned potatoes, cover with water, and bring to a boil. Reduce heat to medium-high, and cook for 12 to 15 minutes or until potatoes are tender and easily pierced with the tip of a knife. Drain potatoes in a colander, rinse with cold water, and drain well again. Transfer potatoes to a large bowl. (Alternatively, you can steam cubed potatoes for 10 minutes or until tender.)

2. In a small bowl, combine Vegan Soy Milk Mayonnaise, apple cider vinegar, Dijon mustard, celery seed, sea salt, and black pepper.

3. Pour mayonnaise mixture over potatoes, and stir gently to coat.

4. Add celery, red onion, green onions, parsley, and dill, and stir gently to combine. Chill for 30 minutes or more to allow flavors to blend.

5. Serve cold or at room temperature.

Variation: You can also prepare this recipe using Yukon Gold or white potatoes, or 4 pounds fingerling potatoes or small new potatoes. For **Golden Potato Salad with Basil Aioli,** replace the red-skinned potatoes with an equal amount of Yukon Gold or Yellow Fin potatoes, replace the mayonnaise mixture with 1½ cups Basil Aioli (recipe in Chapter 22), and omit the parsley and dill.

HOT POTATO

Potatoes should be stored in a cool, dark, well-ventilated place so they don't start to sprout or turn green. You can still use potatoes with these imperfections. Just cut off the offending parts and use the remaining potato in your recipe.

Truly Eggless Egg Salad

A combination of spices infuses crumbled tofu with tons of flavor, and the addition of turmeric gives this veganized egg salad a reminiscent yellow tint.

Yield:	Prep time:	Serving size:
3 cups	10 to 15 minutes, plus 30 minutes chill time	¾ cup

1 lb. firm or extra-firm tofu

1½ TB. lemon juice

1 tsp. onion powder

1 tsp. garlic powder

¾ tsp. sea salt

½ tsp. turmeric

½ tsp. celery seed

¼ tsp. freshly ground black pepper

½ cup Vegan Soy Milk Mayonnaise (recipe in Chapter 22)

⅓ cup celery (including inner leaves), finely diced

¼ cup green onions, white and green parts, thinly sliced

¼ cup chopped fresh parsley

2 TB. prepared pickle relish

1. Squeeze tofu over the sink to remove as much water as possible. Using your fingers, crumble tofu into a medium bowl.

2. Add lemon juice, onion powder, garlic powder, sea salt, turmeric, celery seed, and black pepper. Using a potato masher, mash together tofu and seasonings until well combined. Cover and chill for 15 minutes.

3. Add Vegan Soy Milk Mayonnaise, celery, green onions, parsley, and pickle relish, and stir well to combine. Cover and chill for 15 minutes to allow flavors to blend. The color will also turn more yellow as it chills.

4. Serve as a salad on a bed of greens; use as a filling for sandwiches, wraps, or hollowed out vegetables; or pipe on slices of squash or tomatoes and serve as a side dish or appetizer. Or enjoy with crackers, tortilla chips, toasted pitas, or other flat breads as a snack or appetizer.

Variation: For **Mock Tuna Salad,** replace the turmeric with $\frac{1}{2}$ teaspoon powdered kelp (available at natural foods stores).

Cornucopia Veggie Wraps

Wraps have become a popular lunch option, and in this recipe, they're filled with your choice of spread and multiple layers of fresh vegetables and then folded (rather than rolled) to resemble little vegetable-filled cornucopias.

Yield:	Prep time:	Serving size:
4 wraps	10 to 15 minutes	1 wrap

4 (8-in.) white, whole-wheat, or flavored flour tortillas

Dijon or spicy mustard, vegan cream cheese, Vegan Soy Milk Mayonnaise (recipe in Chapter 22), or Lemon-Garlic Hummus (recipe in Chapter 22), or other bean-based spread

4 leaves loose-leaf lettuce or lettuce, rinsed and patted dry

$\frac{1}{2}$ cup yam, peeled and shredded

$\frac{1}{2}$ cup zucchini, shredded

$\frac{1}{2}$ cup yellow summer squash, shredded

$\frac{1}{2}$ cup carrot, shredded

3 large Roma tomatoes, thinly sliced

1 medium cucumber, thinly sliced

1. In a large skillet over medium heat, warm each tortilla for 1 or 2 minutes per side. (Alternatively, warm tortillas in the microwave for 20 to 30 seconds.)

2. Place 1 tortilla flat on a large cutting board or work surface. Apply desired amount of Dijon mustard over top half of tortilla, leaving a 1-inch border around edges. Place 1 lettuce leaf vertically in center of tortilla so it hangs over top edge slightly. Top with 2 tablespoons yam, 2 tablespoons zucchini, 2 tablespoons summer squash, 2 tablespoons carrot, 3 Roma tomato slices, and 6 cucumber slices in 2 rows.

3. Fold bottom of tortilla up to center, and fold in each side, one overlapping the other, to enclose vegetables. Secure wrap with a toothpick. Repeat assembly procedure for remaining tortillas and ingredients.

4. Serve immediately, or wrap veggie wraps in plastic wrap or parchment paper or put in an airtight container, and refrigerate for up to 3 days.

Variation: Feel free to substitute any of your favorite vegetables, such as shredded beets, spinach, sliced radishes, chopped veggies, or sprouts. You can also add slices of vegan cheese or marinated and baked tofu or tempeh.

HOT POTATO

When purchasing tortillas, be sure to always check the nutrition facts listed on the package, particularly the fat content, which varies greatly from brand to brand. Many manufacturers add excessive amounts of oil to help keep the tortillas softer and easier to roll.

Veggie Hero Sandwiches

These hearty cold sandwiches are great for a packed lunch and are made by layering slices of seitan, vegan mozzarella, and crisp vegetables and then dressing them with olive oil, red wine vinegar, and seasonings.

Yield:	Prep time:	Serving size:
6 sandwiches	5 to 10 minutes	1 sandwich

6 (6-in.) Italian or submarine rolls

6 red-tipped loose-leaf lettuce leaves or other lettuce

1½ lb. Baked Seitan Roast (recipe in Chapter 21), thinly sliced

6 slices vegan mozzarella cheese or other variety

1 medium red onion, thinly sliced

2 large tomatoes, thinly sliced

Olive oil

Red wine vinegar

Sea salt

Freshly ground black pepper

Italian seasonings blend or dried basil and oregano

1. Split Italian rolls in ½ lengthwise, open, and place on a large cutting board or work surface.

2. Layer in Italian rolls, in order, 1 red-tipped lettuce leaf, 4 ounces sliced Baked Seitan Roast, 1 slice vegan mozzarella cheese, several slices red onion, and several slices tomato.

3. Drizzle olive oil and red vinegar over top. Season generously with sea salt, black pepper, and Italian seasonings blend, and serve.

Variation: For added flavor, spread a little spicy or Dijon mustard on the Italian rolls, and season with a little crushed red pepper flakes as well. For **Very Veggie Hero Sandwiches,** replace the sliced Baked Seitan Roast with 1½ cups (1 large) each green and red bell peppers, thinly sliced with ribs and seeds removed, and 1 cup black olives, pitted and sliced.

IN A NUTSHELL

You'll often see versions of these types of layered sandwiches also called subs, hoagies, or grinders on restaurant menus.

Italian Tempeh "Meatball" Sandwiches

Our Sammy's Spicy Tempeh Sausages are shaped into balls and baked to make *tempeh*-based meatless "meatballs," which are then covered in a zesty marinara sauce and mozzarella cheese to create these tasty, hot sandwiches.

Yield:	Prep time:	Cook time:	Serving size:
6 sandwiches	20 to 25 minutes	30 to 40 minutes	1 sandwich

1 batch Sammy's Spicy Tempeh Sausages mixture (recipe in Chapter 19)	6 (6-in.) submarine rolls, other soft rolls, or hot dog buns
Olive oil	Shredded vegan mozzarella cheese or other variety (optional)
1 batch Chunky Marinara Sauce (recipe in Chapter 22)	

1. Preheat the oven to 400°F. Line a cookie sheet with parchment paper.

2. Prepare Sammy's Spicy Tempeh Sausages mixture according to the recipe instructions through step 3. Using your hands or a small scoop, shape mixture into 24 (1¼-inch) balls, and place on the prepared cookie sheet. Using your fingers, rub a little olive oil over top of each "meatball."

3. Bake for 25 to 30 minutes or until "meatballs" are dry to the touch and lightly browned on the outside.

4. Split open submarine rolls, spoon a little Chunky Marinara Sauce on bottom half, add 4 baked "meatballs," top with some additional marinara sauce, and sprinkle with a little shredded vegan mozzarella cheese (if using). Serve immediately.

Variation: For **Spaghetti and Meatless Meatballs,** forego the submarine rolls and use the Chunky Marinara Sauce and Sammy's Spicy Tempeh Sausage Meatballs to top individual servings of cooked spaghetti. Sprinkle a little vegan Parmesan cheese or nutritional yeast flakes over servings as desired.

DEFINITION

Tempeh is a cultured food product made by mixing partially cooked soybeans with a beneficial mold (*rhizosporus oligosporus*) and fermenting it. The result is a firm soybean cake with a marbled appearance, which is why tempeh is often classified as the bleu cheese version of tofu.

Spicy Red Bean Burgers

These protein-packed vegan burgers are made with a spicy and well-seasoned blend of sautéed vegetables, including a fiery jalapeño pepper, red beans, and rolled oats.

Yield:	Prep time:	Cook time:	Serving size:
4 burgers	15 minutes, plus 30 minutes chill time	15 to 20 minutes	1 burger

⅔ cup yellow onion, diced

⅔ cup green bell pepper, ribs and seeds removed, and diced

⅔ cup red bell pepper, ribs and seeds removed, and diced

1 medium jalapeño pepper, ribs and seeds removed, and finely diced

1 TB. olive oil

½ TB. minced garlic

1 tsp. chili powder

½ tsp. dried basil

½ tsp. dried oregano

½ tsp. smoked paprika

½ tsp. seasoning salt or sea salt

½ tsp. freshly ground black pepper

¼ tsp. chipotle chile powder or cayenne

1 (15-oz.) can red beans, drained and rinsed

1½ TB. nutritional yeast flakes

1 TB. ketchup

1 TB. spicy brown or Dijon mustard

⅔ cup rolled oats

¼ cup chopped fresh parsley

4 whole-grain hamburger buns or rolls, split

Lettuce leaves, tomato slices, onion slices, vegan cheese, or toppings of choice

Vegan Soy Milk Mayonnaise (recipe in Chapter 22), ketchup, mustard, or other condiments of choice

1. Line a cookie sheet or large plate with parchment paper, and set aside.

2. In a large nonstick skillet over medium heat, combine yellow onion, green bell pepper, red bell pepper, jalapeño pepper, and ½ tablespoon olive oil. Sauté, stirring often, for 3 minutes.

3. Add garlic, chili powder, basil, oregano, smoked paprika, seasoning salt, black pepper, and chipotle chile powder, and sauté, stirring often, for 2 minutes. Remove the skillet from heat.

4. In a large bowl, combine red beans, nutritional yeast flakes, ketchup, and spicy brown mustard. Using a potato masher or fork, roughly mash red bean mixture.

5. Add sautéed vegetable mixture, rolled oats, and parsley, and stir well to combine.

6. Gently pack red bean mixture into a $\frac{1}{2}$-cup measuring cup using the back of a spoon, flip the cup over onto the prepared cookie sheet, and give the cup a tap to release patty. Using a burger press or your hands, slightly flatten patties. Repeat with remaining red bean mixture, and refrigerate for 30 minutes or more.

7. In a large nonstick skillet over medium heat, heat remaining $\frac{1}{2}$ tablespoon olive oil. In batches, add burger patties to the skillet and cook for 5 to 7 minutes or until well browned. Flip over patties with a spatula, and cook for 5 more minutes or until golden brown and crisp around edges.

8. Serve burgers on whole-grain hamburger buns with lettuce leaves or your choice of toppings and Vegan Soy Milk Mayonnaise or your choice of condiments.

Variation: You can make these burgers in large batches, cook them, and freeze them in an airtight container for up to 3 months. Then simply reheat burgers in the oven or skillet as desired. For **Mexicali Black Bean Burgers,** add $\frac{1}{2}$ cup fresh or frozen cut corn to the sautéed vegetable mixture, replace the red beans with an equal amount of black beans, and replace the parsley with $\frac{1}{3}$ cup chopped fresh cilantro.

IN A NUTSHELL

You can quickly and easily portion out quarter-pounder veggie burgers using a $\frac{1}{2}$-cup measuring cup and then flatten them slightly with your hands or a burger press. A burger press consists of a large ring and hand-grip plunger, and it helps you form well-compacted and uniformly shaped patties. They're sold in most kitchen supply stores.

Portobello Mushroom Burgers with Basil Aioli

Earthy *portobello mushrooms* are a great meatless alternative, especially when they're marinated and cooked burger-style, enhanced with a creamy Basil Aioli and your choice of toppings.

Yield:	Prep time:	Cook time:	Serving size:
4 burgers	15 minutes, plus 15 minutes marinate time	5 to 7 minutes	1 burger

2 TB. balsamic vinegar

2 TB. tamari, shoyu, or Bragg Liquid Aminos

1 TB. olive oil

1 TB. minced garlic

½ tsp. dried basil

½ tsp. dried oregano

¼ tsp. garlic pepper or freshly ground black pepper

4 large portobello mushrooms

4 whole-grain hamburger buns or rolls, split (or 8 slices bread)

Lettuce leaves, onion slices, tomato slices, vegan cheese, and other toppings of choice

1 batch Basil Aioli (recipe in Chapter 22)

1. In a small bowl, combine balsamic vinegar, tamari, olive oil, garlic, basil, oregano, and garlic pepper.

2. Remove stems from portobello mushrooms. Place mushrooms gill side down on a large plate, spoon about 2 teaspoons marinade mixture on each mushroom, flip over mushrooms, spoon more marinade over top, and set aside for at least 15 minutes to marinate.

3. Place a large nonstick skillet over medium heat.

4. Remove mushrooms from marinade and place cap side down in the skillet. Cook for 3 or 4 minutes or until mushrooms begin to soften. Flip over mushrooms with a spatula (gill side down), pour any extra marinade over top, and cook 2 or 3 more minutes or until mushrooms are tender. (Alternatively, cook marinated portobello mushrooms on a hot grill.)

5. Serve mushrooms on whole-grain hamburger buns with lettuce leaves or your choice of toppings and several generous dollops of Basil Aioli.

Variation: For **Margarita Mushroom Burgers,** when portobello mushrooms are tender, flip them cap side up, top each with 1 slice vegan mozzarella cheese, and cover the skillet to melt cheese. Serve on hamburger buns with baby spinach and tomato slices, and top each with several generous dollops of Sun-Dried Tomato Aioli (variation in Chapter 22).

> **DEFINITION**
>
> **Portobello mushroom** are a mature and larger form of the smaller crimini mushroom. Brown, chewy, and flavorful, portobellos are often served as whole caps, grilled, or as thin sautéed slices.

Main and Side Dishes

In This Chapter

- Meatless main dishes
- Creative comfort foods
- International pasta and grain options
- Colorful and delicious side dishes

In Chapter 16, we discussed a few vegan mock meats and protein alternatives you can find in stores. Then in Chapters 19 and 20, we shared a few homemade recipe options, and this chapter gives you a few more to extend your culinary repertoire.

This chapter starts off with sauced, seasoned, and baked tempeh, tofu, and seitan recipes. All these tasty meat-free dinner options or fantastic sandwich fillings can also be added to salads, soups, stews, or cooked grains or pasta.

Legumes are protein-packed stars in these recipes, too. Beans are blended to make tasty quesadillas or simmered Southern-style with leafy greens, chickpeas and veggies meld together into a curry-flavored stew over couscous, and pea pods are tossed into a colorful pasta dish. You also learn how to create your own vegan mac-n-cheese and whip up some tasty rice- and quinoa-based side dishes.

We show you how easy it is to prepare roasted veggies, which can be served as a side or used to make hearty sandwiches when layered between slices of bread or wrapped in tortillas. Or dice them and add them to cooked grains or pasta, with a little vinaigrette, to make a filling meal. We also teach you how to make marvelous mashed potatoes, and how you can transform your mashed spuds in many ways by using different potato varieties, adding additional ingredients such as roasted garlic or shredded vegan cheese, and seasoning with fresh herbs such as dill or rosemary. You also can use leftover mashed potatoes to thicken soups or stews or make quesadillas.

IN A NUTSHELL

Got leftover mashed potatoes? Make Potato Quesadillas! Spoon a generous serving of mashed potatoes on ½ of a flour tortilla, sprinkle on a little nutritional yeast flakes and/or shredded vegan cheese, and fold over tortilla to enclose the filling. Bake at 400°F for 15 minutes or until golden brown and crisp for a low-fat version, or cook in a lightly oiled skillet until browned on both sides and heated through. Serve with your choice of salsa and vegan sour cream.

By the end of this chapter, you will have enough recipes to create many fabulous vegan meals. We encourage you to showcase your new vegan culinary talents by inviting friends or family over for a meal. Positive example is the best teacher. By serving them a delicious and nutritious vegan meal, you can put their minds at ease and also satisfy their curiosity as to what exactly you eat as a vegan. Your diners may even find it hard to believe they're eating a vegan meal!

Ginger-Teriyaki Tempeh or Tofu

Whether you choose to have tempeh or tofu, you're going to love how the homemade tangy teriyaki sauce quickly and easily infuses the slices with tons of flavor as they're oven baked.

Yield:	Prep time:	Cook time:	Serving size:
8 pieces	5 to 10 minutes, plus 20 minutes tofu press time	40 to 45 minutes	2 pieces

2 (8-oz.) pkg. tempeh or 1 lb. firm or extra-firm tofu

¼ cup tamari, shoyu, or Bragg Liquid Aminos

2 TB. brown rice vinegar

1½ TB. toasted sesame oil

1½ TB. brown rice syrup or agave nectar

1½ TB. minced garlic

1½ TB. fresh peeled and minced ginger

1 tsp. dry mustard

½ tsp. crushed red pepper flakes

1. If using tofu, squeeze block of tofu over the sink to remove excess water. Place tofu in a colander in the sink, cover with a plate, place a 28-ounce can on top of the plate, and leave tofu to press for 20 minutes.

2. Preheat the oven to 400°F.

3. Cut pressed tofu in ½ lengthwise, turn each ½ cut side down, and cut each ½ into 4 slices for a total of 8 slices. If using tempeh, skip pressing procedure, and cut each package of tempeh into 4 pieces.

4. Place tempeh or tofu slices in a single layer in a 8×10-inch or larger baking pan. Using a fork, pierce each piece of tempeh or tofu several times along its length, flip over pieces, and pierce other side.

5. In a small bowl, whisk together tamari, brown rice vinegar, toasted sesame oil, brown rice syrup, garlic, ginger, dry mustard, and crushed red pepper flakes. Pour mixture over tempeh or tofu pieces.

6. Bake for 20 minutes. Remove from the oven, flip over pieces with a spatula, and bake for 20 to 25 more minutes or until most of teriyaki sauce mixture is absorbed.

7. Serve hot or cold as a main or side dish, or filling for a sandwich with fresh veggies. Or cut into strips and add to soups, stir-fries, salads, pasta, rice, or grain dishes.

Variation: You could also prepare this dish by cutting the blocks of tempeh or tofu into 1-inch cubes. Mix with teriyaki sauce mixture, and bake according to the recipe instructions.

IN A NUTSHELL

Tofu and tempeh are also delicious when tossed with tamari, olive oil, a little nutritional yeast flakes, and seasonings of choice, and baked until golden brown and crispy around the edges.

Baked Breaded Tofu Cutlets

This healthier, vegan version of fried chicken is made with slices of pressed tofu bathed in a soy buttermilk mixture before being coated with a seasoned breading and then baked until golden brown.

Yield:	Prep time:	Cook time:	Serving size:
16 pieces	30 minutes, plus 20 minutes tofu press time	25 to 30 minutes	2 pieces

2 lb. firm or extra-firm tofu

1¼ cups soy or other nondairy milk

2 TB. lemon juice

1 cup medium-grind yellow cornmeal

½ cup nutritional yeast flakes

1 TB. onion powder

1 TB. garlic powder

1 TB. dried parsley or 2 TB. chopped fresh Italian flat-leaf parsley

2 tsp. dried basil

2 tsp. dried oregano

1 tsp. smoked or sweet paprika

1 tsp. sea salt

½ tsp. freshly ground black pepper

1½ cups whole-wheat or white whole-wheat flour

1. Squeeze blocks of tofu over the sink to remove excess water. Place tofu in a colander in the sink, cover with a plate, place a 28-ounce can on top of the plate, and leave tofu to press for 20 minutes.

2. Preheat the oven to 400°F. Line a cookie sheet with parchment paper or a Silpat liner.

3. Cut each block of pressed tofu in ½ lengthwise, turn each ½ cut side down, and cut each ½ into 4 slices for a total of 8 slices per block or 16 pieces total.

4. In a small bowl, whisk together soy milk and lemon juice, and set aside for 10 minutes to thicken.

5. On a large plate, combine yellow cornmeal, nutritional yeast flakes, onion powder, garlic powder, parsley, basil, oregano, smoked paprika, sea salt, and black pepper.

6. On a small plate, place whole-wheat flour. Working with 1 tofu piece at a time, place tofu into flour, flip over to evenly coat on all sides, and place tofu on a large plate. Stir remaining whole-wheat flour into cornmeal mixture.

7. Dip each floured tofu piece into soymilk mixture and then into seasoned breading mixture, pressing down slightly and flipping over as needed to evenly coat piece on all sides. Place breaded tofu cutlets on the prepared cookie sheet.

8. Bake for 15 minutes or until lightly browned. Remove from the oven, and flip over tofu cutlets with a spatula. Bake for 10 to 15 more minutes or until golden brown. Remove from the oven.

9. Serve 2 pieces per person as a main dish, side dish, or filling for a sandwich with fresh veggies on a bun, roll, or in a tortilla with a creamy sauce or some Vegan Soy Milk Mayonnaise (recipe in Chapter 22). Or cube them and add to soups, stews, salads, pasta, rice, or grain dishes.

Variation: For bite-size nuggets, cut each block of pressed tofu into 1-inch cubes, bread, and bake according to the recipe instructions. Then serve them with ketchup, a mixture of agave nectar and mustard, or other dipping sauce of choice. For **Bold and Spicy Breaded Tofu Cutlets,** in the breading mixture, replace dried basil and oregano with 2 teaspoons chili powder, ½ teaspoon ground cumin, and ¼ teaspoon chipotle chile powder or ⅛ teaspoon cayenne. Then serve with barbecue sauce.

HOT POTATO

Watch out for unnecessary fat! You can fry the breaded tofu in a little olive oil for a crispier crust, but be sure to drain it well and blot off any excess oil before eating.

Baked Seitan Roast

Firm and chewy seitan is a great-tasting, cholesterol-free alternative to meat. This seitan roast can be sliced and served as a main dish plain or with Groovy Onion Gravy (recipe in Chapter 22) or used in your favorite recipes.

Yield:	Prep time:	Cook time:	Serving size:
1 (8×4-inch) roast	5 to 10 minutes	60 to 75 minutes	2 or 3 slices

¾ cup yellow onion, finely diced

1 TB. olive oil

2 TB. minced garlic

1½ TB. fresh peeled and minced ginger

3 cups low-sodium vegetable broth or water

⅓ cup nutritional yeast flakes

¼ cup tamari, shoyu, or Bragg Liquid Aminos

2 TB. toasted sesame oil

1 TB. onion powder

1 TB. garlic powder

1 tsp. dried thyme

1 tsp. rubbed (dried) sage

½ tsp. sea salt

½ tsp. black pepper

3 cups vital wheat gluten

⅔ cup whole-wheat flour

1. Preheat the oven to 350°F. Lightly oil an 8×4-inch loaf pan.

2. In a medium nonstick skillet over medium heat, combine yellow onion and olive oil. Sauté, stirring often, for 5 minutes.

3. Add garlic and ginger, and sauté, stirring often, for 2 minutes. Remove the skillet from heat, and allow to cool slightly.

4. Transfer sautéed onion mixture to a blender or food processor fitted with an S blade. Add vegetable broth, nutritional yeast flakes, tamari, toasted sesame oil, onion powder, garlic powder, thyme, rubbed sage, sea salt, and black pepper, and process for 2 minutes or until smooth.

5. Divide wet ingredients, transferring ½ to a small bowl, and set aside; use other ½ to mix seitan.

6. In a large bowl, combine vital wheat gluten and whole-wheat flour. Stir in wet ingredients, a little at a time, until firm dough forms. Using your hands, knead dough in the bowl for 2 minutes. Shape into an 8-inch log, and press it into the prepared loaf pan. Pour ½ of reserved wet ingredients over top of seitan roast.

7. Bake for 45 minutes. Remove pan from the oven, and pour remaining reserved wet ingredients over seitan roast. Reduce oven temperature to 325°F, and bake for 20 to 25 more minutes or until all liquid is absorbed and seitan roast is very firm to the touch. Allow to cool for 10 minutes in the pan.

8. Remove seitan roast from the pan. Use a sharp knife to cut seitan roast into thin slices. Serve sliced seitan as a main dish plain or top with gravy.

IN A NUTSHELL

Dice or cut leftover seitan roast into strips or cubes and add to soups, stews, casseroles, salads, pasta, rice, and grain dishes. Or use it as a filling for sandwiches or wraps.

Curried Vegetable and Chickpea Stew with Lemon Couscous

This Indian-inspired stew is seasoned with a fragrant blend of spices that are combined with aromatic vegetables and chunks of sweet potatoes, zucchini, bell peppers, diced tomatoes, and chickpeas, and served over a lemony couscous.

Yield:	Prep time:	Cook time:	Serving size:
8 cups stew and 4 cups couscous	15 minutes	35 to 40 minutes	1 cup stew and ½ cup couscous

1 cup (1 medium) yellow onion, diced

⅔ cup green bell pepper, seeds and ribs removed, and diced

⅔ cup red bell pepper, seeds and ribs removed, and diced

½ TB. olive oil

1 TB. minced garlic

1 tsp. *curry powder*

1 tsp. ground cumin

½ tsp. ground coriander

¼ tsp. ground cinnamon

1½ tsp. sea salt

1 tsp. freshly ground black pepper

2 cups (2 large) sweet potatoes, diced

1 medium zucchini, quartered lengthwise and sliced

1 (15-oz.) can chickpeas, drained and rinsed

1 (14-oz.) can diced tomatoes, with juice

3 cups low-sodium vegetable broth or water

3 TB. lemon juice

1⅓ cups whole-wheat couscous

1. In a large pot over medium heat, combine yellow onion, green bell pepper, red bell pepper, and olive oil. Sauté, stirring often, for 5 minutes.

2. Add garlic, curry powder, cumin, coriander, cinnamon, 1 teaspoon sea salt, and ½ teaspoon black pepper, and sauté, stirring often, for 2 more minutes.

3. Add sweet potato, zucchini, chickpeas, diced tomatoes, ½ cup vegetable broth, and 1 tablespoon lemon juice, and stir well to combine. Cover, reduce heat to low, and simmer for 20 to 25 minutes or until vegetables are tender.

4. Meanwhile, in a medium saucepan over high heat, bring remaining 2½ cups vegetable broth and remaining 2 tablespoons lemon juice to a boil. Add whole-wheat couscous, remaining ½ teaspoon sea salt, and remaining ½ teaspoon black pepper, and stir to combine. Cover, remove the saucepan from heat, and set aside for 5 minutes to allow couscous to absorb liquid.

5. Uncover and fluff couscous with a fork to loosen grains. Taste stew and adjust seasonings as desired. Serve hot, spooning individual servings of stew over couscous.

Variation: Feel free to prepare this stew with other fresh or frozen vegetables such as eggplant, broccoli, cauliflower, or potatoes. For **Thai-Style Vegetable and Chickpea Stew over Rice,** replace the spices with 1 tablespoon red or yellow curry paste, replace diced tomatoes with 1½ cups coconut milk beverage (or canned coconut milk), and add ¼ cup chopped fresh cilantro. Also, omit the lemon couscous, and instead serve individual servings over cooked brown or basmati rice.

DEFINITION

Curry powder is an Indian spice blend typically made of turmeric, coriander, chiles, cumin, mustard, ginger, fenugreek, garlic, cloves, salt, and any number of other spices, all ground together. It comes in various colors, from bright yellow to deep red, and different levels of heat, from mild to extra hot. It also contains many powerful antioxidants and anti-inflammatory compounds.

Variation: For **Gluten-Free Mac-n-Cheese,** use corn and quinoa elbows or other gluten-free shaped pasta, and use Gluten-Free Vegan Cheezy Sauce (variation in Chapter 22).

> **DEFINITION**
>
> **Smoked paprika** is a variety of Spanish paprika. Smoked paprika is made from mature pimento peppers that are dried, naturally smoked over oak-wood fires, and stone-ground to a fine, powdery consistency. It has a deep red color with a slightly smoky and bittersweet flavor.

Veggie Lo Mein

You can easily make this popular Chinese take-out dish at home by tossing cooked spaghetti with a tangy tamari and brown rice vinegar–based sauce and a colorful blend of crisp veggies.

Yield:	Prep time:	Cook time:	Serving size:
10 or 11 cups	10 to 15 minutes	10 minutes (depending on pasta variety)	1½ cups

12 oz. whole-wheat spaghetti or other variety

⅓ cup tamari, shoyu, or Bragg Liquid Aminos

⅓ cup *brown rice vinegar*

3 TB. toasted sesame oil

3 TB. unbleached cane sugar or brown rice syrup

2 TB. minced garlic

2 TB. fresh peeled and minced ginger

1 tsp. crushed red pepper flakes

½ tsp. freshly ground black pepper

1 cup (¼ medium head) napa or other green cabbage, shredded

1 cup (¼ medium head) red cabbage, shredded

⅔ cup carrots, shredded

⅔ cup red bell pepper, ribs and seeds removed, and diced

½ cup fresh or thawed frozen pea pods, cut in ½ diagonally

½ cup green onions, white and green parts, thinly sliced

½ cup chopped fresh cilantro

⅓ cup toasted peanuts or 2 TB. raw or toasted sesame seeds

1. Fill a large saucepan ⅔ full of water, and bring to a boil over medium-high heat. Add whole-wheat spaghetti, and cook, stirring occasionally, according to the package directions or until al dente. Remove the saucepan from heat. Drain spaghetti in a colander, but do not rinse.

2. Meanwhile, in a large bowl, whisk together tamari, brown rice vinegar, toasted sesame oil, unbleached cane sugar, garlic, ginger, crushed red pepper flakes, and black pepper. Add spaghetti, and using a pair of tongs, toss well to coat.

3. Add napa cabbage, red cabbage, carrots, red bell pepper, pea pods, green onions, cilantro, and peanuts, and toss well to combine. Serve hot, cold, or at room temperature as main or side dish as desired.

Variation: For **Tempeh and Veggie Lo Mein,** add 3 pieces Ginger-Teriyaki Tempeh (recipe earlier in this chapter), roughly chopped or cut into small strips.

DEFINITION

Brown rice vinegar is vinegar produced from fermented brown rice, water, and koji (a beneficial type of mold), or from unrefined rice wine (sake) and water. It's popular in Asian-style dishes.

Savory Mixed Rice Pilaf

This pilaf is made with a combination of sautéed aromatic vegetables, a mixed rice and grain blend, and seasonings with a bit of parsley for added color.

Yield:	Prep time:	Cook time:	Serving size:
5 or 6 cups	7 to 10 minutes	50 to 55 minutes	1 cup

1 cup (1 medium) yellow onion, diced

1 cup (2 large stalks) celery (including inner green leaves), diced

1 TB. olive oil

1½ cups mixed wild rice and grain blend of choice

2 TB. minced garlic

1 TB. toasted sesame oil

1½ tsp. dried thyme

1 tsp. rubbed (or dried) sage

1 tsp. sea salt

½ tsp. freshly ground black pepper

3 cups water or low-sodium vegetable broth

1 bay leaf

½ cup green onions, white and green parts, thinly sliced

⅓ cup chopped fresh Italian flat-leaf parsley

1½ TB. tamari, shoyu, or Bragg Liquid Aminos

1. In a large saucepan over medium heat, combine yellow onion, celery, and olive oil. Sauté, stirring often, for 3 minutes.

2. Add mixed wild rice and grain blend, garlic, toasted sesame oil, thyme, rubbed sage, sea salt, and black pepper and sauté, stirring often, 2 more minutes.

3. Add water and bay leaf, increase heat to high, and bring to a boil. Cover, reduce heat to low, and simmer for 40 to 45 minutes or until mixed rice blend is tender and all liquid is absorbed. Remove from the heat, and remove and discard bay leaf.

4. Fluff mixed rice blend mixture with a fork to loosen grains. Add green onions, Italian flat-leaf parsley, and tamari, and stir gently to combine.

5. Serve hot as a side dish, or use as a filling for baked winter squashes or other vegetables.

Variation: For **Mushroom Mixed Rice Pilaf,** add 1½ cups crimini or other mushrooms, cut in ½ and thinly sliced, to the sautéing onion mixture.

IN A NUTSHELL

When making a pilaf, you sauté the uncooked rice or grain in a little oil alone or with some aromatic vegetables first, which adds a slightly nutty flavor and also helps the rice retain its shape during the simmering process.

Mexicali Quinoa

Quinoa is combined with red onions, green bell pepper, jalapeño pepper, diced tomatoes with green chiles, and seasonings to create a spicy side dish.

Yield:	Prep time:	Cook time:	Serving size:
5 or 6 cups	10 to 15 minutes	30 to 35 minutes	1 cup

¾ cup red onion, diced

¾ cup green bell pepper, ribs and seeds removed, and diced

½ TB. olive oil

1 medium jalapeño pepper, ribs and seeds removed, and finely diced

1½ TB. minced garlic

1½ cups quinoa

1 (14-oz.) can fire-roasted diced tomatoes with green chiles, with juice

1 cup low-sodium vegetable broth or water

½ TB. chili powder

½ TB. dried oregano

1 tsp. ground cumin

1 tsp. smoked or sweet paprika

¾ tsp. sea salt

½ tsp. freshly ground black pepper

¼ tsp. chipotle chile powder, cayenne, or hot pepper sauce

⅓ cup green onions, white and green parts, thinly sliced

⅓ cup chopped fresh cilantro or Italian flat-leaf parsley

1. In a large saucepan over medium heat, combine red onion, green bell pepper, and olive oil. Sauté, stirring often, for 3 minutes.

2. Add jalapeño pepper and garlic, and sauté, stirring often, for 1 minute.

3. Place quinoa in a fine-mesh sieve, and rinse well under running water for 1 minute.

4. Add quinoa, fire-roasted diced tomatoes, vegetable broth, chili powder, oregano, cumin, smoked paprika, sea salt, black pepper, and chipotle chile powder to the saucepan. Increase heat to high, and bring to a boil. Cover, reduce heat to low, and simmer for 22 to 25 minutes or until quinoa is tender and all liquid is absorbed.

5. Stir in green onions and cilantro, and remove from heat.

6. Fluff quinoa with a fork to loosen grains. Taste and adjust seasonings as desired. Serve hot.

Variation: For **Mexicali Millet,** replace quinoa with an equal amount of millet.

> **HOT POTATO**
>
> Quinoa is covered with a bitter-tasting coating called saponin that acts as a natural insect repellent. Remove this nasty-tasting coating by rinsing quinoa under running water. So before adding quinoa to a recipe, you should check it for bits of dirt and debris in a fine-mesh sieve and then give it a good rinse.

Mean Greens and Beans

Greens and beans are a winning combination of fiber, low-fat protein, calcium, and iron, and this recipe features an assortment of leafy greens and creamy butter beans.

Yield:	Prep time:	Cook time:	Serving size:
5 or 6 cups	15 to 20 minutes	30 minutes	1 cup

1 medium green bell pepper, ribs and seeds removed, and diced

1 cup (1 medium) yellow onion, diced

1 TB. olive oil

2 TB. minced garlic

1 cup low-sodium vegetable broth or water

1 bunch collard greens, stems removed, and roughly chopped

1 bunch green or purple kale, stems removed, and roughly chopped

1 bunch rainbow Swiss chard, stems removed, and roughly chopped

2 (15-oz.) cans butter beans or other beans, drained and rinsed

1½ TB. nutritional yeast flakes

½ TB. dried thyme

1 tsp. crushed red pepper flakes

¾ tsp. sea salt

½ tsp. freshly ground black pepper

¼ tsp. cayenne

Hot red pepper sauce (optional)

1. In a large stock pot over medium heat, combine green bell pepper, yellow onion, and olive oil. Sauté, stirring often, for 5 to 7 minutes or until vegetables are soft and lightly browned.

2. Add garlic, and sauté, stirring often, for 1 minute.

3. Add vegetable stock, increase heat to high, and bring to a boil. Add collard greens, green kale, and rainbow Swiss chard to the pot in batches, covering the pot between batches to help greens wilt.

4. Add butter beans, nutritional yeast flakes, thyme, crushed red pepper flakes, sea salt, black pepper, and cayenne, and stir well to combine. Cover, reduce heat to low, and simmer for 15 to 20 minutes or until greens are tender.

5. Taste and adjust seasonings as desired. Serve hot, garnishing individual servings with hot pepper sauce (if using).

Variation: Substitute other greens such as spinach, turnip greens, mustard greens, and beet greens, and for a heartier dish serve over cooked rice, quinoa, or other grains. For **Bayou Black-Eyed Peas and Greens,** replace butter beans with 2 (15-ounce) cans black-eyed peas, drained and rinsed, and serve over cooked rice.

IN A NUTSHELL

In the South, it's customary to enjoy your greens and beans with a little something to sop up the juices, such as biscuits and cornbread. Find vegan recipes for both of these in Chapter 23.

Stir-Fried Vegetables with Cashews

In this Asian-inspired recipe, vegetables are stir-fried until crisp-tender and then given a slightly salty and smoky finish with the addition of tamari, toasted sesame oil, and buttery cashews.

Yield:	Prep time:	Cook time:	Serving size:
8 or 9 cups	15 to 20 minutes	25 to 30 minutes	1½ cups

½ TB. peanut or other oil

2 cups (1 lb.) broccoli, cut into florets

1 medium red bell pepper, ribs and seeds removed, and cut into 1-in. strips

1 cup (1 medium) yellow summer squash or zucchini, cut into 1-inch strips

1 cup crimini or shiitake mushrooms, thinly sliced

1 cup (1 medium) red or yellow onion, cut into ½ moons

1 cup (2 large) carrots, thinly sliced diagonally

4 cups (½ bunch) bok choy or other leafy greens, stems removed, and cut chiffonade

1 cup fresh or frozen pea pods, cut in ½ diagonally

1 TB. minced garlic

1 TB. fresh peeled and minced ginger

1 tsp. crushed red pepper flakes

½ tsp. freshly ground black pepper

½ cup green onions, white and green parts, thinly sliced

⅓ cup chopped fresh parsley or cilantro

⅓ cup toasted cashews

2 TB. tamari, shoyu, or Bragg Liquid Aminos

1 TB. brown rice vinegar

½ TB. toasted sesame oil

1. In a large nonstick skillet or wok over medium-high heat, heat peanut oil. When hot, add broccoli, red bell pepper, yellow summer squash, crimini mushrooms, red onion, and carrots, and sauté, stirring often, for 3 minutes.

2. Add bok choy, pea pods, garlic, ginger, crushed red pepper flakes, and black pepper, and sauté, stirring often, for 2 minutes.

3. Add green onions, parsley, toasted cashews, tamari, brown rice vinegar, and toasted sesame oil, and stir gently to combine. Remove skillet from the heat.

4. Taste and adjust seasonings as desired. Serve hot as a side dish or over cooked rice or other grains as a main dish.

Variation: Feel free to prepare this recipe with other fresh or frozen veggies such as cauliflower, eggplant, cabbage, or green beans. For **Teriyaki Tofu and Veggie Stir-Fry,** add 1½ cups Ginger-Teriyaki Tofu (recipe earlier in this chapter), cut into 1-inch cubes.

IN A NUTSHELL

When making a stir-fry, cut and assemble all your ingredients ahead of time. Also preheat the oil before adding the vegetables or other ingredients, and be sure to constantly stir the ingredients to help them cook quickly and prevent them from sticking.

Rustic Roasted Vegetables

You're encouraged to eat plant-based foods from every color of the rainbow for good health, and these tasty oven-roasted vegetables will help you do just that!

Yield:	Prep time:	Cook time:	Serving size:
10 to 12 cups	15 minutes	30 to 40 minutes	1 cup

1 medium eggplant, cut into 2-in. cubes

1 large or 2 medium zucchini, quartered lengthwise and sliced 1-in. thick

1 large or 2 medium yellow summer squash, quartered lengthwise and sliced 1-in. thick

1 large red or yellow onion, cut from end to end into ½-in.-thick ½ moons

1 large green bell pepper, ribs and seeds removed, and cut into 1-in. cubes

1 large red or orange bell pepper, ribs and seeds removed, and cut into 1-in. cubes

2 TB. nutritional yeast flakes

2 TB. minced garlic

2 TB. olive oil

1½ TB. chopped fresh rosemary or ½ TB. dried

1½ TB. chopped fresh thyme or ½ TB. dried

1 tsp. dried basil

1 tsp. dried oregano

1 tsp. sea salt

½ tsp. freshly ground black pepper

1. Preheat the oven to 425°F. Line a cookie sheet with parchment paper or a Silpat liner.

2. In a large bowl, combine eggplant, zucchini, yellow summer squash, red onion, green bell pepper, red bell pepper, nutritional yeast flakes, garlic, olive oil, rosemary, thyme, basil, oregano, sea salt, and black pepper. Toss well to thoroughly coat vegetables. Transfer vegetable mixture to the prepared cookie sheet, and spread into a single layer.

3. Bake for 20 minutes. Remove from the oven. Stir vegetables with a spatula, and spread into a single layer again. Bake for 10 to 15 more minutes or until vegetables are just tender and slightly browned in places.

4. Transfer vegetables to a large bowl or platter. Taste and adjust seasonings as desired. Serve hot, cold, or at room temperature as a side dish, part of a main dish, or diced and added to pasta, rice, or grain dishes. They're also great served as a sandwich, on rolls or bread, with a creamy or tahini-based sauce, or with a little additional olive oil and red wine vinegar.

Variation: Get creative by throwing in an assortment of your own favorite veggies. For **French-Style Roasted Vegetables,** omit the rosemary, thyme, basil, and oregano, and replace them with 1½ tablespoons herbes de Provence.

IN A NUTSHELL

Roasting brings out the delicate sweetness of vegetables, and the carmelization of the natural sugars on the skins and cut surfaces add a rich, earthy flavor to dishes. Winter squashes and root vegetables are especially delicious when roasted. Use other herbs and spices to vary and intensify flavors even more.

Mouthwatering Mashed Potatoes

Practically any variety of potatoes can be used for making mashed potatoes, but buttery Yukon Golds are our first choice, and they come out ultra creamy when mashed with a little soy milk and nonhydrogenated margarine.

Yield:	Prep time:	Cook time:	Serving size:
6 cups	10 to 15 minutes	15 to 20 minutes	1 cup

3 lb. (8 or 9 large) Yukon Gold potatoes, peeled and cut into 2-in. cubes

¾ to 1 cup soy or other nondairy milk

2 TB. nonhydrogenated margarine or olive oil

1 tsp. sea salt

½ tsp. freshly ground black pepper or white pepper

1. In a large pot, place Yukon Gold potato cubes, cover with water, and bring to a boil over high heat. Reduce heat to medium-high, and cook for 15 to 20 minutes or until potatoes are tender. Remove from heat. Reserve 1 cup cooking liquid, drain potatoes in a colander, and return cooked potatoes to the pot.

2. Add soy milk, nonhydrogenated margarine, sea salt, and black pepper, and using a potato masher, mash potatoes until as smooth or chunky as desired, adding a little reserved cooking liquid as needed to achieve desired consistency.

3. Taste and add additional seasonings or margarine as desired. Serve hot, alone, or topped with Groovy Onion Gravy (recipe in Chapter 22), or use as desired in your favorite recipes.

Variation: For **Herbed Mashed Potatoes,** add either 3 or 4 tablespoons fresh or 1 or 2 tablespoons dried herbs (such as thyme, dill, parsley, and/or rosemary) to the finished mashed potatoes.

IN A NUTSHELL

If you prefer your mashed potatoes chunky or with a few lumps, use an old-fashioned hand potato masher. If you prefer very creamy mashed potatoes, use a mixer (not a food processor) on low speed to whip the potatoes to your desired consistency. You can make mashed potatoes ahead of time and keep them warm in a covered casserole in a 250°F oven or in a slow cooker on the low setting.

Amazing Accompaniments

In This Chapter

- Super sauces and gravy
- Soy milk–based mayonnaise and aioli
- Tahini-enhanced dressing and hummus
- Chunky and rich marinara sauce

Looking to add a little pizzazz to your sandwich or meal? We all can benefit from a little help every now and then, and sometimes your culinary creations could use a little assistance in their preparation. In this chapter, you'll find recipes meant to embellish, complement, and enhance the flavors of your final dish—or "accompaniments," as we like to call them. You'll notice they're used as a component in several other recipes in this book as well.

We've included what we consider some must-haves for any vegan, such as sauces, condiments, spreads, and even gravy. Feel free to use a little or a lot of them to your heart's (or taste buds') desire. Throughout these pages, we give you several suggestions for using these accompaniments, and we're sure you'll come up with several others on your own.

Vegan Cheezy Sauce

With the help of nutritional yeast and a few other ingredients, you can easily make a cheezy-tasting sauce perfect for topping your favorite vegan dishes.

Yield:	Prep time:	Cook time:	Serving size:
1½ cups	5 minutes	5 minutes	¼ cup

½ cup nutritional yeast flakes

3 TB. whole-wheat or other flour

4 tsp. arrowroot

½ tsp. sea salt

½ tsp. dry mustard

½ tsp. garlic powder

¼ tsp. smoked or sweet paprika

1½ cups soy or other nondairy milk

1 TB. olive oil

1. In a medium saucepan, whisk together nutritional yeast flakes, whole-wheat flour, arrowroot, sea salt, dry mustard, garlic powder, and smoked paprika.

2. Add soy milk and olive oil, and whisk until very smooth. Set over low heat, and cook, whisking often to avoid lumps, for 3 to 5 minutes or until thickened. Remove the saucepan from heat.

3. Serve hot as a sauce, or allow to cool for use as a dip or spread. Store in an airtight container in the refrigerator for up to 5 days. Reheat in a saucepan as desired.

Variation: For **Gluten-Free Vegan Cheezy Sauce,** omit the whole-wheat flour and arrowroot and replace with 2 tablespoons cornstarch.

IN A NUTSHELL

This vegan version of cheese sauce has an endless array of uses, from a sauce over vegetables, pasta, or grain dishes, to an addition to soups or stews, or as an accompaniment to main dishes. You can even use it to make a yummy vegan Mac-n-Cheese (recipe in Chapter 21)!

Vegan Soy Milk Mayonnaise

Most natural foods stores and many grocery stores carry vegan mayonnaise in both refrigerated and nonrefrigerated varieties, but it's so easy to make your own using this soy milk–based recipe.

Yield:	Prep time:	Cook time:	Serving size:
2 cups	5 minutes	3 minutes	1 tablespoon

½ cup water

3 TB. cornstarch

¾ cup soy milk

½ TB. Dijon mustard

½ TB. nutritional yeast flakes

1 tsp. agave nectar

1 tsp. sea salt

1 tsp. onion powder

½ tsp. garlic powder or garlic granules

½ cup olive oil

1 TB. apple cider vinegar

1 TB. lemon juice

1. In a small saucepan over high heat, combine water and cornstarch. Cook, whisking often, for 2 or 3 minutes or until thickened. Remove the saucepan from heat.

2. In a blender, blend soy milk, Dijon mustard, nutritional yeast flakes, agave nectar, sea salt, onion powder, and garlic powder for 30 seconds.

3. Add cornstarch mixture, and process for 30 seconds. Scrape down the sides of the container with a spatula.

4. With the blender running, through the feed tube (or remove the lid), slowly add olive oil, followed by apple cider vinegar and lemon juice, and process for 1 minute.

5. Use immediately or cover and refrigerate. Mayonnaise will thicken slightly after being chilled. Use as a condiment for sandwiches or wraps, as an ingredient in salad dressing or dips, and in your other favorite recipes. Store mayonnaise in an airtight container in the refrigerator for up to 2 weeks.

Variation: For a small amount of **Vegan Dijonnaise,** add an additional 3 tablespoons Dijon mustard or spicy brown mustard to 1 cup Vegan Soy Milk Mayonnaise.

IN A NUTSHELL

You can use this vegan mayonnaise recipe measure for measure in place of regular mayonnaise in your favorite recipes, as a spread for sandwiches, and as the base for dressings or sauces.

Basil Aioli

Aioli is an emulsified sauce typically made of garlic, olive oil, and egg that has a similar consistency to mayonnaise. In this vegan version, we use our Vegan Soy Milk Mayonnaise as the base and add some garlic and fresh basil to amp up the flavor.

Yield:	Prep time:	Serving size:
2 cups	5 minutes	1 tablespoon

1½ cups Vegan Soy Milk Mayonnaise (recipe earlier in this chapter)

1 cup fresh basil leaves, tightly packed

6 large cloves garlic

2 TB. nutritional yeast flakes

1 TB. lemon juice

1. In a blender or food processor fitted with an S blade, process Vegan Soy Milk Mayonnaise, basil, garlic, nutritional yeast flakes, and lemon juice for 1 minute.

2. Scrape down the sides of the container with a spatula, and process for 30 more seconds or until smooth and basil is finely chopped.

3. Serve with crackers, bread slices, or assorted raw vegetables for a snack or appetizer, or use as a condiment for sandwiches, wraps, or roasted vegetables. Store aioli in an airtight container in the refrigerator for 5 to 7 days.

Variation: For **Sun-Dried Tomato Aioli,** only use ½ cup basil leaves. Soak ½ cup sun-dried tomato pieces in hot water for 15 minutes or until softened, and process with the other aioli ingredients.

IN A NUTSHELL

Freshly squeezed lemon juice and other citrus juices have a superior flavor to bottled versions. Fresh lemon juice will keep for several days in the refrigerator. You can also squeeze large amounts of lemon juice and freeze 1- and 2-tablespoon portions in ice-cube trays. Transfer the solid cubes to an airtight container or zipper-lock bag, and store them in the freezer for use as needed.

Tahini Dressing

Raw tahini and flaxseed oil are both rich in omega-3s and give this salad dressing a luscious creaminess that's enhanced by the zesty tang of apple cider vinegar and fresh garlic and ginger.

Yield:	Prep time:	Serving size:
1½ cups	5 minutes	2 tablespoons

¾ cup water

¼ cup raw *tahini*

¼ cup flaxseed oil

¼ cup apple cider vinegar

3 TB. chopped fresh Italian flat-leaf parsley

1½ TB. fresh peeled and minced ginger

1 TB. minced garlic

1 TB. tamari, shoyu, or Bragg Liquid Aminos

1. In a blender or food processor fitted with an S blade, process water, raw tahini, flaxseed oil, apple cider vinegar, Italian flat-leaf parsley, ginger, garlic, and tamari for 1 minute.

2. Scrape down the sides of the container with a spatula, and process for 30 more seconds or until completely smooth.

3. Transfer to an airtight container, and use immediately, or refrigerate to thicken. Use as a dressing for salads and slaws, or as a sauce over cooked veggies, pasta, or grains. Store tahini dressing in an airtight container in the refrigerator for 5 to 7 days.

Variation: For **Curried Tahini Dressing,** add 1 teaspoon curry powder.

DEFINITION

Tahini is a thick paste made from ground sesame seeds. Available in both raw and roasted varieties, tahini is often used in Middle Eastern cuisine and features prominently in hummus, baba ghanouj, soups, salad dressings, and more.

Lemon-Garlic Hummus

By blending together chickpeas, tahini, olive oil, lemon juice, garlic, and some spices, you can create a rich and creamy *hummus*.

Yield:	Prep time:	Serving size:
4 cups	5 minutes	¼ cup

2 (15-oz.) cans chickpeas, drained and rinsed

⅓ cup lemon juice

6 to 8 large cloves garlic

3 TB. water

2 TB. raw tahini

2 TB. olive oil

1 tsp. ground cumin

½ tsp. sea salt

¼ tsp. freshly ground black pepper

¼ cup chopped fresh Italian flat-leaf parsley

1. In a food processor fitted with an S blade, process chickpeas, lemon juice, garlic, water, raw tahini, olive oil, cumin, sea salt, and black pepper for 1 or 2 minutes until smooth and creamy.

2. Scrape down the sides of the container with a spatula, add Italian flat-leaf parsley, and process for 30 more seconds. Taste and add more seasonings or lemon juice as desired.

3. Serve with pita bread or assorted raw vegetables for a snack or appetizer, or use as a filling for sandwiches, wraps, or hollowed-out or sliced vegetables. Store hummus in an airtight container in the refrigerator for 5 to 7 days.

Variation: You can vary hummus tremendously by adding additional ingredients and changing the spices and oil used. For **Roasted Garlic Hummus,** replace the fresh garlic cloves with 8 roasted garlic cloves (see Groovy Onion Gravy recipe in this chapter for instructions), and replace the olive oil with 1½ tablespoons toasted sesame oil.

DEFINITION

Hummus is a purée of chickpeas with tahini, olive oil, lemon juice, garlic, herbs, and seasonings, also called hummus bi tahini. Hummus originated in the Middle East and Mediterranean. The word comes from the Arabic word for chickpea, known also as the ceci or garbanzo bean.

Groovy Onion Gravy

Never again go without gravy at a family dinner or holiday celebration! In less than 10 minutes, you can prepare this savory vegan gravy you can serve over mashed potatoes, grains, main dishes, and even biscuits!

Yield:	Prep time:	Cook time:	Serving size:
4 cups	5 minutes	10 minutes	¼ cup

⅔ cup whole-wheat flour

1 cup (1 medium) yellow onion, diced

1 TB. olive oil

1 TB. minced garlic

4 cups low-sodium vegetable broth or water

½ cup nutritional yeast flakes

2 TB. tamari, shoyu, or Bragg Liquid Aminos

1½ tsp. rubbed (dried) sage

1 tsp. sea salt

½ tsp. freshly ground black pepper

1. In a medium saucepan over low heat, cook whole-wheat flour, stirring constantly, for 2 or 3 minutes or until lightly browned and fragrant. Transfer browned flour to a medium bowl, and set aside.

2. In the same saucepan over medium heat, combine yellow onion and olive oil, and sauté, stirring often, for 3 to 5 minutes or until soft.

3. Add garlic, and sauté, stirring often, for 1 minute.

4. Add vegetable broth, nutritional yeast flakes, tamari, rubbed sage, sea salt, and black pepper to browned flour, and whisk well to combine. Add wet ingredients to sautéed onion mixture. Whisk well to combine, and continue to cook mixture, whisking constantly, for 2 or 3 minutes or until thickened. Taste and adjust seasonings as desired.

5. Serve gravy on top of your favorite vegetables, mashed potatoes, biscuits, or main dishes. Or use it to make sauces for casseroles or add to soups or stews. Store gravy in an airtight container in the refrigerator for up to 5 days.

Variation: For **Creamy Onion Gravy,** add ½ cup soy milk or other nondairy milk to the finished gravy, along with an additional 1½ tablespoons nutritional yeast flakes to lighten the color and flavor.

> **IN A NUTSHELL**
>
> If you like your gravy smooth, purée the finished gravy or strain it through a sieve to remove the onion pieces. You can also make this gravy in large batches, portion it into servings, and freeze it. Then just simply thaw and reheat before using.

Chunky Marinara Sauce

This easy marinara sauce is made with the classic combination of onions, garlic, and canned tomatoes, with fresh basil and parsley added for an authentic Italian flavor.

Yield:	Prep time:	Cook time:	Serving size:
4 cups	5 minutes	15 to 20 minutes	½ cup

1 cup (1 medium) yellow onion, diced

1 TB. olive oil

2 TB. minced garlic

1 tsp. dried oregano

¾ tsp. sea salt

½ tsp. freshly ground black pepper

1 (14-oz.) can crushed tomatoes, with juice

1 (14-oz.) can diced tomatoes, with juice

1 bay leaf

¼ cup chopped fresh basil

3 TB. chopped fresh Italian flat-leaf parsley

1 TB. nutritional yeast flakes (optional)

1. In a medium or large saucepan over medium heat, combine yellow onion and olive oil. Sauté, stirring often, for 5 to 7 minutes or until soft.

2. Add garlic, oregano, sea salt, and black pepper, and sauté, stirring often, for 1 minute.

3. Stir in crushed tomatoes, diced tomatoes, and bay leaf, reduce heat to low, and simmer, stirring occasionally, for 8 to 10 minutes or until tomatoes have broken down a bit.

4. Remove and discard bay leaf. Stir in basil, Italian flat-leaf parsley, and nutritional yeast flakes (if using). Remove the saucepan from heat.

5. Use as a sauce for pasta, lasagna, pizza, or other dishes, or on sandwiches. Store sauce in an airtight container in the refrigerator for up to 5 days.

Variation: For a more intense, slow-cooked-flavored **Robust Marinara Sauce,** use 1 (14-ounce) can each fire-roasted crushed tomatoes and diced tomatoes, with juice, instead, and add ¼ cup red wine (such as Chianti, burgundy, or merlot).

> **IN A NUTSHELL**
>
> Italians are famous for their tomato-based sauces. Knowing how to make a good marinara sauce is an essential skill for any aspiring cook—especially for those who love to eat pasta and pizza!

Baked Goods and Sweet Treats

In This Chapter

- Tips for successful vegan baking
- Baking biscuits, cornbread, and muffins
- Fun fruit snacks
- Sweet vegan cookies, pies, and cakes

Being a great cook or chef takes skill and requires practice. But when it comes to cooking, the process can be more forgiving when you're altering a recipe or making it up as you go along; adding an extra dash here or handful there won't necessarily have a dramatic impact on the end result.

But that's not the case with baking. Baking is more of a precise science, like chemistry in the kitchen. Vegan baking can be a bit trickier than the heavily egg- and dairy-laden baked goods and desserts. Egg alternatives provide the height and texture to cakes, breads, and cookies. Exact measurements of leaveners and their triggering ingredients are necessary to ensure the proper end result.

The ratio between dry and wet ingredients determines if you have a dry- or moist-tasting product. You can swap ingredients in certain instances, but keep the ratio in mind when playing around with substitutions. Additional ingredients such as chocolate chips, dried fruits, or nuts usually have less impact, and you can vary the amounts to suit your tastes.

You can find some vegan baked goods in grocery and natural foods stores, but they may not meet all your quality standards. If you want to survive as a vegan and satisfy your sweet tooth on your own terms, you're going to have to learn to be a vegan baker. However, there's no need to be intimidated! Just follow along with us, roll up your sleeves, and get baking!

In this chapter, we give you recipes for vegan baked goods, sweet treats, and desserts. Vegan baked goods may be indulgences, but in general, they are lower in fat, sugar, and calories than their egg and dairy counterparts. Also, these vegan recipes use more wholesome ingredients and provide a little something extra, instead of just filling you with empty calories and fat.

IN A NUTSHELL

Having a well-stocked pantry helps you bake when the urge hits you. Buy commonly used baking items in bulk to save money and eliminate excess packaging. Be sure to store your dry goods in airtight containers to keep them fresh and free of pests, and label them appropriately to avoid any confusion later on.

Soy Buttermilk Biscuits

Clabbering soy milk by combining it with something acidic, such as lemon juice, creates a vegan buttermilk, which give these Southern-style biscuits a great flavor.

Yield:	Prep time:	Cook time:	Serving size:
12 (2-inch) biscuits	10 minutes	10 to 12 minutes	1 biscuit

1 cup soy or other nondairy milk

2 TB. lemon juice

2 cups whole-wheat pastry flour

1½ TB. aluminum-free baking powder

½ tsp. sea salt

¼ cup safflower or other oil

1. Preheat the oven to 400°F. Line a cookie sheet with parchment paper or a Silpat liner.

2. In a small bowl, combine soy milk and lemon juice. Set aside to thicken for 5 minutes.

3. In a medium bowl, combine whole-wheat pastry flour, aluminum-free baking powder, and sea salt.

4. Using a pastry blender, a fork, or your fingertips, work in safflower oil until mixture resembles coarse crumbs. Add soy milk mixture, and stir just until combined. Using your hands, gather dough up into a ball in the bowl.

5. Transfer dough to a floured surface. Using your hands, knead dough for 1 minute. Roll or pat dough to a ½-inch thickness. Using a 2-inch biscuit cutter or glass, cut out 12 biscuits. Carefully transfer them to the prepared cookie sheet.

6. Bake for 10 to 12 minutes or until golden brown on the bottom and around the edges. Serve biscuits hot, either plain, with jam, or split and topped with gravy.

Variation: For **Sweet Biscuits,** add 2 tablespoons unbleached cane sugar to the dry ingredients. Then mix together some fresh-cut fruits such as berries, peaches, and plums; sprinkle them with a little additional sugar; and leave them to macerate for a while. Then use the biscuits and macerated fruit to make vegan shortcakes!

DEFINITION

Clabbering is a souring process done by combining soy milk (or other nondairy milk) with a little lemon juice or vinegar. When left to sit for a few minutes, the soy milk will sour and thicken slightly. Sometimes this mixture is referred to as vegan buttermilk because it can be used as a measure-for-measure replacement for buttermilk in recipes.

Vegan Cornbread

In the time it takes to preheat your oven, you can mix the batter for this maple syrup–sweetened cornbread. This recipe makes enough cornbread to feed a hungry family, but you can also cut the ingredient amounts in half and bake in a 9-inch pan instead.

Yield:	Prep time:	Cook time:	Serving size:
1 (9×13-inch) pan	5 minutes	20 to 25 minutes	1 piece

2½ cups medium-grind yellow cornmeal	1½ cups soy or other nondairy milk
2 cups whole-wheat pastry flour	1½ cups water
3 TB. aluminum-free baking powder	⅓ cup maple syrup
½ tsp. sea salt	⅓ cup safflower or other oil
	1 tsp. vanilla extract (optional)

1. Preheat the oven to 375°F. Lightly oil a 9×13-inch baking pan.

2. In a large bowl, combine yellow cornmeal, whole-wheat pastry flour, aluminum-free baking powder, and sea salt.

3. In a medium bowl, whisk together soy milk, water, maple syrup, safflower oil, and vanilla extract (if using). Add wet ingredients to dry ingredients, and stir until just combined.

4. Transfer batter to the prepared pan. Bake for 20 to 25 minutes or until a toothpick inserted in the center comes out clean. Allow to cool slightly before cutting into 12 pieces. Serve warm or at room temperature.

Variation: For **Corn Muffins,** pour the prepared cornbread batter into lightly oiled or paper-lined 12-cup muffin tins, filling them ⅔ full, and bake at 425°F for 15 to 20 minutes or until lightly browned around the edges.

HOT POTATO

Store your cornmeal in an airtight container in the refrigerator or freezer to prevent it from going rancid or attracting bugs. It can last for several months this way. Also, use organic, non-GMO (non–genetically modified) cornmeal whenever possible.

Bakery-Style Berry Muffins

These muffins are packed with juicy berries and make for a great breakfast treat or snack. A sprinkling of *turbinado sugar* gives them a sweet crunch on top.

Yield:	Prep time:	Cook time:	Serving size:
12 muffins	5 to 7 minutes	18 to 22 minutes	1 muffin

1 cup soy or other nondairy milk

2 TB. lemon juice or apple cider vinegar

2 cups whole-wheat pastry flour

¼ cup plus 1 TB. turbinado sugar

1 tsp. aluminum-free baking powder

1 tsp. baking soda

¼ tsp. sea salt

⅓ cup sunflower or other oil

1 tsp. vanilla extract

1½ cups fresh or frozen blueberries, blackberries, raspberries, sliced strawberries, or mixed berries of choice

1. Preheat the oven to 375°F. Lightly oil a 12-cup muffin tin, line with paper liners, or use silicone muffin cups.

2. In a small bowl, combine soy milk and lemon juice. Set aside to thicken for 5 minutes.

3. In a large bowl, combine whole-wheat pastry flour, ¼ cup turbinado sugar, aluminum-free baking powder, baking soda, and sea salt.

4. Add soy milk mixture, sunflower oil, and vanilla extract, and stir until just blended. Gently fold in blueberries.

5. Fill prepared muffin cups ¾ full, and sprinkle tops with remaining 1 tablespoon turbinado sugar. Bake for 18 to 22 minutes or until lightly browned and a toothpick inserted in the center comes out clean. Allow muffins to cool slightly in the pan and then transfer to a rack to cool as desired.

6. Serve warm or at room temperature. Store extra muffins in an airtight container or zipper-lock bag at room temperature.

Variation: For **Cranberry-Walnut Muffins,** replace the berries with an equal amount fresh or frozen cranberries, and evenly sprinkle ½ cup chopped walnuts over top of batter.

DEFINITION

Turbinado sugar is sugar made from the juice extracted from unrefined raw cane sugar, which is then spun in a centrifuge or turbine (hence its name). It has a very fine texture and a slight molasses flavor and can be used to replace light brown sugar. You might be familiar with the most commonly sold brand of turbinado sugar—Sugar in the Raw.

Flavorful Fruit Snacks

These naturally sweetened dried fruit–and-nut treats travel well, are great for snacking and providing quick energy, and are perfect for raw foodists, as well as those trying to avoid refined sugars and sweeteners.

Yield:	Prep time:	Serving size:
14 to 16 pieces	10 minutes	2 pieces

¾ cup raisins

¾ cup raw walnuts

¾ cup pitted medjool dates

¾ cup dried apricots

¾ cup shredded unsweetened coconut, plus more for rolling

2 TB. orange juice

Zest of 1 medium orange

1. In a food processor fitted with an S blade, pulse raisins, raw walnuts, medjool dates, and dried apricots several times to roughly chop, and then process for 1 or 2 minutes to finely chop.

2. Add coconut, orange juice, and orange zest, and process for 1 or 2 minutes or until mixture comes together to form a ball.

3. Place some shredded coconut on a plate and set aside.

4. Dampen your hands with water, roll fruit mixture into 14 to 16 (1-inch) balls, and roll fruit balls in shredded coconut. Store fruit snacks in an airtight container or zipper-lock bag in the refrigerator or freezer.

Variation: For **Cranberry-Pecan Snacks,** replace the dried apricots, coconut, and orange juice with 1½ cups raw walnuts, 1½ cups pitted medjool dates, 1½ cups dried cranberries, and zest of 1 medium orange. Shape into balls, but do not roll in coconut.

HOT POTATO

Many dried fruits are preserved with sulfites, so be sure to buy organic and unsulfured dried fruit. Also, always wash citrus fruits before zesting them, and be sure to use organic fruits for zesting to avoid getting a little pesticide residue along with your zest.

Oatmeal Trail Mix Cookies

These chewy oatmeal cookies are lightly spiced; sweetened with your choice of agave nectar or maple syrup; and enhanced with a trail mix blend of nuts, seeds, and dried fruits.

Yield:	Prep time:	Cook time:	Serving size:
2½ to 3 dozen cookies	10 minutes	15 to 18 minutes	2 cookies

2½ cups whole-wheat pastry flour

2 cups old-fashioned or regular rolled oats

1 tsp. ground cinnamon

¾ tsp. ground ginger or cardamom

¾ tsp. baking soda

½ tsp. aluminum-free baking powder

½ tsp. sea salt

⅔ cup almond or other nondairy milk

⅔ cup agave nectar or maple syrup

½ cup sunflower or other oil

½ TB. vanilla extract

1½ cups trail mix blend

1. Preheat the oven to 375°F. Line 2 cookie sheets with parchment paper or Silpat liners.

2. In a large bowl, combine whole-wheat pastry flour, old-fashioned rolled oats, cinnamon, ginger, baking soda, aluminum-free baking powder, and sea salt. Add almond milk, agave nectar, sunflower oil, and vanilla extract, and stir well to combine. Stir in trail mix.

3. Portion cookie dough using a 1½-inch scoop or by heaping tablespoonfuls onto the prepared cookie sheets, spacing them 2 inches apart. Flatten each cookie slightly with wet fingers.

4. Bake for 15 to 18 minutes or until golden brown on the bottom and around the edges. Remove from the oven. Let cool slightly before transferring to a rack to cool completely. Store cookies in an airtight container at room temperature.

Variation: Feel free to replace the trail mix blend with your favorite variety of dried fruit, nuts, and seeds. For **Raisin-Walnut Oatmeal Cookies,** replace the trail mix blend with ⅔ cup raisins and ⅔ cup raw or toasted walnuts, roughly chopped.

HOT POTATO

Choose a trail mix blend that contains an assortment of dried fruit, nuts, and seeds. If it contains large nut pieces, roughly chop them before adding them to the cookie batter.

Wheat-Free Hemp Chocolate-Chip Cookies

If you're sensitive to wheat, you're going to love these cookies made with barley and oat flour, hemp seeds, and chocolate chips.

Yield:	Prep time:	Cook time:	Serving size:
2½ to 3 dozen cookies	10 minutes	12 to 14 minutes	2 cookies

3 TB. water

1 TB. ground flaxseeds or flaxseed meal

¾ cup nonhydrogenated margarine

⅔ cup unbleached cane sugar

⅔ cup light brown sugar, packed

2 tsp. vanilla extract

1½ cups barley flour

1½ cups oat flour

1 tsp. baking soda

1 tsp. aluminum-free baking powder

½ tsp. sea salt

1½ cups vegan chocolate chips

⅓ cup raw hemp seeds

1. Preheat the oven to 375°F. Line 2 cookie sheets with parchment paper or Silpat liners.

2. In a large bowl, combine water and flaxseeds. Let sit for 5 minutes.

3. Add nonhydrogenated margarine, unbleached cane sugar, brown sugar, and vanilla extract, and stir together until light and creamy.

4. Add barley flour, oat flour, baking soda, aluminum-free baking powder, and sea salt, and stir well to combine. Stir in chocolate chips and raw hemp seeds.

5. Portion cookie dough using a 1½-inch scoop or by heaping 1 tablespoonfuls onto the prepared cookie sheets, spacing them 2 inches apart.

6. Bake for 12 to 14 minutes or until golden brown on the bottom and around the edges. Remove from the oven. Let cool slightly before transferring to a rack to cool completely. Store cookies in an airtight container at room temperature.

Variation: For **Mint Chocolate-Chip Cookies,** use only 1 teaspoon vanilla extract, add ½ teaspoon peppermint extract, and omit the hemp seeds.

Maca Bars

You'll be pleasantly surprised by the buttery, caramel-like flavor of these bar cookies that results from combining vegan margarine, sweet brown sugar, vanilla and almond extracts, and malty-flavored maca powder.

Yield:	Prep time:	Cook time:	Serving size:
1 (9-inch) pan or 8 or 9 pieces	10 minutes	25 to 30 minutes	1 piece

3 TB. water	1 cup whole-wheat pastry flour
1½ TB. Ener-G Egg Replacer	3 TB. *maca powder*
⅓ cup nonhydrogenated margarine, melted	1 tsp. aluminum-free baking powder
1 cup light brown sugar, packed	¼ tsp. baking soda
1 tsp. vanilla extract	½ tsp. sea salt
½ tsp. almond extract	⅓ cup raw almonds, roughly chopped

1. Preheat the oven to 350°F. Lightly oil a 9-inch baking pan.

2. In a medium bowl, combine water and Ener-G Egg Replacer, and whisk vigorously for 1 minute or until very frothy (like beaten egg whites).

3. Add nonhydrogenated margarine, brown sugar, vanilla extract, and almond extract, and stir well to combine. Add whole-wheat pastry flour, maca powder, aluminum-free baking powder, baking soda, and sea salt, and stir well to combine. Stir in chopped raw almonds.

4. Transfer batter to the prepared pan. Bake for 25 to 30 minutes or until a toothpick inserted in the center comes out clean. Allow to cool slightly before cutting into 8 or 9 pieces. Serve warm or at room temperature.

Variation: For **Butterscotch Maca Bars,** replace the brown sugar with an equal amount of packed muscavado sugar, replace the almond extract with an additional ½ teaspoon vanilla extract, and omit the almonds.

> **DEFINITION**
>
> **Maca powder** is made from a root vegetable, also known as Peruvian ginseng, that grows in the mountain plateaus of the Andes. When added to foods, maca powder imparts a slightly malty, butterscotch flavor, and is quite often used in raw food desserts and sweet treats.

Chewy Walnut Brownies

Blended bananas are used as a replacement for eggs and to add moisture to the batter for these rich and fudgy brownies topped with chopped walnuts.

Yield:	Prep time:	Cook time:	Serving size:
1 (9×13-inch) pan or 12 pieces	10 minutes	30 to 40 minutes	1 piece

1 (12-oz.) pkg. vegan chocolate chips	½ tsp. sea salt
¼ cup nonhydrogenated margarine	⅔ cup walnuts
1½ cups whole-wheat pastry flour	3 medium bananas, peeled and cut into 2-in. pieces
1 cup unbleached cane sugar	
½ tsp. aluminum-free baking powder	1 tsp. vanilla extract

1. Preheat the oven to 350°F. Lightly oil a 9×13-inch baking pan.

2. In the top of a double-boiler, combine chocolate chips and nonhydrogenated margarine, and heat until thoroughly melted. Remove from the heat, and set aside. (Alternatively, melt mixture in a microwave-safe bowl in the microwave, heating for 30-second increments until chocolate chips just begin to melt, and stir until smooth.)

3. In a large bowl, combine whole-wheat pastry flour, unbleached cane sugar, aluminum-free baking powder, and sea salt.

4. In a food processor fitted with an S blade, pulse walnuts several times to finely chop. Transfer chopped walnuts to a small bowl, and set aside.

5. Place bananas and vanilla extract in the food processor, and process for 2 minutes. Scrape down the sides of the container with a spatula, and process for 1 more minute or until smooth.

6. Add banana purée and melted chocolate-chip mixture to dry ingredients, and stir well to combine. Transfer batter to the prepared baking pan. Sprinkle chopped walnuts over top, and using your hands, gently press them into batter.

7. Bake for 30 to 40 minutes or until center is set. Allow to cool completely, at least 1 hour, before cutting into 12 pieces.

Variation: For **Frosted Walnut Brownies,** don't sprinkle chopped walnuts prior to baking. Instead, immediately after removing the brownies from the oven, sprinkle an additional ½ cup vegan chocolate chips over the top. When they've melted, gently spread them with a knife to completely cover the top of the brownies. Sprinkle the chopped walnuts over the top, and allow frosting to set completely before cutting brownies.

IN A NUTSHELL

It's best to allow brownies to cool completely, and use a sharp knife to cut them into uniform squares. To greatly increase their flavor and texture, we suggest making these brownies several hours or even a day in advance of serving them.

Whole-Wheat Pastry Dough

You can use this pastry dough to make piecrusts for sweet and savory pies, turnovers, tarts, and even quiche.

Yield:	Prep time:
enough for 2 (9-inch) piecrusts	5 minutes, plus 30 minutes chill time

3 cups whole-wheat pastry flour

¼ cup unbleached cane sugar

1 tsp. sea salt

⅔ cup nonhydrogenated margarine

¼ to ⅓ cup cold water

1. In a large bowl, combine whole-wheat pastry flour, unbleached cane sugar, and sea salt.

2. Using a pastry blender, a fork, or your fingertips, work nonhydrogenated margarine into dry ingredients until mixture resembles coarse crumbs. Drizzle in cold water, a little at a time, and mixing gently until a soft dough forms.

3. Gather pastry dough into a ball, divide in half, and flatten each half into a disc. Wrap each disc with plastic wrap, and refrigerate for 30 minutes or more.

4. Place each chilled dough disc between 2 (12×16-inch) pieces of parchment paper for easier rolling out and transferring to pans. Bake as directed in your recipe.

Variation: For a **Prebaked Pie or Tart Crust,** roll pastry out to a 12-inch circle (⅛-inch thick), place 1 rolled-out pastry dough in a 9-inch pie pan, and flute edges as desired. (Alternatively, use a lightly oiled 9-inch tart pan with a removable bottom, and press to cover bottom and sides of the tart pan.) Bake at 350°F for 10 to 15 minutes or until lightly browned and set.

IN A NUTSHELL

Chill your pastry dough to make it easier to roll out. When cooled, the fats in the dough harden and form layers throughout the dough, giving a pleasant flavor and texture when baked. It also allows the gluten in the dough to relax and not get overworked, which could result in a heavy crust instead of a crisp and flaky one. You can also roll out the pastry dough on a floured work surface and brush off the excess flour before placing in the baking pan. Rolling the dough between pieces of parchment paper is much easier and prevents sticking.

Favorite Fruit Pie

This recipe provides instructions for using our Whole-Wheat Pastry Dough to make a double-crusted fruit pie. To encourage your culinary creativity, you get to decide what fruits and spices to use in the filling.

Yield:	Prep time:	Cook time:	Serving size:
1 (9-inch) pie or 8 pieces	20 minutes	40 to 45 minutes	1 piece

5 cups berries or halved fruit, or 6 cups thinly sliced fruit

⅔ cup plus 1 TB. unbleached cane sugar

¼ cup tapioca starch

2 tsp. lemon juice

1 tsp. vanilla or other flavored extract (optional)

1 tsp. ground cinnamon

½ to ¾ tsp. ground cardamom, ground ginger, freshly grated nutmeg, or additional spice(s) of choice

1 batch Whole-Wheat Pastry Dough (recipe earlier in this chapter)

1 TB. soy or other nondairy milk

1. Preheat the oven to 350°F.

2. In a large bowl, combine berries or fruit, ⅔ cup unbleached cane sugar, tapioca starch, lemon juice, vanilla extract (if using), cinnamon, and additional spice(s), and set aside.

3. For easier rolling, place each chilled Whole-Wheat Pastry Dough disc between 2 (12×16-inch) pieces of parchment paper, and roll each into a 12-inch circle (⅛-inch thick).

4. Work with 1 rolled crust at a time, and set the other aside. Remove and discard top sheet of parchment paper. Flip crust into a pie pan, and remove and discard remaining parchment paper.

5. Spoon fruit filling into bottom crust. Remove and discard top sheet of parchment paper from second crust. Flip second crust over top of fruit filling, and remove and discard remaining parchment paper. Trim overhanging edge of both crusts about 1 inch from the outer edge of the pie pan. Gently press down on outer edges to seal, and flute edges as desired.

6. Using a knife, cut 3 or 4 slits into top crust. Brush top crust with soy milk, and sprinkle remaining 1 tablespoon unbleached cane sugar over top.

7. Bake for 40 to 45 minutes or until crust is lightly browned. Remove from the oven. Allow pie to cool for at least 1 hour before cutting.

8. Serve warm or at room temperature, plain, with a dollop of vegan whipped topping or Tofu Mousse and Crème Topping (see next recipe), or with scoops of nondairy ice cream as desired.

Variation: For **Crumb-Topped Fruit Pie,** omit the top pastry dough, and sprinkle a mixture of ½ cup unbleached cane sugar, ⅓ cup whole-wheat pastry flour, and ½ teaspoon ground cinnamon, with ¼ cup nonhydrogenated margarine worked in over fruit filling.

IN A NUTSHELL

In pie recipes, you're often instructed to "flute edges" to give a decorative edge border to your pie crust. You can do this quickly and easily by pressing the tines of a fork into the pastry dough all the way around the outer edge. For a fancier fluted edge, push the outer edge of pastry dough in with the thumb and index finger of one hand, while pressing toward it with the index finger of your other hand.

Tofu Mousse or Crème Topping

Using a food processor, you can transform a block of *silken tofu* into a luscious and creamy mousse or topping for your favorite vegan desserts.

Yield:	Prep time:	Serving size:
3 cups	5 minutes, plus 1 hour chill time	⅔ cup as mousse or 2 or 3 tablespoons as topping

2 (12-oz.) pkg. firm or extra-firm silken tofu	½ cup unbleached cane sugar, agave nectar, maple syrup, or brown rice syrup
	2 tsp. vanilla extract

1. In a food processor fitted with an S blade, process silken tofu, unbleached cane sugar, and vanilla extract for 1 minute. Scrape down the sides of the container with a spatula, and process for 1 or 2 more minutes or until very smooth and creamy.

2. Transfer tofu mousse or crème topping to an airtight container, and refrigerate for 1 hour.

3. Serve as a topping for fruit, granola, pies, cakes, and desserts—or enjoy all on its own.

Variation: For **Chocolate or Carob Mousse,** add 2 cups melted vegan chocolate or carob chips, and only use $\frac{1}{3}$ cup sweetener of choice. For **Tofu Cream Pie,** fill a prebaked graham cracker crust or Prebaked Pie or Tart Crust (variation earlier in this chapter) with tofu mousse or any of its variations, and refrigerate for several hours before cutting. Alternatively, bake the pie at 350°F for 30 to 35 minutes and allow to cool completely before cutting. Garnish with fresh fruit, chopped nuts, shredded unsweetened coconut, or chopped chocolate.

DEFINITION

Silken tofu is made from soybeans and has a creamy, velvety-smooth texture. The process for making silken tofu differs slightly from regular tofu in that the soy milk curds and excess water are not separated during production. Depending on the silken tofu's final texture, it's labeled soft, firm, or extra-firm. Silken tofu is often blended for making sauces, salad dressings, beverages, desserts, and baked goods.

Vegan New York–Style Tofu Cheesecake

The filling for this tofu-based cheesecake is flavored with a generous amount of vanilla and fresh lemon juice and zest, and includes a veganized version of the classic New York–style sweetened sour cream topping.

Yield:	Prep time:	Cook time:	Serving size:
1 (9-inch) cheesecake or 12 pieces	10 minutes, plus several hours chill time	45 to 50 minutes	1 piece

1 (7-oz.) pkg. amaranth graham crackers	1 cup plus 2 TB. unbleached cane sugar
1 tsp. ground cinnamon	2 TB. pure vanilla extract
¼ cup nonhydrogenated margarine	3 TB. fresh lemon juice
2 lb. extra-firm tofu	Zest of 2 large lemons
	⅓ cup vegan sour cream

1. Preheat the oven to 350°F. Lightly oil a 9-inch springform pan.

2. In a food processor fitted with an S blade, process graham crackers and cinnamon for 1 minute to crush to fine crumbs.

3. Add nonhydrogenated margarine, and process for 1 minute. Using your hands, firmly press crust mixture into the bottom of the prepared springform pan.

4. Wipe out food processor with a clean towel.

5. Squeeze tofu blocks over the sink to remove as much excess water as possible from each block. Using your fingers, crumble tofu into the food processor. Add 1 cup unbleached cane sugar, vanilla extract, lemon juice, and lemon zest, and process for 3 minutes.

6. Scrape down the sides of the container with a spatula, and process for 2 more minutes or until smooth and creamy. Pour filling into crust, and smooth with a spatula. Bake for 40 minutes.

7. Meanwhile, in a small bowl, combine sour cream and remaining 2 tablespoons unbleached cane sugar.

8. After cheesecake has baked for 40 minutes, remove it from the oven. Spread topping over cheesecake, leaving a 1-inch border around the edges. Bake for 7 more minutes or until topping's sheen changes from shiny to slightly dull. Do not allow to brown.

9. Remove from the oven. Allow to cool to room temperature, place springform pan on a large plate, and refrigerate for several hours, preferably overnight. Loosen sides of cheesecake with a knife, and remove ring from the springform pan. Dip a knife in warm water before cutting into 12 pieces and serving.

Variation: For a lighter-textured version, replace 1 pound tofu with 2 (8-ounce) containers vegan cream cheese. For **New York–Style Tofu Cheesecake with Berries,** add 1 cup fresh or frozen berries to the filling.

HOT POTATO

Most graham crackers labeled "honey grahams" are not suitable for vegans. Health Valley Amaranth Graham Crackers are vegan and contain 70 percent organic ingredients. If you can't find these where you live, try looking for a vegan animal cracker or vanilla-, lemon-, spice-, or chocolate-flavored plain cookie you can crush to make crumbs for the crust.

Lemon-Vanilla Cake with Creamy Vegan Buttercream Frosting

This moist, golden cake is flavored with a generous amount of lemon juice and vanilla and is topped with a light and fluffy, buttercream frosting.

Yield:	Prep time:	Cook time:	Serving size:
1 (9×13-inch pan) or 12 pieces	15 to 20 minutes	20 to 25 minutes	1 piece

3 cups whole-wheat pastry flour	¼ cup safflower or other oil
1½ cups unbleached cane sugar	3 TB. vanilla extract
1 TB. baking soda	2 TB. apple cider vinegar
½ tsp. sea salt	½ cup nonhydrogenated margarine
¾ cup water	3 cups vegan powdered sugar
¾ cup plus 1 TB. lemon juice	2 TB. soy or other nondairy milk

1. Preheat the oven to 350°F. Lightly oil a 9×13-inch baking pan.

2. In a large bowl, combine whole-wheat pastry flour, unbleached cane sugar, baking soda, and sea salt.

3. In a medium bowl, whisk together water, ¾ cup lemon juice, safflower oil, 2½ tablespoons vanilla extract, and apple cider vinegar. Add wet ingredients to dry ingredients, and whisk well to combine.

4. Pour cake batter into the prepared pan. Bake for 20 to 25 minutes or until a toothpick inserted in the center comes out clean. Remove cake from oven, and allow cake to cool completely before frosting.

5. In a large bowl, and using an electric mixer on medium speed, beat nonhydrogenated margarine for 1 minute.

6. Add powdered sugar, soy milk, remaining 1 tablespoon lemon juice, and remaining ½ tablespoon vanilla extract, and beat for an additional 2 or 3 minutes or until light and fluffy. Using a knife or small spatula, decoratively apply frosting to top of cake. Cut into 12 pieces, and serve.

Variation: For **Lemon-Vanilla Cupcakes,** lightly oil or line with paper liners 2 (12-cup) muffins tins, fill each muffin cup ¾ full with cake batter, and bake for 20 to 22 minutes. Cool cupcakes completely before frosting.

HOT POTATO

Lemons at room temperature (or warmer) release more of their juice more easily than ones straight from the refrigerator. Rolling or pounding a lemon on a hard surface before juicing can also help free those juices. An average-size lemon typically yields 1 or 2 teaspoons grated zest and 2 or 3 tablespoons juice.

Pineapple Upside-Down Cake

With this popular cake, the assembly procedure is reversed, and the sugary-sweet pineapple topping is placed in the bottom of a cast-iron skillet and then topped with a cake batter flavored with coconut yogurt and pineapple juice.

Yield:	Prep time:	Cook time:	Serving size:
1 (10-inch) cake or 8 pieces	15 to 20 minutes	35 to 40 minutes	1 piece

¼ cup nonhydrogenated margarine	1 (6-oz.) container plain or vanilla coconut yogurt
⅔ cup light brown sugar, packed	2 TB. safflower or other oil
1 (20-oz.) can sliced pineapple, with juice	1 tsp. vanilla extract
⅓ to ½ cup pecan halves	2 cups whole-wheat pastry flour
2 TB. water	⅔ cup unbleached cane sugar
1 TB. Ener-G Egg Replacer	2 tsp. baking soda
¾ cup reserved pineapple juice	¼ tsp. sea salt

1. Preheat the oven to 375°F.

2. In a 10-inch cast-iron skillet over low heat, melt nonhydrogenated margarine. Stir in brown sugar, and remove the skillet from heat.

3. Arrange pineapple rings on top of brown sugar mixture, and place 1 pecan half in center of each slice.

4. In a large bowl, combine water and Ener-G Egg Replacer, and whisk vigorously for 1 minute or until very frothy (like beaten egg whites).

5. Add reserved pineapple juice, coconut yogurt, safflower oil, and vanilla extract to egg replacer, and whisk well to combine. Add whole-wheat pastry flour, unbleached cane sugar, baking soda, and sea salt, and whisk well to combine.

6. Pour batter over pineapple slices. Bake for 35 to 40 minutes or until a toothpick inserted in the center comes out clean. Allow to cool for 5 minutes.

7. Loosen sides of cake with a knife. Place a large plate on top, and invert cake. Serve warm or at room temperature, cut into 8 pieces.

Variation: For **Island Pineapple Upside-Down Cake,** replace the pecan halves with whole cashews, and sprinkle ¼ cup shredded unsweetened coconut over the pineapple slices prior to topping with cake batter.

HOT POTATO

We recommend using a cast-iron skillet to make this cake, because it prevents the margarine from burning. Plus, the heatproof handle makes it easier to invert the cake. If you don't have one, you can use another similar ovenproof skillet or a 9-inch baking pan.

Mocha Almond Cake

A combination of brewed coffee, chocolate almond milk, cocoa powder, and cinnamon give this cake a rich, dark chocolate flavor, and sliced almonds provide a decorative touch and a bit of crunch.

Yield:	Prep time:	Cook time:	Serving size:
1 (8-inch pan) or 8 pieces	5 to 10 minutes	45 to 50 minutes	1 piece

½ cup cold coffee	1 tsp. apple cider vinegar
½ cup chocolate almond or other nondairy milk	1½ cups whole-wheat pastry flour
½ cup agave nectar or maple syrup	½ cup cocoa powder
6 oz. firm or extra-firm silken tofu	1 tsp. aluminum-free baking powder
3 TB. safflower or other oil	¾ tsp. baking soda
1 tsp. vanilla extract	½ tsp. ground cinnamon
1 tsp. almond extract	¼ tsp. sea salt
	½ cup raw sliced almonds

1. Preheat the oven to 350°F. Lightly oil an 8-inch springform pan or baking pan.

2. In a blender or food processor fitted with an S blade, process cold coffee, chocolate almond milk, agave nectar, silken tofu, safflower oil, vanilla extract, almond extract, and apple cider vinegar for 1 or 2 minutes or until smooth.

3. Add whole-wheat pastry flour, cocoa powder, baking powder, baking soda, cinnamon, and sea salt, and process for 1 minute. Scrape down the sides of the container with a spatula, and process for 30 more seconds or until smooth.

4. Reserve 3 tablespoons raw almonds for top of cake, and stir remaining into cake batter. Transfer cake batter to the prepared springform pan, and sprinkle reserved almonds on top. Bake for 45 to 50 minutes or until a toothpick inserted in the center comes out clean. Allow cake to cool for 15 minutes.

5. Loosen sides of cake with a knife, remove ring from the springform pan (if using), and allow cake to cool completely before cutting into 8 pieces and serving.

Variation: For **Mocha Almond Carob Cake,** use carob-flavored nondairy milk, and replace the cocoa powder with an equal amount of raw or roasted carob powder.

IN A NUTSHELL

The Mayan culture was the first to use raw cacao beans to flavor foods and beverages and to make into chocolate.

Vegan Lifestyle Choices

Being a vegan is about much more than not eating animals; it encompasses multiple aspects of your life choices. Veganism is a lifestyle. The more experienced and aware you become as a vegan, the more you'll discover new and hidden animal-based items in your life.

In the final chapters of this book, we offer advice on buying vegan beauty and household products, finding cruelty-free clothing, and caring for companion animals.

Body Care and Personal Items

In This Chapter

- Avoiding animal testing
- A look at vegan cosmetics
- Choosing body-care products
- Vegan brushes and sponges

The products that go on your body, used for personal care in a variety of ways, are just as important to vegans as those products that go in it. As you might imagine, now that you're trying to live your life as cruelty-free as possible, you'll have to consider some issues when it comes to buying, using, and applying things such as shampoo, soap, makeup, and even dental floss.

In this chapter, we take a look at some of the issues surrounding these and other personal-care items, ranging from the presence of animal ingredients to the practice of testing products on animals, and to those items that pose a risk to humans as well as animals.

Animal Testing Issues

Being a cruelty-free vegan consumer as much as possible means being informed and making wise purchasing decisions. When it comes to stocking the contents of your makeup case or your hair- and skin-care products, the most serious issue to be aware of is animal testing, also known as vivisection.

Many new products are routinely tested on living, unanesthetized animals in laboratory environments. These tests are carried out in the name of consumer safety by many cosmetics, personal care, pharmaceutical, and household goods manufacturers.

Animal testing is a heavily debated issue, but it shouldn't be. There really isn't any logical argument for animal testing in any instance. The rabbits, mice, rats, cats, frogs, and guinea pigs used in these tests don't share enough in common with humans, in terms of genetic makeup, to provide accurate enough data as to how humans would react to the same substance. What applies to a rat or a cat doesn't necessarily apply to humans when viewed from a physiological perspective.

Even the chimpanzee, which is a 99 percent match for human DNA, doesn't work for accurately testing human responses to medications, cosmetics, and cleaners. Their systems react differently, based on the simple fact that despite how closely related we are, we are still two completely different species. Knowing how a chimp, rabbit, or cat reacts to the exposure to any given substance does not guarantee a human's system will react in the same way.

VEGAN VOICES

Animal studies are done for legal reasons and not for scientific reasons. The predictive value of such studies for man is meaningless.

—Dr. James D. Gallagher, director of medical research, Lederle Laboratories, *Journal of the American Medical Association,* March 14, 1964

Purchase products that say "no animal testing," and also look for the cruelty-free bunny logo. Many companies are aware of their customers' sensitivities to these issues and go out of their way to include such labeling on their product packaging. They know these consumers can be very loyal and will spread the word to others, thus increasing their sales and customer base. To be sure you don't accidentally buy a product tested on animals, you can go online and find lists of companies that test on animals. See stopanimaltests.com, which is affiliated with PETA (People for the Ethical Treatment of Animals), for lots of helpful information.

Because animal testing isn't mandatory in most cases and due to growing public outcry over these practices, some companies are doing away with animal testing altogether. Instead, they're using actual human cells and tissues, artificial skin and eyes, and even computers to carry out the same scenarios in testing product safety.

The only reason the practice continues is because of a company's fear of being sued due to personal injury as a result of its product. Rather than use animal testing to prove its products are safe for human use, perhaps such companies should start with better, more natural ingredients that don't cause harm in the first place.

Don't Mess Up Your Makeup

As the sayings go, beauty is in the eye of the beholder, and beauty is only skin deep. These may be clichés, but everyone really is beautiful in his or her own way. Some choose to let their natural beauty shine through with just a simple cleansing and maybe some moisturizer, while others like to give their natural beauty a little assistance with lotions, toners, masks, cosmetics, and other concoctions.

When it comes to applying something to your skin and your face in particular, it's important to pay attention to ingredients. Many hidden animal ingredients are used in the making of cosmetics and other beauty products.

Bet you didn't know that fish scales are sometimes used to give lipsticks, nail polishes, and hair products an iridescent sparkle. Or that crushed beetles are used to tint blushes, lip liners, and lipsticks, and crushed silkworm cocoons are included to give your face powder a smooth finish. Sounds like the makings of a potion made by the wicked witch, not something for a cover girl!

IN A NUTSHELL

Avoiding all the animal ingredients that may be lurking in your beauty products can be tough, so educate yourself. You can find the names of commonly used animal ingredients online. PETA has a very informative list at peta.org/living/vegetarian-living/animal-ingredient-guide.aspx.

You don't have to pay a lot of money to help yourself look more beautiful or appealing, vegan style. It's easy for creative vegans to use simple kitchen ingredients to make homemade beauty products. Use coconut oil as a lotion, hair treatment or conditioner, or even as a lip gloss. Use oatmeal as a facial or body scrub to loosen dry skin, and avocados to moisturize it. If you want to learn more about how to make your own natural beauty products, check out your local library, bookstore, or the internet for some great books and ideas.

If you want to purchase vegan cosmetics, you can find them in all price ranges and in many retailers, drug stores, natural foods stores, online, and direct from the company. Be aware, though, as with all products that contain better-quality and cruelty-free ingredients, you get what you pay for, and some of the better products do cost a bit more. These are some companies that make cosmetics and beauty care products suitable for vegans.

- Aveda
- Beauty Without Cruelty
- Ecco Bella
- Herbs of Grace
- Kiss My Face

- Merry Hempsters
- No Miss
- Urban Decay
- Zia
- Zuzu Luxe

Once you discover the products you truly love, use the most, and can't do without, you can search out alternative ways to purchase them to save money. Try to take advantage of specials and sales, buy company direct, or purchase in large quantities or bulk.

Personal-Care Items

Store shelves are flooded with so many personal-care products—toothpastes, mouthwashes, lotions, moisturizers, shaving creams, shampoos, conditioners, soaps, body washes, perfumes, body sprays, powders, and scrubs. Be sure to read the packaging and labels on these products before buying them because they, too, can contain many obvious and not-so-obvious animal-based ingredients.

Many of the top perfume manufacturers use animal musk in their perfumes. Scent glands of civets, relatives of the mongoose, produce the musk, and these glands are painfully squeezed and drained every week or two to collect the musk. Musk deer are also used in the collection of animal musk, and they have been hunted to near extinction for their scent glands. Be sure to avoid any products that contain natural or even synthetic musk, as much painful animal testing and musk collection went into the development of the synthetic form of musk.

Vegans try to avoid animal ingredients, but they also try to avoid ingredients that cause harm to themselves, others, and the environment. Besides animal ingredients, many personal-care products also contain substances that can be harmful to your health. For instance, many deodorants contain aluminum, which may have links to Alzheimer's. Toothpastes may contain fluoride, which is toxic and responsible for thousands of accidental poisoning cases each year.

As you become an educated consumer, feel free to share the information with others who may be unaware. You may even save a life in the process.

Taking Care of Your Smile

You brush, floss, rinse, and go to the dentist regularly and are pretty much doing everything you can to take good care of your teeth. But are you really? Now that you've gone vegan, at least you know drinking lots of cow's milk isn't the way to get a winning smile. You know the calcium in tofu and leafy greens can do a lot more to strengthen your teeth and bones, and the fiber present in these foods requires you to properly and fully chew it, which is good for your molars and jaw muscles. But are you buying the right vegan products to keep your teeth strong and healthy and your breath fresh?

Try to buy toothpastes and mouthwashes that contain natural cleaners, whiteners, and fresheners, like those made with natural abrasives (such as calcium carbonate), salts, herbs, and botanicals to help scrub away food particles, plaque, and film. Keep in mind that minty freshness is always best when it comes from a natural source like peppermint or spearmint, not a numbered chemical compound.

What about fluoride? Is it friend or foe? The practice of adding fluoride to consumer products, using it in dentistry practices, and adding it to our drinking water are highly controversial and often-debated topics. Many would be surprised to learn that fluoride is a hazardous toxic waste, a by-product of phosphate-based fertilizer and aluminum production. Some studies have shown that the claims of fluoride's positive effects on dental health are unfounded and that it's actually harmful to your health and the environment. The same fluoride that's classified as a poison and can scorch and kill crops and pollute the air on contact is being regularly added to drinking water and oral-care products. Avoid the poison on your toothbrush, and seek out nonfluoridated toothpastes instead.

IN A NUTSHELL

You can also make your own tooth-polishing powder by mixing baking soda, a little hydrogen peroxide, and sea salt. This mixture also whitens your teeth over time and improves the health of your gums.

Also, check your dental floss, as most are coated in beeswax or petroleum-based products. Eco-DenT GentleFloss is a good vegan and cruelty-free dental floss. It uses a blend of essential oils, herbs, and plant waxes and even comes in a plastic-free, biodegradable and recyclable box. Eco-DenT also makes several other vegan and cruelty-free oral hygiene products. You can find natural toothpastes in tubes and powdered form, as well as unwaxed dental floss in most retailers and natural foods stores.

Handling Hair Care

Having healthy skin, nails, and hair depends on a diet rich in B vitamins, especially biotin. Biotin-rich foods such as leafy greens, whole-grains, and beans form the basis of a vegan diet. For a tremendous impact on your outward appearance, get plenty of biotin-rich foods in your diet. Oils high in essential fatty acids—such as omega-rich flax, hemp, avocado, and soybean oils—are also great internal and external lubricants and conditioners.

Eating a well-balanced diet helps give your hair a healthy shine and luster, provides it with moisture, makes it stronger, and reduces hair breakage and loss. Diet helps your hair's inner beauty come shining through, but helping nature along a little doesn't hurt either. Just try to avoid the use of harsh chemical-based products that strip away your hair's natural moisture, leaving dry, brittle, damaged, or fly-away hair.

Read product packaging and labels, and analyze the quality and types of ingredients in your hair-care products. Look for natural and organic ingredients first and foremost, and avoid long chemical names you're unfamiliar with, as they may be harsh chemicals or derived from animals. Some common animal-based ingredients that find their way into hair products and other beauty items include the following:

- Collagen
- Honey and bee-based products
- Hydrolyzed animal protein
- Lanolin

- Milk protein
- Nonvegetable glycerin
- Shark and fish oils
- Silk protein

For a complete list of animal ingredients in both personal-care products and food items, see the excellent and comprehensive book *Animal Ingredients A to Z*, compiled by the E. G. Smith Collective. It's available in libraries and bookstores across the United States.

HOT POTATO

Sodium laurel sulfate and one of its variations, sodium laureth sulfate, are the most common foaming agents used in shampoos and other foaming personal-care products. The good news is that it's chemically derived from coconuts, not from animal ingredients. The bad news is that there's quite a bit of controversy surrounding its safety. Some believe it causes hair loss, skin rashes and irritation, and even cancer. Do some research before selecting products that contain sodium laurel sulfate or sodium laureth sulfate.

After being sure a product does not have any unwanted ingredients, you can move on to looking for some of the ingredients you do want. Herbals and botanicals are wonderful for fragrance, to clean the scalp, and to moisturize. Which ones to choose depend on to whom the product is geared. Flowery scents containing botanicals such as chamomile, lavender, roses, geranium, passion flower, and citrus are often considered feminine scents, while those like clary sage, rosemary, thyme, and tea tree oil are more often considered masculine scents.

More natural conditioners and other styling products have been hitting the market with many of those same natural ingredients and fragrances, along with moisturizing oils and extracts from avocados, soybeans, sea vegetables, jojoba, and nuts and seeds like almonds, macadamias, pumpkin, sunflower, and flaxseeds. Grain-based proteins from wheat, oats, corn, and rice are also added to give the hair strength. Many products are also vitamin fortified.

Soap ... It's Time to Come Clean

We all know that using soap is supposed to make you clean, and the antibacterial varieties are even supposed to kill germs. So why, then, would so many soap companies use slaughterhouse by-products to make a product that's supposed to get you clean? Tallow, the rendered fat from cows and sheep, is used to make many popular brands of soaps, foods, and even candles. Many of the biggest manufacturers rely heavily on the use of tallow as a base for their soaps.

Besides tallow, many of the massively produced brands of soap contain synthetic chemicals, colorants, and fragrances that can be irritating to skin, especially the delicate facial area. Rashes, dry patches, itching, and blistering—these are all common skin reactions to chemical ingredients in soaps. Many liquid soaps contain harsh antibacterial and antifungal ingredients that can wash away not only the germs, but your body's natural oils as well. This can leave your skin feeling dry and irritated.

What is a vegan to do to get all clean and sudsy? Look for vegetable glycerin–based soaps or oil-based soaps made with coconut, olive, almond, sunflower, soybean, and hemp oils and sometimes *shea butter*. Note that if a soap doesn't specifically list vegetable glycerin, there's a good chance the glycerin used is derived from animal sources. Most vegan oil-based soaps provide better moisturizing benefits to your skin, result in less clogged pores, and cause fewer skin irritations and breakouts than the conventional tallow-based soaps.

> **DEFINITION**
>
> **Shea butter** is derived from the shea nut, which grows in many parts of Africa. It's used in the treatment of minor skin problems and irritations such as eczema, dermatitis, psoriasis, sunburn, or sun damage, and to soothe dry skin, scalps, and lips. It can be used alone or blended with other ingredients to make hair and skin products, including pomades, salves, lotions, cosmetics, soaps, shampoos, conditioners, and other hair- and personal-care products.

Saving Your Skin

Having soft, smooth skin depends on having proper moisture and lubrication both inside and out. Start by eating a well-balanced vegan diet containing plenty of nuts, seeds, and healthy oils to provide a little natural protective lubrication from the inside out.

For those who have a beauty regimen, many vegan options exist in the form of tonics, toners, moisturizers, cleansers, and makeup removers. If you like to have a skin-care system in place to keep yourself looking young and radiant, you can find several great vegan products by Beauty Without Cruelty, Dessert Essence, and Jason. Need a lotion to rub on dry elbows or after shaving? When selecting one, be sure to read the labels to ensure an all-vegan product; lanolin, fish oils, and silk and animal proteins are added to many skin products unnecessarily.

Brushes and Sponges

Now that you know how to pick out vegan beauty products, you're all set to apply and use them. Uh-oh, wait a minute—take a look at that comb, brush, or sponge you're going to use to style or apply the products. Is it made using animal products?

For centuries, hair combs and brush handles were traditionally made with bone, tortoise shells, mother of pearl, abalone, or even ivory tusks. Animal hair, mostly boar hair, was and is still commonly used to make the bristles of hair and makeup brushes. Many men's brushes used to apply shaving cream are made with badger's hair because it is softer and gentler on the face.

Fortunately, you don't have to buy an animal-based brush or comb to groom yourself. Many manufacturers make wood- or plastic-handled combs and brushes that are quite sturdy, long-lasting, and suitable for vegans. You also can find natural or man-made bristles made from nylon or natural fibers. Many retailers sell vegan-friendly hair combs and brushes. In most discount retailers and natural foods stores, as well as through online sources, you can readily find EcoTools, a collection of vegan bath tools, cosmetics accessories, and makeup brushes from earth-friendly and cruelty-free materials.

Natural sponges may look like they're dried plants because of all their tiny pores, nooks, and crannies, but a sponge is really a multicelled form of sea animal—a living, eating, water- and oxygen-filtering creature that wants nothing more than to be left alone to live its life. These amazing creatures can anchor themselves to rocks, plants, and other underwater debris or stand free against the ebb and flow of the tide and water currents.

IN A NUTSHELL

Having evolved more than half a billion years ago, sponges, also known as porifera, are among the earliest known forms of animal life in existence. They eat plankton and other tiny particles that pass through their body's filtration system. Sponges are hermaphrodites, which means each individual sponge contains both male and female elements.

You can purchase cellulose sponges, made primarily from wood fiber, for use in your household and other cleaning tasks. For applying your makeup, check out synthetic, foam-based sponges available at most retailers.

To clear up any potential confusion, pumice doesn't come from a spongelike animal; rather, it's a piece of volcanic rock. Loofahs, which are also often mistaken for sponges, are actually made from a particular species of dried squash. They help loosen and remove dead skin cells, so use them and scrub to your heart's content. You don't have to give up your loofah once you go vegan!

Vegan-Friendly Sources

You can find vegan cosmetics and personal products in many retailers, in natural foods stores, from the manufacturers directly, and via online shopping sources. To guarantee that what you're using is truly cruelty free and vegan, shop from vegan merchant websites such as veganstore.com or veganessentials.com. A few quality producers of vegan products include these:

- ABBA
- Aubrey Organics
- Avalon
- Beauty Without Cruelty
- Desert Essence
- Earth Science

- Ecco Bella
- Jason
- Lamas Beauty

- Nature's Gate
- Paul Penders

As a consumer, you have the option of deciding whether or not to support companies that make mostly animal-based products and only a few vegan products or those that strive to create an all-vegan or veg-friendly product line. How and where you spend your money is a personal decision that often depends on how much of it you have available to spend, so the decision is yours to make.

The Least You Need to Know

- Animal testing is a serious issue involving many body-care products, and you should take great care to avoid purchasing those that utilize it.
- Cosmetics often contain animal ingredients or have been tested on animals, so be sure of what you're buying and from whom you're buying it.
- Be sure to read the labels of body-care products before buying them, as they can contain many obvious and not-so-obvious animal-based ingredients.
- Natural sponges are actually animals, not plants, and cosmetic, shaving, and hair brushes are sometimes made with animal hair bristles. Vegans avoid all these items.
- You can purchase vegan, cruelty-free body- and personal-care items in many retailers, natural foods stores, and online.

Dressing to Impress

Chapter

25

In This Chapter

- Avoiding vegan-unfriendly materials
- Understanding the cruelty of leather and wool
- Shopping for animal-free clothing
- Veganizing shoes and accessories
- Putting compassion in fashion

As a new vegan, you've undoubtedly put a lot of time and effort into eliminating animal-based foods and ingredients from your diet and other aspects of your life. But what about the contents of your closet and your dresser drawers? Some vegan-unfriendly items are likely hanging or folded in there. In this chapter, we turn our attention to your wardrobe and the various issues associated with it.

Many traditional clothing items derive either wholly or in part from animals, so a vegan really has to be aware of what he or she chooses to wear. Walking into a clothing store and picking out the first thing that appeals to you generally isn't an option. Going shopping for clothing usually involves reading labels and being an informed consumer. Let's take a look at some of the common clothing items vegans avoid, as well as some of the ones they seek out.

"I Wouldn't Be Caught Dead in That!"

In some respects, the issue of what to wear as a vegan is a pretty simple one. Vegans don't wear animal skin, fur, or anything else produced by an animal. The idea is that those items belong to the animals, who had to suffer and eventually die to provide them, and it's both undesirable and wrong to wear them as clothing. Common animal-based clothing materials to avoid include fur, feathers, shells, silk, wool, leather, suede, and other skins taken from animals.

Leather and Suede

The most common animal clothing you encounter will undoubtedly be leather and its roughly buffed variation, suede. Throughout the world, all sorts of animals are used to make leather goods and garments, but in the United States, most leather comes from cattle. Leather is used for a variety of clothing and household purposes, and most of it is a by-product of the animal food industry. Animals who are primarily raised as livestock and intended for food or milk production are shared among many different industries at the end of their lives. The skin or hide of many animals are used to make most of the leather goods we encounter so often in our daily lives. Equally disturbing and cruel is the fact that calfskin and sheepskin comes from calves and baby sheep that are killed just for their soft young skin, as are snakes used to acquire snakeskin for shoes and purses.

Leather manufacturers around the world sometimes use skins from other animals such as cats, dogs, horses, pigs, goats, sheep, snakes, alligators, and deer in the production of their leather products. When purchasing animal-skin products, especially discount merchandise produced in other countries, you could get any of these skins as part of a leather or suede purse, shoes, or clothing. Truth-in-labeling laws are virtually nonexistent for leather products.

Factory farming has a negative impact on the environment through waste runoff and the clearing of forests for grazing land, but the environmental impact doesn't stop at the end of an animal's life. The *tanning* industry uses substances such as formaldehyde, mineral salts, coal tars, arsenic, lead, cyanide-based dyes, and chromium. When released into the environment, these substances contaminate water and negatively impact the health of humans and nonhumans alike.

> **DEFINITION**
>
> **Tanning** is the process of turning animal hide into pliable, finished leather through exposure to various chemicals, preservatives, and dyes.

Hairy Business

When it comes to obtaining and wearing animal skins, the inherent cruelty is obvious. The cruelty isn't as apparent to some people when it comes to materials such as wool or other animal hair, for which animals aren't always directly killed in the production.

The idea that animals are not harmed in the shearing processes of commercial wool production is a myth. Animal hair used as clothing fibers is generally only acquired after the animals involved have endured tremendous amounts of suffering throughout all aspects of the process.

For sheep used in the production of wool, large sections of skin around the tail area are often intentionally sliced off without the use of anesthesia. This "mulesing" is done to prevent maggot infestation from flies that are attracted to their specially bred thick folds of skin covered in unnaturally thick amounts of wool. The idea is that the scarred skin that will grow in its place will be more resistant to infestation.

Angora rabbits used in the production of angora wool, for use in sweaters and other clothing items, also have it bad. In between shearings, they spend all their time in tiny cages, where the delicate pads of their feet become easily cut on the rough wire mesh of their cages and often become ulcerated and infected. Male angora rabbits are usually killed at birth due to their hair's lower growth rate. Females are the gender of choice for angora production because they produce up to 80 percent more wool.

Animal Accents

When shopping for clothes or accessories, let your eyes, nose, and fingers be your guide. That's right, ogle the texture or grain, take a whiff, and give the fabric a good rub between your fingers. You'll almost instantly be able to tell if it's made of animal or man-made materials. Next, check the label for the material content. These simple prescreening steps can serve you well when shopping in thrift or secondhand stores, when tags and labels are often missing from the garments.

Be sure to fully inspect items before you buy because sometimes animal-based ingredients are hidden or not mentioned on the label. For instance, a little fur or leather trim could be lurking on a coat or shoes, or down feathers or wool quilting could be inside your parka.

Vegan Clothing Options

Today, clothing made from natural and man-made fabrics is widely available. Natural cloth fabrics such as hemp, linen, cotton, bamboo, and other natural fiber blends are soft, lightweight, and snuggly, and are made into shirts, sweaters, pants, socks, and even shoes. Companies such as Ecolution, Of The Earth, Eco Dragon, Patagonia, Hemptown, and Sweetgrass make it easy to find styles and fashions to suit all tastes. You can also purchase jackets and coats made from these same natural fibers or from man-made nylon, polyester, rubber, synthetic Ultrasuede, microfiber, and polar fleece.

Clothing made from natural fibers tends to breathe better and keep you cooler, which makes it ideal for warmer weather conditions. Man-made fibers tend to trap in warmth and keep out air, so they're better for colder climates and temperatures. For those in need of warm sweaters, coats, scarves, and mittens, there's no need to fret over not wearing wool, angora, or cashmere any more. Popular fleece and microfiber fabrics are oh-so-soft, cozy, and insulating!

> **IN A NUTSHELL**
>
> Pesticides are used in heavy concentrations on many fiber crops, especially cotton. Be a wise shopper and search out organic sources whenever possible for your clothing, footwear, and accessory needs. Earth-friendly alternatives to cotton are available. Hemp and bamboo, for example, often don't require the use of pesticides and other chemicals, especially when grown organically.

Veganizing Your Wardrobe

Buying secondhand items from consignment shops, boutiques, thrift stores, or even garage sales is a great way to get some inexpensive vegan duds to help revamp and veganize your wardrobe quickly and affordably. You'll need to do a bit of searching, and you might be amazed at what you find. You may even stumble upon organic cotton, hemp, or linen items for only a few dollars.

For those times when you want something brand new, you'll usually have more luck finding vegan clothing at discount retailers that stock more man-made and cloth-based products than at larger department stores, which tend to carry a lot more leather, suede, wool, and fur items. With a little effort, you should be able to find quality vegan apparel ranging from bargain-basement to high-end designer labels. And good news! Several designers such as Stella McCartney, Calvin Klein, Anne Klein, Genevieve Gaelyn, and Atom Cianfarani have pledged to not use animal materials in their designs!

It's also a good idea to check your local community for shops and boutiques that sell fair trade clothing items. These are more ethical alternatives to those items mass produced by cheap labor. The internet can provide a wealth of sources for fair trade and conventionally produced vegan clothing. Ethicalwares.com is a great site run by vegans. It sells fair trade items, music, accessories, shoes, clothing, and much more.

Putting on Pleather

Vegans and nonvegans alike have embraced pleather, faux (fake) fur, and other synthetically derived animal skin look-alikes. Such items are particularly popular among veg-conscious celebrities, musicians, fashion models and designers, and those who want to dress trendy or flashy without having to buy the farm or add to the suffering that happens on it.

HOT POTATO

The drawback to pleather and other petroleum-derived synthetic fabrics is that their production and disposal are not environmentally friendly. Whenever possible, you should choose natural fibers over man-made ones, but when there's no other alternative, many feel it's better than contributing to the suffering of living, feeling creatures.

Pleather is short for "plastic leather"; it has become quite popular because it's much more affordable than animal-based leather and can be just as durable, pliable, easily dyed, and useful as any animal's skin. It's used in the production of boots, shoes, wallets, purses, hats, coats, jackets, vests, pants, shirts, undergarments, and other gear. It's also used to make car and bicycle seats, upholstery, and sports equipment. Vinyl and polyester are also commonly used to make much of the same outerwear and gear.

Designers Genevieve Gaelyn and Atom Cianfarani, creators of the Gaelyn and Cianfarani fashion label, have developed an Earth-friendly clothing material they use in some of their creations. It's handcrafted from recycled bicycle inner tubes and is often mistaken for leather.

Friend or Faux?

The creation of faux furs came about for several reasons but primarily out of the desire to find a more affordable alternative to animal furs. In addition, many animal welfare organizations have been busy spreading the word about the cruelty involved in wearing fur. As a result, more and more people are opting to wear faux furs instead of the real thing. They're more affordable, fashionable, and definitely a much more humane and politically correct option.

You can find faux fur fashions at most retailers, in department stores and boutiques, on the web, and even in the private collections of many top fashion designers. The wide variety of faux fur selections available may surprise you. Naturally, you can expect to find imitations of all sorts of furs, with their natural hues and striking patterns or spots, as the basis of garments or as adornments on collars and cuffs.

However, some vegans are so opposed to the thought of wearing animal skins or fur that they even avoid look-alike items that resemble animal products. To do so makes them feel odd, and it can also send the wrong message that wearing animal skins is desirable. If the item looks realistic enough, many people might assume you're actually wearing leather or fur, and you'll then be a walking billboard for wearing those items.

Shoes and Accessories

Most people have one or more pairs of leather shoes in their closet when they go vegan. It's only natural, as most of us, when growing up, were told about the importance of buying shoes that last, and getting a good value for our money meant buying leather shoes. This applies to dress shoes, work shoes, boots, sandals, and athletic shoes of all kinds—even ice skates.

As a new vegan, you'll probably need to replace much of your footwear. But don't despair. You can easily find durable shoes made from natural and man-made materials in the form of canvas, hemp, linen, cotton, nylon, rubber, polyester, acrylic, vinyl, and even recycled materials. Most retailers and department stores carry nonleather shoes, although you may have to do a bit of searching to find them among the leather stuff. Selection varies from season to season; more nonleather styles tend to be available in the summer months.

IN A NUTSHELL

Major discount and department stores and national shoe chains such as Payless ShoeSource normally carry many man-made selections in all styles, such as dress shoes, sneakers, boots, and sandals. This makes buying nonleather shoes relatively easy and inexpensive from coast to coast.

After getting your shoes in order, check out your other accessories, including purses, bags, luggage, and other gear you may have for hauling, carrying, and traveling. Such pieces are often made from leather. Replacing any leather or wool gloves, hats, or scarves with cloth or synthetic alternatives is quite easy. You can purchase cloth, straw, metal, vinyl, pleather, and nylon-based purses, bags, and luggage to replace any animal-skin products. As for leather belts, many man-made versions are available and suitable for vegans.

Don't forget to check your jewelry box; you may have to do a bit of thinning out there as well. Many earrings, necklaces, rings, bracelets, and other jewelry items can contain obvious animal ingredients. Leather and suede are often used for bands, ties, clasps, and accents on watches, necklaces, and bracelets. Feathers, shells, pearls, abalone, and pieces of bone are often parts of earrings, necklaces, hats, and even hair accessories.

What's wrong with pearls, you may ask? Well, when an irritant like a piece of sand gets inside an oyster's shell, a special liquid called nacre is secreted over it to lessen the pain of having it scratch against its soft tissue. Cultured pearls are those created as a result of human intervention. In the process, oysters are forcibly opened, an incision is made, and a bead or other irritant is placed inside. The oysters are kept in cages until the irritant-turned-pearl has reached the desired size.

Compassion in Fashion

By now you should know that animals don't have to suffer so you can put clothes on your back. You indeed can have compassion in fashion, and we have women to thank for pushing the envelope and helping make widespread change. In particular, the influential Lady Muriel Dowding wasn't content to stand idly by when confronted with the animal cruelty she encountered in her everyday life. During the 1950s in London, she was very active in antivivisection campaigns and as an animal rights advocate in the House of Lords. She did whatever she could to effect positive change on behalf of animals.

Lady Dowding traveled in many influential circles and was appalled at seeing people wearing fur coats and accessories. She encouraged clothing manufacturers that didn't use animal-based products to proudly say so, and in doing so, she developed a "Beauty Without Cruelty" tag for positively describing and promoting such companies' cruelty-free clothing production.

Beauty Without Cruelty began as a simple tag to signify that no animal had to suffer in the production of the garment bearing the label. Later it became the name of Lady Dowding's cosmetics company, which was one of the first of its kind to employ no animal testing and ensure animal-free ingredients. It still continues to make many fine products suitable for vegans.

Marcia Pearson, former top fashion model, is now the founder of the nonprofit organization Fashion with Compassion. She was greatly influenced by the work of Lady Dowding. After finally meeting face-to-face, the two of them got together and decided to use their celebrity status to help popularize the concepts of compassion in fashion and cruelty-free living. They organized fashion shows and other events to showcase new options in cruelty-free products and clothing items. This started a snowball effect, and now many celebrities eagerly voice their concerns about animal rights, environmental, and vegan/vegetarian issues.

The Least You Need to Know

- Vegans avoid all clothing, accessories, and footwear derived from animal-based sources, including leather, wool, silk, feathers, shells, and bone.
- Many people don't realize the suffering and cruelty involved with bringing leather and wool products to our wardrobes.
- Natural and man-made clothing materials suitable for vegans include cotton, linen, hemp, bamboo, polyester, acrylic, nylon, vinyl, and pleather.
- Replacing leather shoes and accessories is relatively easy, due to the widespread availability of nonleather alternatives.

Other Things to Consider

In This Chapter

- Finding and removing animal-based products from your home
- Exposing gelatin in film and other products
- Veganizing your candles
- Feeding dogs and cats a vegan diet

Throughout this book, we've taken a look at many different issues that surround living as a vegan, from gracefully handling family meals to knowing how to replace the animal ingredients in your recipes. As with everything else in life, being armed with a little bit of knowledge about the issues can make them a lot easier to deal with and can increase your chances of success as a vegan.

This final chapter focuses on a few additional things you need to consider as you continue your voyage into veganism, from down-filled comforters and pillows, to taking vegan photos, to lighting cruelty-free candles, to having vegan dogs and cats!

Household Items

If you look closely enough around your home, you'll undoubtedly find animal products lurking in the unlikeliest of places. Be on the lookout for sheets and bedspreads made of silk, as well as pillows and comforters that contain down, usually derived from geese or ducks. You can donate these items to a homeless shelter or other charitable organization because these types of items are always needed. Replace them with man-made and natural fiber options made of cotton, bamboo, polyester, etc.

If you're an artist or into home improvement, double-check your paint brushes because typically those used for fine art are usually animal hair–based and taken from a variety of animals, including sables, squirrels, hogs, camels, oxen, ponies, and goats. Also, brushes used for oil-based house paints and solvent-thinned finishes are usually made from hog bristles, sometimes called China bristles. A variety of synthetic art brushes are now available.

IN A NUTSHELL

The most popular brand of glue used at home and school today, Elmer's, actually contains no animal products. In fact, it would be pretty hard for you to find an animal-based glue for everyday use in the home. And according to the U.S. Postal Service, the glue used on stamps is vegan and also kosher. The glue used on envelopes is usually free of animal ingredients as well, so you now have no excuse for not writing to your mother!

Gelatin is another animal-based substance you'll encounter quite often in your household items, often without even knowing it. Gelatin is used in everything from golf balls to help them roll straight, to the binder used in attaching the abrasive particles to sandpaper, to the glossy coating used on some wallpapers and playing cards. It helps put the crinkle in crepe paper, the shine in glossy papers, and adds to the strength of rag-based papers like the paper money in your wallet or the blueprints for your new home.

You may be surprised to learn that gelatin has been used in the production of photographic film since around 1870. Without exception, all modern film contains gelatin, including the rolls and instant self-developing films, film used for taking medical x-rays, and the kind of film traditionally used to shoot Hollywood movies.

Fortunately, most of us have switched over to digital cameras. Digital photography is an easy and fun way to avoid the gelatin issue while still being able to exercise the Ansel Adams or Margaret Bourke-White inside you. Most movies are filmed completely digitally as well, which has greatly reduced the need for gelatin-based film. For vegan artists, amateur and professional photographers, and others who still like to dabble in film-based photography, some companies have responded to customer demand for animal-free alternatives and have started to make gelatin-free rolls of film. With a bit of searching, you even can find companies that process film without the use of gelatin.

One note of caution: glossy photographic paper can often contain a gelatin coating. This goes for the professional stuff as well as the kind you can purchase for your home printer. Stick with matte (nonglossy) paper unless you know for sure gelatin wasn't used in the glossing process.

These few examples show how animal products are used in everyday household items. It's easy to become overwhelmed when faced with the seeming omnipresence of nonvegan products and ingredients in your everyday life, but relax. Being vegan means doing the best you can to eliminate the use and abuse of animals in your life. It's not an easy task, due to the fact that by-products of the animal foods industry are virtually everywhere. Just do your best, and feel good about making whatever positive changes you can. Every little bit truly does help, and your actions can have a pro-vegan ripple effect on the world around you in unimaginable ways!

Cleaning Products

The biggest issue with products used to clean sinks, toilets, floors, carpet, baths, and windows is that of animal testing and the presence of toxic ingredients. Just like products used to clean our bodies, many household cleaning products also undergo a great deal of senseless animal testing. The best thing you can do to avoid cleaning products that have been tested on animals is to look for a cruelty-free logo and the phrase "no animal testing" on package labels.

Also, check out the ingredients to avoid harsh chemicals, detergents, and dyes, and purchase products that contain biodegradable and environmentally friendly ingredients. Luckily for conscientious consumers, alongside the conventional cleaners you can also find eco-friendly products to clean your clothes, dishes, bathrooms, kitchens, and floors in most retailers, grocery stores, and natural foods stores. A few notable natural and cruelty-free brands to look for include: Bi-O-Kleen, Citra-Sol, Dr. Bronner's, Earth Friendly Products, Ecover, Mountain Green, Planet, and Seventh Generation.

IN A NUTSHELL

Some progressive cleaning products contain natural and organic ingredients such as herbal extracts, essential oils, citrus blends, and vinegar.

You can also make your own household cleaners using simple ingredients like vinegar, baking soda, and lemon juice. Find more tips for making homemade cleaners online or in the excellent book, *How It All Vegan!* by Sarah Kramer and Tanya Barnard. (See govegan.net or Appendix B for details.)

Flickering Light

What could possibly not be vegan about something as simple as lighting and enjoying a candle? Well, let's take a look at that match you're planning on using to light it. Most matches use gelatin to bind all the incendiary chemicals together to form the match head. Does that mean you have to go back to rubbing two sticks together to make a flame? Not at all. Just use a lighter.

But wait, before you light your candle with that lighter, are you sure the candle's wick doesn't contain lead? As recently as 2003, when a small percentage of all candles sold in the United States were found to contain lead-cored wicks, a federal ban was put in place. Zinc is another common component of metal-cored wicks, but unfortunately, this may not be a safe alternative, as recent studies have shown zinc-based wicks can cause problems of their own. To be completely sure you're safe, use nonmetallic wicks made from natural fibers like hemp or cotton.

IN A NUTSHELL

The Romans developed the first wick-based candles, which were made from tallow derived from sheep or beef suet. These early candles burned dirty and left a lingering odor. Since the development of paraffin wax in the mid-1800s, the production of pure tallow candles is a rarity. Still, tallow and its derivatives are sometimes used as ingredients in modern candles, either in the wax itself or as a base for additives.

Mind Your Beeswax

For vegans, a major problem with candles is that many of them are made either entirely, or partially, from beeswax. Beeswax is a substance secreted from the abdomen of bees to help form the storage units within the hive, or honeycomb. The honeycomb can contain honey, pollen, or eggs, depending on the particular need. In winter months, the larvae and others in the colony use the honeycomb for food.

When beekeepers collect honey, they smoke the bees out of the hive and slice away the honey-rich honeycomb. After removing the honey, they melt down and purify the honeycomb to form beeswax. Then they mix in scents and other substances and pour the beeswax into molds of all shapes and sizes and form many varieties of candles.

Candles made from paraffin wax, a by-product of the crude oil refinement process, are the most common, cheaper alternative to beeswax candles. Unfortunately, these are not an ideal alternative because burning paraffin candles has a lot of drawbacks, too. They produce a lot of dirty soot while they burn, along with many of the same harmful and carcinogenic toxins that are released when burning diesel fuel. And because it is not possible to mix scented, natural essential oils with paraffin wax in the candle-making process, the industry has developed artificial, petroleum-based scents that release even more undesirable chemicals and soot into the air you breathe.

Fortunately, healthier vegan alternatives to both beeswax and paraffin-based candles are available. Let's take a look at some of them.

Soy Candles and Other Sources of Light

Candles based on plant oils such as soy, palm, or hemp are a safer alternative to petroleum-based candles. These burn just as well as the other kinds—even better in some ways—and don't release harmful toxins and loads of black soot into the air.

Soy candles, made from soy wax, have been growing in popularity and are becoming a viable vegan alternative to beeswax and paraffin. Soy wax is produced by adding hydrogen to soy oil molecules in a process similar to that used to create hydrogenated vegetable oils. Although hydrogenated oils, or trans fats, are terribly unhealthy to eat, they make for really good, relatively clean-burning, candles. Just don't eat them, and you'll be fine!

Candles made from palm, hemp, and other plant oils and waxes, alone or in combination, have also become more available in recent years. Like soy candles, these are also nontoxic, cleaner-burning vegan alternatives to conventional candles.

HOT POTATO

Like many quality items that are good for you and the environment, alternative wax candles can be pricier than the cheap conventional kind. They're generally also longer burning, so you usually get your money's worth while treating yourself, the earth, and your fellow creatures more kindly in the process.

Another vegan alternative to beeswax and paraffin is the humble, old-fashioned oil-based lamp. Some pretty nifty modern versions are available these days, and often they can run on olive and other vegetable oils. If you get a few small oil lamps with some organic hemp or cotton wicks, they can easily and inexpensively take the place of candles for many years, if not decades.

Vegan Dogs and Cats?

When it comes to animal companions and how to properly care for them, vegans need to be concerned about all the same things nonvegans are concerned about. But some issues are specific to vegans, such as what constitutes an optimal diet for their animal companions. Because vegans don't like to support animal foods industries, especially factory farming, they're often dismayed at the prospect of having to continue to buy those products for their dogs and cats.

HOT POTATO

The meats used in commercial pet foods are often substandard and can even be harmful to your furry friends. There's no mandatory government testing of these meats for safety before they end up in your friend's bowl.

New vegans often want to know if it's safe to feed their faithful companions a vegan diet, foregoing all animal foods. The answer, depending on the species in question, is a qualified yes. Let's take a look at the two most popular nonherbivorous companion animals, dogs and cats.

Dogs are omnivores that eat both animal and plant foods in their diets. Experts agree that a proper meatless diet, high in protein and other essential nutrients, can easily supply dogs of all breeds and sizes with everything they require to stay healthy and happy. A number of commercial vegetarian dog foods are available, both moist and dry. Some of the more popular brands are Evolution Diet, Natural Life, Natural Balance, Wysong, and Nature's Recipe. It's also easy to make homemade vegan food for your canine pal, so check the web or your local library for recipe ideas.

Unlike dogs, cats are carnivores and have different nutritional needs. They cannot fulfill all their nutritional requirements on a plant-based diet alone, without supplementation. Most important among the nutrients cats need is the amino acid taurine, found only in animal tissue. Without it, cats can go blind and experience a wide range of other health problems. A synthetic form of taurine is regularly supplemented in conventional nonvegan cat foods as well, because most of the taurine originally present in meat is destroyed during the cooking process. It's also vital to supplement vitamins A and D_2, as well as the essential fatty acid arachidonate and a few other nutrients.

Some nutritionally complete prepared vegan cat foods are available in both canned and kibble form. Most notable are those marketed under the Evolution Diet brand. It's also possible to make your own vegan cat food with the help of the right supplementation. A product called Vegecat makes it easy with their supplement blend. You simply mix the powdered Vegecat supplement in with your homemade vegan cat food, and it adds all the taurine and other nutrients your cat needs.

HOT POTATO

Onions are toxic to cats (and dogs, to a lesser extent) and should never be included in any form, whether raw, cooked, or powdered, in any of your cat's food. Compounds called sulfoxides and disulfides destroy red blood cells, which leads to anemia. Garlic contains the same harmful compounds, but in lesser amounts.

Feeding your cat a vegan diet involves having faith in the bioavailability of the supplemented forms of the needed nutrients, so it's a decision you shouldn't make lightly. It should also be noted that many people feel the only appropriate diet for carnivores like felines is raw meat, which is what they would naturally eat in the wild. However, the internet is full of success stories of vegan cats, and we recommend you do a little research on the topic yourself before coming to any conclusions.

We recommend you check with your veterinarian for additional information and advice about feeding your dog, cat, or other companion animals a vegan diet.

We hope this book has shown you how living a vegan lifestyle can help put the compassion you feel toward others into action and be one of the most rewarding things you can do. By going vegan, you are giving a gift, not only to animals, but to yourself as well, and soon you'll see all the benefits adding up. You'll feel healthier and happier, and before you know it, you'll have a glow that will shine from the inside out. Plus, you'll feel good knowing you're helping make a positive difference in the world around you by no longer eating an animal-based diet or using animal products in your life.

Going vegan can have a ripple effect on all parts of your life and the lives of those around you, and your decision to make changes in your lifestyle choices could help others have the courage to do so in their own life as well!

The Least You Need to Know

- Animal-based ingredients are found in many products in the home, in many different forms. Don't let it overwhelm you; just do the best you can to eliminate and replace them with vegan alternatives.

- Using a digital camera and sharing photos electronically is a viable vegan alternative to using conventional gelatin-based photographic film.

- Search out companies that employ cruelty-free products for processing and printing photos, and beware of glossy photo paper, which often contains gelatin.

- Candles based on plant oils—such as soy, palm, and hemp—are healthier vegan alternatives to those made from beeswax or paraffin.

- Dogs can easily thrive on a meatless diet, while vegan cats require supplementation of nutrients such as taurine, vitamins A and D_2, and others. Check with your vet for advice on feeding your companion animals a vegan diet.

Glossary

arrowroot A starch obtained from the tubers of the tropical herb *Maranta arundinacea*. It's used primarily as a thickener, but arrowroot tubers are sometimes also eaten whole as a vegetable. *Arrowroot* is derived from the Arawak word *aru-aru*, meaning "meal of meals."

bioavailability The proportionate amount or level of a certain nutrient contained within a specific food that's actually used or utilized by the body.

brown rice vinegar Vinegar produced from fermented brown rice, water, and koji (a beneficial type of mold), or from unrefined rice wine (sake) and water, which is popular in Asian-style dishes.

clabbering A souring process done by combining soy milk (or other nondairy milk) with a little lemon juice or vinegar, which, when left to sit for a few minutes, will cause the soy milk to sour and thicken slightly. Sometimes this mixture is referred to as vegan buttermilk because it can be used as a measure-for-measure replacement for buttermilk in recipes.

coconut water The clear liquid found inside young green coconuts. It's mild and sweet in flavor and rich in electrolytes, making it the perfect natural sports drink.

compassion The emotional and sympathetic awareness of another's distress, combined with the motivation and desire to alleviate that distress.

crimini mushroom A relative of the white button mushroom that's brown in color and has a richer flavor. The larger, fully grown version is the portobello. *See also* portobello mushroom.

curry powder A ground blend of rich and flavorful spices used as a basis for curry and many other Indian-influenced dishes. Common ingredients include hot pepper, nutmeg, cumin, cinnamon, pepper, and turmeric. Some curry can also be found in paste form.

enzyme A protein that acts as a catalyst for specific biochemical reactions of other substances, and does so without the enzyme itself being destroyed or altered in the process. Each enzyme is designed to initiate a specific response with a specific result, as in digestion of food. Enzymes are vital to the body for achieving and sustaining optimal health.

enzyme inhibitor Present in the seeds or nuts of plants to aid in self-preservation, an enzyme inhibitor protects the seed so it has a better chance to germinate and reach full maturity before being gobbled up.

essential amino acid Our bodies' key protein-building blocks; they must come from dietary sources. Essential amino acids include histidine, isoleucine, leucine, lysine, methionine, phenylalanine, threonine, tryptophan, and valine.

essential fatty acid Fatty acid made of alpha-linoleic acid and linoleic acid, which are necessary for the formation and maintenance of cells. Commonly referred to as omega-3 and omega-6 fatty acids, these classes compete for dominance within your body. Having a greater proportion of one over the other can increase your risks for chronic diseases.

farfalle The Italian word for "butterflies" describes pasta of the same shape. The pasta is made from rectangular strips of pasta with zigzag or pinked edges and is crimped in the center. The shape is also often called bow ties.

gelatin (also *gelatine*) A gelling agent made from boiling the connective tissues and skins of animals. It's used in the manufacturing of many products used for consumption and personal use, including foods, beverages, beauty products, pills, and even photographic film.

hummus A purée of chickpeas with tahini, olive oil, lemon juice, garlic, herbs, and seasonings, also called hummus bi tahini. Hummus originated in the Middle East and Mediterranean. The word comes from the Arabic word for chickpea, known also as the ceci or garbanzo bean.

kudzu (also **kuzu**) A starch-based thickening product made from the tuber of the kudzu plant. In Japan and throughout much of Asia, the leafy foliage is cooked like other greens, and the large tubers are used as a thickening agent. The quick-growing vine was brought from Japan to the southern United States, where it's referred to as "the vine that ate the South" because it now covers nearly 7 million acres of land.

lacto-ovo vegetarian A vegetarian who also includes dairy (*lacto*) and eggs (*ovo*) in his or her diet.

lignan A variety of phytoestrogen, similar to isoflavones, that helps regulate estrogen production in the human body. Lignans have been shown to have cancer-fighting properties that can help inhibit or prevent the growth of breast, colon, and prostate cancers.

maca powder A powder made from a root vegetable, also known as Peruvian ginseng, that grows in the mountain plateaus of the Andes. When added to foods, maca powder imparts a slightly malty, butterscotch flavor. It's used quite often in raw food desserts and sweet treats.

milk In its Standards of Identity, the U.S. Food and Drug Administration (FDA) defines milk as "lacteal secretions from mammals." This term is also commonly used to describe milklike liquids made from plant-based sources, like soy, coconut, oats, rice, hemp seeds, almonds, and other nuts and seeds.

miso A thick, pastelike condiment made from fermenting soybeans with salt and koji (a beneficial type of mold), often in combination with other beans or grains like chickpeas, barley, or rice. Miso ranges from sweet, mild, and mellow with a light beige color, to strong and rich with earthy dark-brown or red tones.

nutritional yeast flakes Inactive yeast that has a nutty, almost cheeselike flavor, commonly used as an imitation cheese flavoring for foods and in the production of nondairy cheese products. It's an excellent product for vegans to use to attain their recommended daily dose of vitamin B_{12}. Do not confuse it with active yeast, the type used for making breads and baked goods.

oxalate An organic acid that occurs naturally in leafy greens, berries, nuts, black tea, and other foods.

phytoestrogen A naturally occurring plant compound similar to estradiol, the most potent form of human estrogen. The effects of phytoestrogens are not as strong as most estrogens, and they are very easily broken down and eliminated. They help regulate the estrogen levels in your body.

portobello mushroom A mature and larger form of the smaller crimini mushroom. Brown, chewy, and flavorful, portobellos are often served as whole caps, grilled, or as thin sautéed slices. *See also* crimini mushroom.

preeclampsia A condition involving hypertension, retention of fluids, protein loss, and excessive weight gain during pregnancy. Preeclampsia occurs in at least 2 percent of all pregnancies in the United States.

preventive medicine   The field of medicine concerned primarily with helping healthy people stay healthy and providing the tools and information needed to keep disease at bay. It explores the environmental and dietary effects on disease and health and works to determine the root causes instead of reaching for quick fixes.

quinoa   Commonly referred to as a supergrain, this small and ancient seed is high in protein, essential amino acids, fiber, calcium, and many vitamins and minerals.

selenium   A rare mineral, closely related to sulfur, with a distinctive red-gray metallic appearance. In small amounts, it's an essential mineral for mammals and higher plants. In larger amounts, it's toxic. Selenium helps stimulate metabolism and protect against the oxidizing effects of free radicals. These days, most selenium is produced and obtained as a by-product of the copper-refining process.

shea butter   Derived from the shea nut, which grows in many parts of Africa, shea butter is used in the treatment of minor skin problems and irritations. It can be used alone or blended with other ingredients to make various hair and skin-care products.

silken tofu   A food made from soybeans that has a velvety-smooth and creamy texture. The process for making silken tofu differs slightly from regular tofu, in that the soy milk curds and excess water are not separated during production. Depending on the silken tofu's final texture, it's labeled soft, firm, or extra-firm. Silken tofu is often blended for making sauces, salad dressings, beverages, desserts, and baked goods.

smoked paprika   A variety of Spanish paprika made from mature pimento peppers that are dried, naturally smoked over oak-wood fires, and stone-ground to a fine, powdery consistency. It has a deep red color with a slightly smoky and bittersweet flavor.

tahini   A thick paste or butter made from ground sesame seeds. It's often used in Middle Eastern cuisine and features prominently in hummus, baba ghanoush, soups, salad dressings, and many other dishes.

tanning   The process of turning animal hide into pliable, finished leather through exposure to various chemicals, preservatives, and dyes.

tempeh   A cultured food product made by mixing partially cooked soybeans with a beneficial mold (*Rhizosporus oligosporus*) and fermenting it. The result is a firm soybean cake with a marbled appearance, which is why tempeh is often classified as the blue cheese version of tofu.

turbinado sugar   Sugar made from the juice extracted from unrefined raw cane sugar, which is then spun in a centrifuge or turbine (hence its name). It has a very fine texture and a slight molasses flavor. It can also be used to replace light brown sugar. You might be familiar with the most commonly sold brand of turbinado sugar, Sugar in the Raw.

turmeric   A spicy, pungent yellow root that's dried and finely ground to a powder for use in many dishes, especially Indian cuisine, for color and flavor. Turmeric is the source of the yellow color in many prepared mustards and curry powder.

uncooking   The art of preparing or processing raw foods in ways that do not involve the use of heat hotter than 115°F. This leaves vital nutrients and enzymes in the food intact.

veg-friendly   Having an understanding of the basics of vegan and vegetarian dietary guidelines and philosophies and providing vegan or vegetarian options.

vegan   A person who excludes all animal foods and ingredients from his or her daily dietary intake and who also avoids using any animal-based items and any form of animal exploitation or suffering in all other aspects of life.

vegetarian   A person who chooses to exclude animal flesh from his or her daily dietary intake.

vital wheat gluten   A powdered form of dehydrated pure wheat gluten. It's often mixed with liquids and seasonings and used to make seitan and its many meat analogue variations. Find it in bulk bins or packaged in most grocery and natural foods stores. It's sometimes also known as instant gluten flour.

Resources

Now that you've begun your journey into veganism, where do you turn for information and support on a wide variety of vegan-related issues? Many books, websites, organizations, and other resources can provide the information you need to help maintain your cruelty-free approach to life. This appendix helps you get started in the right direction!

Books

Nowadays, you can find loads of books on a wide range of topics related to vegan living—and that's good news for new vegans! The following sections list some of the books we think will help you the most, in addition to those we mentioned throughout this book. Happy reading!

Vegan Issues

Adams, Carol J. *Living Among Meat Eaters: The Vegetarian's Survival Handbook.* Continuum International Publishing Group, 2003.

Blair, Linda, and Sunny J. Harris. *Going Vegan!* Sunny Harris and Associates, Inc., 2001.

E. G. Smith Collective. *Animal Ingredients A to Z: Third Edition.* AK Press, 2004.

Lappé, Frances Moore. *Diet for a Small Planet, 20th Anniversary Edition.* Ballantine Books, 1991.

Marcus, Erik. *Meat Market: Animals, Ethics, and Money.* Brio Press, 2005.

———. *Vegan: The New Ethics of Eating, Revised Edition.* McBooks Press, 2000.

Melina, Vesanto, and Brenda Davis. *Becoming Vegan: The Complete Guide to Adopting a Healthy Plant-Based Diet.* Book Publishing Company, 2000.

Robbins, John. *Diet for a New America: How Your Food Choices Affect Your Health, Happiness and the Future of Life on Earth.* H. J. Kramer, 1998.

———. *The Food Revolution: How Your Diet Can Help Save Your Life and Our World.* Conari Press, 2001.

Stepaniak, Joanne. *Being Vegan.* Lowell House, 2000.

———. *The Vegan Sourcebook.* Lowell House, 1998.

Cooking and Uncooking

Atlas, Nava. *Vegan Express.* Broadway Books, 2008.

———. *Vegan Holiday Kitchen: More Than 200 Delicious, Festive Recipes for Special Occasions.* Sterling, 2011.

Bennett, Beverly Lynn. *The Complete Idiot's Guide to Vegan Slow Cooking.* Alpha Books, 2012.

———. *Vegan Bites.* Book Publishing Company, 2008.

Bennett, Beverly Lynn, and Julieanna Hever, MS, RD, CPT. *The Complete Idiot's Guide to Gluten-Free Vegan Cooking.* Alpha Books, 2011.

Bennett, Beverly Lynn, and Ray Sammartano. *The Complete Idiot's Guide to Vegan Cooking.* Alpha Books, 2008.

Bergeron, Ken. *Professional Vegetarian Cooking.* John Wiley and Sons, 1999.

Brill, Steve. *The Wild Vegan Cookbook: A Forager's Culinary Guide (in the Field or in the Supermarket) to Preparing and Savoring Wild (and Not So Wild) Natural Foods.* Harvard Common Press, 2010.

Brotman, Juliano, and Erika Lenkert. *Raw: The Uncook Book: New Vegetarian Food for Life.* HarperCollins, 1999.

Grogan, Bryanna Clark. *World Vegan Feast: 200 Fabulous Recipes from Over 50 Countries.* Vegan Heritage Press, 2011.

Hagler, Louise. *Tofu Quick and Easy.* Book Publishing Company, 2001.

Klaper, Michael, MD, and Gentle World. *The Cookbook for People Who Love Animals.* Gentle World, 1990.

Kramer, Sarah, and Tanya Barnard. *How It All Vegan!: Irresistible Recipes for an Animal-Free Diet.* Arsenal Pulp Press, 1999.

Long, Linda. *Great Chefs Cook Vegan.* Gibbs Smith, 2011.

McCarty, Meredith. *Sweet and Natural: More Than 120 Sugar-Free and Dairy-Free Desserts.* St. Martin's Press, 2001.

McDougall, John A., MD, and Mary McDougall. *The McDougall Quick and Easy Cookbook: Over 300 Delicious Low-Fat Recipes You Can Prepare in Fifteen Minutes or Less.* Penguin Group/Plume Books, 1999.

Newkirk, Ingrid, and PETA. *Compassionate Cook: Please Don't Eat the Animals.* Warner Books, 1993.

Raymond, Jennifer. *The Peaceful Palate: Fine Vegetarian Cuisine.* Book Publishing Company, 1996.

Robertson, Robin. *1,000 Vegan Recipes.* John Wiley & Sons, Inc., 2009.

———. *Vegan Planet: 400 Irresistible Recipes with Fantastic Flavors from Home and Around the World.* Harvard Common Press, 2003.

Stepaniak, Joanne. *The Ultimate Uncheese Cookbook: Delicious Dairy-Free Cheeses and Classic "Uncheese" Dishes.* Book Publishing Company, 2003.

Tucker, Eric, and John Westerdahl. *Millennium Cookbook: Extraordinary Vegetarian Cuisine.* Ten Speed Press, 1998.

Walker, Norman W. *Fresh Vegetable and Fruit Juices: What's Missing in Your Body? Revised Edition.* Norwalk Press/Book Publishing Company, 2008.

Health and Nutrition

Barnard, Neal, MD. *Breaking the Food Seduction: The Hidden Reasons Behind Food Cravings—and 7 Steps to End Them Naturally.* St. Martin's Griffin, 2004.

———. *Food for Life: How the New Four Food Groups Can Save Your Life.* Three Rivers Press, 1994.

———. *21-Day Weight Loss Kickstart: Boost Metabolism, Lower Cholesterol, and Dramatically Improve Your Health.* Grand Central Life and Style, 2011.

Campbell, T. Colin, PhD, and Thomas M. Campbell II. *The China Study.* Benbella Books, 2005.

Diamond, Harvey, and Marilyn Diamond. *Fit for Life.* Warner Books, 1987.

Elliot, Rose. *The Vegetarian Mother and Baby Book: Completely Revised and Updated.* Pantheon, 1996.

Hever, Julieanna, MS, RD, CPT. *The Complete Idiot's Guide to Plant-Based Nutrition.* Alpha Books, 2011.

Klaper, Michael, MD. *Pregnancy, Children, and the Vegan Diet.* Gentle World, 1988.

———. *Vegan Nutrition: Pure and Simple.* Gentle World, 1987.

Lyman, Howard. *Mad Cowboy: Plain Truth from the Cattle Rancher Who Won't Eat Meat.* Touchstone, 1998.

McDougall, John A., MD, and Mary McDougall. *The McDougall Program for a Healthy Heart: A Life-Saving Approach to Preventing and Treating Heart Disease.* Penguin Group/Plume Books, 1998.

Ornish, Dean, MD. *Dr. Dean Ornish's Program for Reversing Heart Disease.* Random House, 1990.

———. *Eat More, Weigh Less.* HarperCollins, 1995.

Pavlina, Erin. *Raising Vegan Children in a Non-Vegan World: A Complete Guide for Parents.* VegFamily, 2003.

Saunders, Kerrie K., PhD. *The Vegan Diet as Chronic Disease Prevention: Evidence Supporting the New Four Food Groups.* Lantern Books, 2003.

Stepaniak, Joanne, and Vesanto Melina. *Raising Vegetarian Children: A Guide to Good Health and Family Harmony.* Contemporary Books/McGraw-Hill, 2002.

Villamagna, Dana, MSJ, and Andrew Villamagna, MD, MSc. *The Complete Idiot's Guide to Vegan Eating for Kids.* Alpha Books, 2010.

Animal Advocacy

Newkirk, Ingrid. *Making Kind Choices: Everyday Ways to Enhance Your Life Through Earth- and Animal-Friendly Living.* St. Martin's Griffin, 2005.

———. *250 Things You Can Do to Make Your Cat Adore You.* Fireside, 1998.

People for the Ethical Treatment of Animals. *PETA 2006 Shopping Guide for Caring Consumers: A Guide to Products That Are Not Tested on Animals.* PETA, 2006.

Singer, Peter. *Animal Liberation.* HarperCollins/Ecco, 2002.

Kids' Books

Bass, Jules, and Debbie Harter. *Herb, the Vegetarian Dragon*. Barefoot Books, 1999.

Roth, Ruby. *That's Why We Don't Eat Animals: A Book About Vegans, Vegetarians, and All Living Things*. North Atlantic Books, 2009.

Tofts, Hannah. *I Eat Vegetables!* Zero to Ten, 2001.

Vignola, Radha. *Victor, the Vegetarian: Saving Little Lambs*. Aviva! 1994.

———. *Victor's Picnic: With the Vegetarian Animals*. Aviva! 1996.

Zephaniah, Benjamin. *The Little Book of Vegan Poems*. AK Press, 2002.

———. *School's Out: Poems Not for School*. AK Press, 1997.

Websites

Vegan websites abound online, and the following links help you successfully navigate your way through vegan cyberspace. They're arranged by category for your surfing pleasure. Don't forget to use a good search engine to help you discover new vegan sites of your own!

Vegan Issues

EarthSave International
earthsave.org

Erik Marcus
erikmarcus.com

Famous Vegetarians / Famous Vegans
famousveggie.com

Friends of Animals
friendsofanimals.org

Go Vegan with Bob Linden
goveganradio.com

Grassroots Veganism with Joanne Stepaniak
vegsource.com/jo

John Robbins
johnrobbins.info

People for the Ethical Treatment of Animals (PETA)
peta.org

Vegan.com
vegan.com

Vegan Outreach
veganoutreach.com

Vegan Village
veganvillage.co.uk

VegSource
vegsource.com

Vegetarian Resource Group
vrg.org

vegTV
vegtv.com

Vegetarians in Paradise
vegparadise.com

Vegan Cooking

Beverly Lynn Bennett's "The Vegan Chef"
veganchef.com

Robin Robertson's Global Vegan Kitchen
robinrobertson.com

Hungry Vegan Blog
hungryvegan.blogspot.com

Vegan Cooking
vegancooking.com

International Vegetarian Union's Recipes
ivu.org/recipes

VegWeb
vegweb.com

Living and Raw Foods
living-foods.com

Vegetarian Resource Group's Recipes
vrg.org/recipes

Vegan Publications

American Vegan
americanvegan.org/magazine.htm

VegNews
vegnews.com

The Vegan
vegansociety.com/about/publications/
vegan-magazine

Restaurant Directories

HappyCow's Vegetarian Guide
happycow.net

VegDining
vegdining.com

Vegan Merchants

Alternative Outfitters
alternativeoutfitters.com

Beauty Without Cruelty
beautywithoutcruelty.com

Different Daisy
differentdaisy.com

Food Fight! Grocery
foodfightgrocery.com

Pangea's The Vegan Store
veganstore.com

Vegan Essentials
veganessentials.com

Vegan Goodies and Treats

Allison's Gourmet
allisonsgourmet.com

Alternative Baking Company
alternativebaking.com

Edward and Sons
edwardandsons.com

Endangered Species Chocolate
chocolatebar.com

Frey Vineyards
freywine.com

Health and Nutrition

Dr. McDougall's Health and Medical Center
drmcdougall.com

Institute for Plant Based Nutrition (IPBN)
plantbased.org

Julieanna Hever, MS, RD, CPT
toyourhealthnutrition.com

Michael A. Klaper, MD
doctorklaper.com

Neal D. Barnard, MD
nealbarnard.org

Physicians Committee for Responsible Medicine (PCRM)
pcrm.org

Pregnancy and Children

Parenting and Family at VegSource
vegsource.com/talk/parenting

Vegan Family House
veganfamily.co.uk

VegFamily
vegfamily.com

Animal Companions

Vegancats.com
vegancats.com

VegePet
vegepet.com

Organizations

For those looking to become more involved with animal rights advocacy or looking for a vegan support group, here is a list of organizations that can help.

American Anti-Vivisection Society
aavs.org

American Vegan Society
americanvegan.org

Compassion Over Killing
cok.net

EarthSave International
earthsave.org

Farm Animal Rights Movement (FARM)
farmusa.org

Farm Sanctuary
farmsanctuary.org

Food Not Bombs
foodnotbombs.net

Friends of Animals
friendsofanimals.org

Gentle Barn
gentlebarn.org

International Vegetarian Union
ivu.org

North American Vegetarian Society (NAVS)
navs-online.org

People for the Ethical Treatment of Animals
peta.com

Toronto Vegetarian Association
veg.ca

Vegan Action
vegan.org

Vegan Outreach
veganoutreach.com

Vegan Society
vegansociety.com

Vegetarian Resource Group
vrg.org

Vegetarians International Voice for Animals (Viva!)
viva.org.uk

Index